Nutrition and Disease Update

Cancer

1-25

11-172

Nutrition and Disease Update

Cancer

Editors

Kenneth K. Carroll
University of Western Ontario
London, Ontario

David Kritchevsky
Wistar Institute
Philadelphia, Pennsylvania

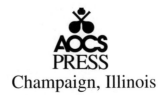

AOCS
PRESS

Champaign, Illinois

AOCS Mission Statement

To be a forum for the exchange of ideas, information and experience among those with a professional interest in the science and technology of fats, oils and related substances in ways that promote personal excellence and provide for a high standard of quality.

Library of Congress Cataloging-in-Publication Data

Nutrition and disease update : cancer / editors, David Kritchevsky,
    Kenneth K. Carroll.
       p.   cm.
    Includes bibliographical references.
    ISBN 0-935315-49-7 (acid-free paper) : $50.00
     1. Cancer—Nutritional aspects. I. Kritchevsky, David.
  II. Carroll, K. K. (Kenneth Kitchener)
  RC268.45.N875   1994
  616.99' 4071—dc20   93-49456
                                                  CIP

Printed in the United States of America with vegetable oil-based inks.

Preface

In 1991 the Life Sciences Research Office (LSRO) and the Federation of American Societies for Experimental Biology (FASEB) undertook preparation of a series of reports evaluating the publicly available scientific evidence regarding certain nutrient–disease relationships. These reports were developed for the Center for Food Safety and Applied Nutrition, Food and Drug Administration (FDA), under the terms of Task Order #9, FDA Contract No. 223-88-2124, as a means of obtaining independent, external scientific data and information on specific topics for which health claims might be made.

The authors and reviewing consultants for the reports were selected by the LSRO, with the concurrence of the LSRO Advisory Committee, which consists of representatives of each constituent society of FASEB. The LSRO staff prepared the index tables and edited the revised reports and tables prior to final approval by the authors and reviewing consultants.

The editors of these reports concluded that this material merited a broad audience, and the American Oil Chemists' Society agreed to publish the reviews relating to heart disease and cancer in two volumes. FASEB and Dr. Kenneth D. Fisher, the LSRO Director, graciously gave permission for use of the original reports and for the inclusion of updates by the authors. These updates provide information from 1991 (when the original reports were prepared) through the present.

These volumes afford the reader concise reviews of recent research on a number of different nutrients and their relationship with cancer and heart disease. They provide an excellent starting point for future research.

Kenneth K. Carroll
David Kritchevsky

Contents

Chapter 1

Dietary Fiber and Cancer

David Kritchevsky, Ph.D.

I. Introduction

A. Background Information

The importance of dietary fiber components in the diet has been recognized for many years but has received increased attention in the past 12 to 15 years. Study of the role of dietary fiber in health and disease was stimulated by the work of Burkitt (1971, 1973a,b) and Painter et al. (1972). These and other investigators hypothesized that the relatively low level of plant fiber in the diets of Western societies predisposed these populations to disease and disorders which differ from those in less developed regions. Interest in this hypothesis has led to a number of laboratory, clinical, and epidemiological studies, suggestions for health benefits of dietary fiber, development of new food products and diets, calls for guidelines on the fiber content and labeling of food products, and revision of nutritional recommendations. However, dietary fiber intake is only one aspect that must be considered in making dietary recommendations and is difficult to address in isolation from the total diet.

Various beneficial health effects have been suggested for dietary fiber, individual components of dietary fiber, and fiber-containing foods. Epidemiological studies and/or clinical trials have been conducted to examine the effects of fiber on glycemic response, lipid metabolism, laxation, diverticular disease, colon cancer, weight loss, and many other conditions. Interpretation of these studies is complicated by differences in the methods used for assessing dietary fiber intake in epidemiological studies and differences in the type and level of fiber components and fiber-containing foods used in clinical trials. The same factors also complicate studies of the potential adverse effects of high amounts of dietary fiber, e.g., altered availability of minerals and trace elements, altered absorption of drugs, changes in bowel function, and others.

1. Definition

Despite increasing public and scientific interest, several problems have impeded research on the health effects of dietary fiber. One major issue has been the absence of a universally accepted definition of dietary fiber. Most definitions encompass a wide variety of compounds with different chemical characteristics and physiological functions.

While the term "crude fiber" has been used for several decades, a universally acceptable definition of dietary fiber has not been achieved. A classification for dietary products and foods was submitted at the XIII International Congress of Nutrition (Spiller and Jenkins, 1986). Four groupings were presented:

a) Whole foods high in fiber,

b) A high-fiber fraction (such as wheat bran) which could be produced without affecting the structure and/or composition of the material as present in the food,

c) Concentrated fibers, such as pectin or cellulose, which have been altered in the course of extraction from food sources and subsequent purification, and

d) Fiber-enriched foods.

Each of these types of product may contain the same amount of a given fiber, but the action of that fiber will be affected by its physical form and by other substances in the food. For example, is the fiber added to a semi-purified diet the same as that fiber in its natural milieu? Is it the same in steric form? Are its interactions with other dietary components the same?

2. Analysis

As might be expected from the diverse chemical constituents, no one analytical methodology has been entirely satisfactory for identification and characterization of the many components of dietary fiber from all sources.

The analysis of dietary fiber is a field still in flux. Marlett (1990) has addressed this problem which has no solution as yet because there are no universally accepted methods of analysis which are based on universally accepted definitions. One major problem lies in the fact that the fiber is an integral part of the foodstuff being analyzed and some of the fiber may be "masked" by its association with other components and nutrients. For example, Marlett et al. (1989) demonstrated that the recovery of soluble fiber is a function of methodology. Thus, pre-treatment with pepsin raises the yield of soluble fiber (percent dry wt. of food) by 48 percent in peas, 71 percent in kidney beans, and 15 percent in oat bran.

The designations of dietary fiber as soluble and insoluble fibers are facile but not totally accurate. Almost all fibers occurring in food are a mixture of the insoluble fibers such as cellulose and hemicellulose and gelling fibers such as pectin. Fibers such as pectin do not form true gels but do increase the viscosity of aqueous solutions. The soluble fibers tend to form gels (pectin, gums) rather than dissolve, as the designation suggests. Thus we are labeling materials by their major component but not total composition, which may be misleading. In general, the brans (wheat, rice, corn, oat) are considered as insoluble fibers but the hypocholesterolemic properties of oat bran are due to its appreciable content of oat gum (β-glucan). An issue that may require more clarification is that food fibers are mixtures whose identity depends in part on analytical methodology used for their identification.

3. Diet–Cancer Relationships

While the overall area of diet and cancer has been of medical concern for many years, intense interest in the lay and medical communities can be dated to 1981 when an exhaustive review by Doll and Peto suggested that 35 percent of cancer deaths (range 10–70 percent) in the U.S. could be attributed to diet. A few years later Peto (1986) reproduced the table which had appeared in the 1981 publication with the heading "Future Perfect" suggesting what might be found in the future. In an accompanying table labeled "Present Imperfect" attribution of cancer causation to diet was revised downward drastically. Instead of suggesting that 35 percent of cancer deaths could be attributable to diet, the figure was 1 percent. In 1960, Higginson and Oettlé suggested that the virtual absence of large bowel cancer in black Africans might be due to an aspect of their diet, specifically dietary bulk. Burkitt (1971) attributed differences in incidence of colon cancer between African and Western populations to dietary fiber intake. Comparisons of fiber intake in populations are really comparisons of fiber-rich foods which contain a number of other materials (carotene, selenium, etc.) which may influence tumorigenesis.

B. Objective and Scope

This review considers the weight of scientific evidence that relates dietary fiber to occurrence of various types of cancer. It reviews and evaluates the literature published since 1987 on relationships between dietary fiber and cancer and compares the conclusions reached with those of previously published exemplary reviews. This review focuses principally on colon and breast cancer in relation to dietary fiber and considers the results of case–control, epidemiologic, and prospective studies of human subjects. Animal studies are cited only when they contribute significantly to understanding the mechanisms of fiber effects in causation of cancer. The review is a component of a series of reports on the interrelationships of dietary components and nutrients with various human diseases.

II. Dietary Fiber and Cancer

A number of noteworthy expert reviews have evaluated and summarized the recent literature on relationships between dietary fiber and cancer; for example, Diet and Health (1989), the National Research Council Committee on Diet, Nutrition and Cancer (NRC, 1982), Peto (1986), the Surgeon General's Report on Nutrition and Health (U.S. Department of Health and Human Services, 1988), and Trock et al. (1990). Most of these reviews have focused on data collected prior to 1988. In general, aggregate data have been equivocal in terms of a protective effect of dietary fiber against cancer. This review, therefore, focuses primarily on papers which have appeared since 1987 relating to fiber intake, colon cancer, and other cancers (Appendix Table).

A. Human Studies

1. Colon Cancer

There have now been several publications in which the findings of ecological and case–control studies have been summarized. It is important to note that the available data are the same but interpretations of reviewers may vary. For instance, Trock et al. (1990) found that the results of Pickle et al. (1984) can be listed under "equivocal support for protective effect of fiber"; whereas, other reviewers (Byers, 1988; Jacobs, 1988) concluded that Pickle's work provided no association between dietary fiber and colon cancer risk. The review by Trock et al. (1990b) went beyond the usual "yes" or "no" ratings and listed data as strongly supporting the protective effect of fiber, moderately supporting it, equivocally supporting it, or not supporting it. As such, these interpretations go beyond the original authors' conclusions.

The LSRO (Pilch, 1987) reviewed data from 18 ecological and 22 case–control studies. The report found fiber to be protective in 66.7 percent of the ecological studies and 36.4 percent of the case–control studies; 27.8 percent of the ecological studies and 40.9 percent of the case–control studies reported no effect; and enhancement was reported in 5.6 percent of the ecological studies and 22.7 percent of the case–control studies. Jacobs (1988) reviewed data pertaining to 24 ecological and 27 case–control studies and generally found protective effects in about half of them and no effect in 40 percent; Bingham (1990) classified the findings from 30 case–control studies conducted between 1969 and 1989 into outcomes relating to fiber, vegetables, cereals, and starch. Protective and non-protective effects (percent) were: fiber 50 and 41; vegetables 63 and 32; cereals 23 and 54; and starch 50 and 50. The results cited above are summarized in Table 1.

4   *David Kritchevsky*

TABLE 1 Association between Fiber Intake and Risk of Colorectal Cancer*

	Authors		
	Jacobs (1988)	Pilch (1987)	Bingham (1990)
Ecological Studies			
No.	24	18	—
Protective (%)	54.2	66.7	—
No effect (%)	41.6	27.8	—
Enhancing (%)	4.2	5.6	—
Case–control			
No.	27	22	22
Protective (%)	44.4	36.4	50.0
No effect (%)	40.7	40.9	40.9
Enhancing (%)	14.8	22.7	9.1

*The numbers reflect studies with several reported outcomes, thus some studies reported separately on total fiber, cereals, etc. There is overlap in the studies reviewed.

It is evident that in the ecological studies there is a bias in favor of a protective effect of fiber; whereas in the case–control studies, findings of effectiveness and non-effectiveness are about equally distributed. In a very thorough review of diet and cancer published in 1988, Rogers and Longnecker stated: "Most epidemiologic studies of fiber or fiber-containing food intake in relation to risk of colorectal cancer are consistent with a very small inverse association or no association."

Thus ecological studies in which populations are compared yield a better correlation than do more precise (but much smaller) case–control studies. Another point to consider is that the current diet of patients with diagnosed colon cancer may be quite different from that ingested before diagnosis. Thus the ecological studies offer diet–disease data on entire populations while case–control studies may report on diets that were dictated by health status and therefore were not typical of prediagnosis food habits.

Graham et al. (1988) reviewed 428 confirmed cases of colon cancer in upstate New York counties and an equal number of controls. There were 225 males and 223 females. When risk was assessed with increasing fat, calories or Quetelet index, there was a significant trend toward increased risk. The p values for trend with fiber alone were 0.97 for men and 0.86 for women. An association with fiber was found only upon a logistic analysis of fiber in conjunction with other nutrients. They found a high fat-low fiber diet carried twice the risk of a low fat-high fiber diet. Their summary states: "Dietary fiber was only equivocally associated with risk."

These investigators also studied rectal cancer in 277 case–control pairs of males and 145 case–control pairs of females in the same area in New York state (Freudenheim et al., 1990a). They found that dietary fiber from vegetables but not from grains was associated with reduced risk. These investigators also analyzed fiber sources as they related to risk in the populations studied for colon and rectal cancer (Freudenheim et al., 1990b; Graham et al., 1988). Using food tables of Paul and Southgate (1978) and Pennington (1976), the investigators analyzed fiber content and composition and concluded that fiber from grain (especially the insoluble fiber) was associated with decreased risk of colon cancer in both males and females and fruit/vegetable fiber was associated with decreased risk in males only. Risk of rectal cancer was negatively associated with intake of fruit/vegetable fiber. The magnitude of negative association was larger after controlling for fat. These findings differ from those of Slattery et al. (1988) who did not find grains to be protective. Whether Slattery et al. controlled for fat intake was not specified.

Slattery et al. (1988) carried out assessment of dietary risk for colon cancer in Utah studying 231 cases and 391 controls. Crude fiber was associated with decreased risk of colon cancer in both males and females. Highest quartiles of intake of fruits/vegetables were also associated with decreased risk in probands of both sexes. Grain intake was not protective. In examining their data on fiber type, risk for "dietary fiber" was higher in the highest quartile of intake than in the two intermediate ones. This suggests the possibility that at highest levels of intake some other interacting dietary factor may be depleted.

In another Utah study (West et al., 1989) 231 colon cancer cases and 391 controls were interviewed. The authors found positive associations with body–mass index, dietary fat, and fiber. Decreased risk was also associated with intake of β-carotene and cruciferous vegetables. Heilbrun et al. (1989) examined diet and colorectal cancer in American Japanese men. Over a 16-year period they identified 102 men with colon cancer and 60 men with rectal cancer who were compared with 361 cancer-free control subjects. Findings of fiber effects were related to fat intake. Thus in men with low fat intake (less than 61 g/d), there was a negative association with dietary fiber intake (p = 0.042). No such association was observed if fat intake exceeded 61 g/d (p = 0.237). They found no association between dietary fiber intake and rectal cancer.

Lee et al. (1989) studied colorectal cancer in Singapore Chinese (203 cases, 405 controls). They saw a protective effect for high intake of cruciferous vegetables and a predisposing effect for a high meat/vegetable ratio. These findings held up when analysis was applied to colon cancer alone. The following were protective for rectal cancer: high intakes of protein, fiber, β-carotene, and vegetables. Gerhardsson de Verdier et al. (1990) studied 352 cases of colon cancer, 217 of rectal cancer, and 512 controls. Test for trend of fiber intake with colon cancer was not significant (p = 0.32) but significance was observed for rectal cancer (p < 0.05). High fiber intake was associated with reduced risk of colon cancer in men and of rectal cancer in both men and women.

Willett et al. (1990) reported on the relation of meat, fat, and fiber intake to colon cancer risk in a prospective study of 88,751 women. They found no significant changes in colon cancer risk associated with total fiber, fruit, vegetable, or cereal fiber. Only fruit fiber showed a consistent trend for reduced risk with increasing intake, but the relationship was not statistically independent of meat intake. As noted for other studies the relative risk at the highest (fifth) quintile of total dietary fiber was 30 percent higher than that for the fourth quintile (0.90 vs 0.69). A positive association with fat was observed.

Recent studies do not clarify effects of fiber on colorectal cancer, but they are helpful for several reasons. They begin to show different effects for right and left colon, and they begin to focus on dietary interactions (Freudenheim et al., 1990a,b; Slattery et al., 1988). For example, the noncellulose polysaccharides, containing mannose and galactose, appeared to protect against cancers in the ascending colons of men; galactose and uronic acid protected the descending colons of women (Slattery et al., 1988). Freudenheim et al. (1990b) reported some evidence that fruit and vegetable fiber seem to protect against cancer of the "distal bowel."

The data indicate no consistent relationship between risk and fiber, whether the fiber be total, crude, cereal, fruit, or grain. This might be corrected somewhat if fiber content were regarded in relation to other nutrients present in the food being analyzed. Animal studies have shown that caloric intake is a major determinant of susceptibility to chemically-induced or spontaneous cancers. Tannenbaum (1945) provided data on this point in the 1940s and recent reports bear it out (Kritchevsky and Klurfeld, 1986). Lyon et al. (1987) have emphasized the importance of considering energy intake in assessing diet and colon cancer.

2. Breast Cancer

Rose (1990) has reviewed the effects of fiber on incidence of breast cancer with emphasis on the influence dietary fiber components or products, such as lignins, might exert on estrogen metabolism. He points out that vegetarians excrete more fecal estrogen than do omnivores and that the opposite is the case for urinary estrogens suggesting that excretion of estrogen via the colon may limit enterohepatic circulation.

Adlercreutz (1990) has also reviewed the data and reports that in a study in Boston (Adlercreutz et al., 1989), the pattern of high plasma estrogen levels, high urinary, and low fecal excretion of estrogen and low urinary excretion of lignans and phytoestrogens was seen in breast cancer cases. He attributes this pattern to a high intake of protein and fat and a concomitant low intake of fiber and grain products. However, in a Finnish study (Adlercreutz et al., 1987, 1988), excretion patterns were similar for cases and controls. Howe et al. (1990a) have published a combined analysis of 12 case–control studies of diet and breast cancer. This mode of data analysis provides a pool of 4427 cases, 434 population or neighborhood controls, and 1754 hospital controls. Relative risk rises significantly with total caloric intake or fat intake, and the most protective effect is seen with markers for vegetable or fruit intake, most notably vitamin C.

Using a different approach, Brisson et al. (1989) examined diet and breast cancer risk using mammographic features as the end point. Positive correlations were seen with total or saturated fat. Significant negative correlations were found with carotenoid and fiber intake.

There are three recently published case–control studies relating to diet and risk of breast cancer (see Appendix Table). Katsouyanni et al. (1988) studied 120 cases and an equal number of controls. They found no evidence for a positive effect of dietary fat or fiber but did find a significant protective effect of vitamin A. Pryor et al. (1989) studied 172 cases and 190 controls in an effort to relate adolescent diet to breast cancer in Utah. The cohort was aged 20–54 years. The authors commented on difficulties in recall of adolescent diets. In the premenopausal group there was a reduced risk of breast cancer between the highest quartile of intake and the other three for crude fiber, grains, and other sources of fiber. In the postmenopausal women risk rose markedly with increasing intake of crude fiber or "other" fiber but was slightly reduced for grains. The designation "grains" alluded to bread and cereal and other fiber relates to all other sources. Van't Veer et al. (1990) studied 133 breast cancer cases and 238 population controls in the Netherlands. The energy-adjusted intake of dietary fiber in the cases (25.4 ± 6.7 g/d) was significantly lower than that of the controls (27.7 ± 7.4 g/d). The most striking correlation was with intake of cereal products.

3. Other Cancers

a. Prostate cancer   Studies of diet and prostate cancer have not focused on fiber per se. Most studies have emphasized intakes of carotene or vitamin A, but these nutrients are often present in fiber-rich foods.

Wilson (1972) has postulated that elevated plasma androgen levels may lead to prostatic hyperplasia and eventually to cancer. Two studies of Seventh-Day Adventist (SDA) and non-SDA men show that the vegans ingest more fiber and excrete more estrogen and testosterone (Pusateri et al., 1990; Ross et al., 1990). This is similar to the argument Adlerkreutz (1990) presents for increased fecal steroid excretion being related to reduced breast cancer risk.

Oishi et al. (1988) studied 100 cases of prostatic cancer, 100 cases of benign prostatic hyperplasia and 100 hospital controls in Japan. Low intakes of β-carotene and vitamin A were correlated with the development of prostate cancer but intake of fiber was not. Severson et al. (1989) examined prospectively the incidence of prostate cancer in 7999 Japanese men followed for 18–21 years. They found 174 cases of prostate cancer. Intakes of rice and tofu were associated with decreased risk and seaweed with increased risk. Le Marchand et al. (1991) have reported on 452 cases of prostate cancer and 899 controls among the multiethnic population of Hawaii. Earlier studies (Kolonel et al., 1987, 1988) had suggested that increased risk was associated with increased vitamin A or β-carotene intake in elderly men. In the new study the β-carotene association is confined to level of intake of papaya (Le Marchand et al., 1991).

b. Miscellaneous cancers   Howe et al. (1990b) studied 249 cases of pancreatic cancer and 505 controls in Canada. Inverse correlations were found for fiber from fruit, vegetables, or cereal. A strong positive correlation was found with total caloric intake. Another Canadian study (Ghadirian et al., 1991) was carried out among French-speaking citizens of Montreal whereas the study of Howe et al. (1990b) was done in Toronto. Examination of 179 cases and 239 controls indicated that the highest positive correlation was found with energy intake. Risk reduction was seen for increasing intake of fiber and β-carotene, but the trends were not significant.

A study of 1244 cases of esophageal and gastric cancers and 1314 controls in north central China suggested increased risk with increased intake of wheat and corn and no elevation of risk connected with decreased intake of fresh fruit or vegetables (Li et al., 1989). The authors suggested a genetic component of cancer susceptibility was present in the population.

Lung cancer in Chinese women in Hong Kong was studied by Koo (1988). The probands had never smoked so that was not a confounding factor. Higher consumption of leafy green vegetables, carrots, tofu, fresh fish, and fresh fruit appeared protective.

4. Conclusion

Except for colon cancer, interest in fiber effects on cancer risks has been minimal. The foregoing studies suggest some influences of fiber on breast cancer; there is a report of inverse correlation between fiber intake and pancreatic cancer (Howe et al., 1990b); and there seems to be no link between fiber and risk of prostate cancer.

B. Animal and Biomedical Studies

1. Animal Studies

While there has been a plethora of studies in animals, the results are difficult to interpret with regard to human effects. These problems in assessing results of animal experiments relating to fiber and colon cancer have been pointed out (Kritchevsky, 1983). Studies are carried out in rats of different strains; they are given different carcinogens or the same carcinogen by different routes of administration; and the diets range from commercial to semipurified. In general, however, the only fiber which has been relatively consistent in its protective effect is wheat bran. Wheat bran leads to a consistent reduction in incidence of experimentally induced colon cancer. For example, Cohen et al. (1991) have shown that wheat bran (10 percent) will reduce incidence of N-nitrosomethylurea-induced mammary tumors by 27 percent when added to a high- (23.5 percent) fat diet and by 25 percent when added to a low- (5 percent) fat diet. The high-fat diet is 43 percent more co-carcinogenic than the low-fat diet. This is the first report of the efficacy of dietary fiber in an animal model for mammary cancer. The results of another study (Klurfeld et al., 1991) confirmed a fairly large body of data indicating that wheat bran is protective against 1,2-dimethylhydrazine-induced colon tumors compared with cellulose and showed that the combination of wheat bran with caloric restriction is more protective than wheat bran in an ad libitum diet.

2. Biomedical Studies of Markers of Colon Cancer Risk

Studies of the effects of dietary fiber on human fecal bile acid excretion were reviewed in the LSRO report (Pilch, 1987). There are a few recent studies relating to metabolic or other markers associated with increased risk of colon cancer. Hoff et al. (1986) carried out a double-blind study in which endoscopic screening for polyps was combined with a dietary survey. They found a relationship between polyp presence or polyp size and estimated total dietary fiber in men ($p = 0.06$). Intake of cruciferous vegetables was negatively correlated with polyp number and extent of dysplasia in adenomas. Allinger et al. (1989) reported that a shift from low- to high-fiber intake reduced total concentrations of soluble fecal fatty acids and deoxycholic acid, both of which may have risk factor significance. In another study, the diets of subjects with familial polyposis were supplemented with 13.5 g/d of wheat bran for 8 wk with the result that the thymidine-labeling index of biopsied mucosal cells was reduced significantly (Alberts et al., 1990).

Using enzyme activity as a marker of cell proliferation, Calvert and Reicks (1988) studied the thymidine kinase specific activity of colonic mucosa of rats fed various fibers for 4 weeks. A diet containing 5 percent guar gum lowered the index by 17 percent, and one containing 10 percent wheat bran reduced it by 33 percent. When the diet contained 5 percent carrageenan, the index was increased 3.8-fold.

C. Discussion

1. Dietary Interactions

High-fiber foods contain an array of the carbohydrate polymers which are included in the term "fiber," as well as a number of other macro- and micronutrients, all of which may possess important biological properties. An important aspect of diets containing high levels of fiber-containing foods is the displacement of other foods. As a consequence, certain nutrition-related effects may result from what has been displaced, or there may be combined effects of fiber and fiber-displaced nutrients. It is difficult to separate fiber effects from those of other active substances in foods, such as β-carotene which is found in vegetables. There are a few studies in which analysis of the fiber has been carried out, but results are not consistent. For example, the work of Heilbrun et al. (1989) and Lee et al. (1989) suggests interaction between the fiber component of the diet and other factors which have not been identified. Slattery et al. (1988) found that in males and females in Utah, the odds ratio (OR) for risk of colon cancer at the highest quartile of starch intake was greater than at the third quartile. Grain intake provided a similar picture for Utah females. These findings suggest an optimum level for some foods which, when exceeded, may increase rather than decrease risk of colon cancer. Similar data on other cancers are lacking.

2. Summary of Certain Associated Factors in the Cancer–Fiber Relationship

a. Basis of association between dietary fiber and cancer   The ingredient, dietary fiber is a food component or may be added to foods. Whether the observed effects are due strictly to the fiber or to other components of the fiber-rich food or to a combination of these remains to be determined.

b. Level of intake for a beneficial effect   There is no agreed-upon measure as to the level of intake at which beneficial effects related to cancer are observed. The supporting data are far from unanimous. Furthermore, whether the effects of fiber are due to the fiber per se, accompanying substances, or displacement of fat and/or calories from the diet by fiber has not been established with certainty.

c. Optimal level of consumption and duration of effect   There are suggestions as to optimum level of intake for "better health" (e.g., normal bowel function) but not for prevention of disease. The FASEB review (Pilch, 1987) suggested that dietary fiber intake be linked to caloric intake and proposed an intake of 10–13 g/1000 kcal. There are no data relating to transience of a fiber effect although this is amenable to experimental testing.

d. Applicability to total U.S. population   Generalization of available scientific information to the entire U.S. population is difficult because data to support strongly the concept that fiber is protective are insufficient and there were few reports on subjects below 25 and over 65 years old. Presumably persons at high risk such as those with a family history of cancer would benefit most. Further, it is not clear as to whether the protective effects observed in some studies are the result of the fact that most high-fiber diets are low-fat diets. In addition, accumulating evidence suggests that caloric intake is a strong risk factor. For example, Lyon et al. (1987) concluded: "Total energy intake must be evaluated before attempting to assign a causal role to any food or nutrient that may be postulated to play a role in colon cancer."

e. Significant food sources of dietary fiber   Significant dietary sources of fiber (general) are whole grains, legumes, fruits, vegetables, and nuts. In addition, isolated fibers such as wheat and oat bran are added to various foodstuffs and prepared food products.

f. Influence of other dietary, nutritional, or health factors   In a marginally or undernourished population, high fiber intake may lead to trace mineral deficiency. This might also be the case in specific sections of our population (old people, children) (Pilch, 1987).

g. Safety concerns about reasonable or high levels of consumption   In general, reasonable consumption of a high-fiber diet poses no real health threat and may lead to less calorically dense diets. Sigmoid volvulus and persorption have been reported, but these are rare even in underdeveloped populations ingesting a high-fiber diet. Excessive consumption of fiber supplements is more likely to result in intestinal problems or poor absorption of trace minerals than would be expected from a high-fiber diet.

h. Difference in efficacy among food sources and supplements   Most of the cancer studies are based on retrospective dietary data and not on effects of isolated fibers. The only material which has been tested as fiber is wheat bran which in concentrated bulk is probably very little different from its native state. Although the bran, per se, may not differ from its native state, the total diet composition and associated nutritional effects may vary if bran is consumed as an additive to non-cereal foods compared with diet composition when bran is consumed in whole grain cereals. Wheat bran is a complex mixture which contains several types of fiber, some protein and fat, and trace minerals.

i. Critical gaps in knowledge   Questions which have not been answered satisfactorily are:

1) Is the putative beneficial effect a result of fiber or another component of the fiber-rich food such as β-carotene? That is, what are the contributions of fiber versus other plant components to lowering cancer risk?

2) If it is fiber, which one(s)? What are the relative contributions of specific categories of fiber types or fiber-rich foods to measurable beneficial effects?

3) Is it higher fiber or lower fat? To what extent can the putative protective effects of fiber be separated from the effects of reduced fat intake?

4) If fiber is shown to be actively protective, what should be the dosage to protect against various types of cancer?

3. Overall Summary

Various beneficial effects have been suggested for foods rich in dietary fiber including reduction of blood cholesterol levels and the risk of developing coronary atherosclerosis. Whole foods high in fiber, high-fiber fractions such as wheat bran, concentrated fibers such as pectins or cellulose, and fiber-enriched foods are types of fiber-containing products.

Interpretation of data is hampered by a number of factors such as the lack of a generally accepted definition of dietary fiber and limited knowledge of the physiological effects, mechanisms of action, and the effects of interactions with other dietary components of various types of dietary fiber. Moreover, simple, reliable methods for rapid and accurate qualitative and quantitative assessment of fiber in foods are not available. Consequently, the accuracy of most estimates of dietary fiber intakes is limited.

Major reviews of data collected prior to 1988 have generally shown the data for a possible effect of dietary fiber against cancer to be equivocal. Publications since 1987 that are evaluated in this report again showed no robust, consistent effect for protection against colorectal cancer; however, results of seven of nine cited studies associated decreased risk with increased intakes of dietary fiber. One study showed decreased risk when high-fiber was combined with low-fat, and one large, prospective, cohort study found no significant association between risk and intake of total fiber, fruits, vegetables, and cereals.

Three recent investigations examined biomedical markers of colon cancer risk. In one, a trend toward fewer and smaller colorectal polyps was observed with increasing total dietary fiber in subjects at high risk for colorectal cancer, and intake of cruciferous vegetables was negatively correlated with polyp number and degree of dysplasia in adenomas. Another study showed reduced concentrations of soluble fecal fatty acids and deoxycholic acid with high-fiber intakes, and a third study reported reduced thymidine labeling in biopsied colorectal mucosal cells in familial polyposis patients given a wheat bran supplement.

For breast cancer, three recent reviews are noteworthy. In relation to the circulating estrogen theory of the etiology of breast cancer, one review concluded that vegetarians (1) excrete more fecal estrogen, thus reducing enterohepatic circulation and (2) have a higher urinary excretion of lignans, a family of compounds formed in the intestine from fiber-associated precursors. A second review noted that breast cancer patients had high plasma estrogen levels, high urinary and low fecal excretion of estrogen, and low urinary excretion of lignans and phytoestrogens, all associated with high intakes of proteins and fat and low intakes of fiber-rich foods and grain products. A third review was a meta-analysis of 12 case–control studies of diet and breast cancer which suggested a protective effect of vegetables, fruit, and vitamin C.

Three of four reports of recent investigations associated decreased risk with increased intakes of carotenoids and fiber, or with crude fiber and grains, or cereals. The fourth study found no association between fiber and risk of breast cancer. Decreased risk of prostatic cancer with higher intakes of fiber was inferred from the circulating hormone hypothesis in one study and from higher intakes of rice and tofu in another study. In a third investigation, risk appeared to increase with high consumption of papaya, or, in a fourth study, with increased intake of β-carotene or vitamin A. A fifth study found no association between fiber and prostate cancer.

Decreased risk of pancreatic cancer was associated with increased intakes of fruit, vegetables, and cereal in one study; in another, a nonsignificant trend toward decreased risk with higher intakes of fiber and β-carotene was reported. Results of a large case–control study of esophageal and stomach cancer in China suggested an increased risk with higher intakes of wheat and corn but no increased risk with low intakes of fresh fruit and vegetables. Risk of lung cancer in nonsmoking women in Hong Kong was inversely associated with consumption of leafy green vegetables, carrots, tofu, and fresh fruit.

In animal studies, the only fiber source which has been relatively consistent in its protective effect against chemically induced colon tumors is wheat bran. One recent study shows it to protect against mammary tumors as well. In addition, diets containing guar gum or wheat bran lowered the thymidine kinase specific activity of rat colonic mucosa by 17 percent and 33 percent respectively compared with controls.

The Surgeon General's Report (U.S. Department of Health and Human Services, 1988) stated, "While inconclusive, some evidence suggests that an overall increase in intake of foods high in fiber might decrease risk for colon cancer," and "Limited information is available on the types of dietary fiber that might protect against cancer. Research will have to define the importance of various fiber compounds relative to risk for specific cancers."

The National Research Council (1989) report states, "Diets high in plant food—i.e., fruits, vegetables, legumes, and whole grain cereals—are associated with a lower occurrence of coronary heart disease and cancer of the lung, colon, esophagus, and stomach," and, "Epidemiologic and clinical studies indicate that a diet characterized by high-fiber foods may be associated with a lower risk of CHD, colon cancer, diabetes mellitus, diverticulosis, hypertension, or gallstone formation, but there is no conclusive evidence that it is dietary fiber, rather than the other components of vegetables, fruit, and cereal products, that reduces the risk of those diseases," and, "In general, the evidence for a protective role of dietary fiber per se in CHD, colon and rectal cancers, stomach cancer, female gynecologic cancers, diabetes, diverticulosis, hypertension and gallstones is inconclusive."

The present review of the recent literature leads to similar conclusions. Resolutions of the weight of scientific evidence will require separation of dietary fiber–cancer relationships and differentiation of specific fiber effects from those attributable to the whole food. Until this is done, the weight of scientific evidence must be viewed as inconclusive.

D. General Conclusions

The Surgeon General's Report, "Nutrition and Health" (1988) concluded that high-fiber diets are associated with lower rates of some types of cancer. The conclusion is non-specific and the data from studies noted in the appendix table of the present report are far from unanimous on this point. The NRC report, "Diet and Health" (1989), echoes the earlier NRC report (1982) which noted that findings were provocative, but insufficient to be conclusive. A critical review of the recent scientific literature leads to a similar conclusion. The subject is a very complex nutritional problem. Resolution of the issues involved will require separation of dietary fiber–cancer relationships and differentiation of specific fiber effects from the general ones attributable to the whole food (fiber, macronutrients, vitamins, minerals, total energy, etc.). Until this is done, the weight of scientific evidence must be viewed as inconclusive.

III. Bibliography*

Adlercreutz, H. 1990. Diet, breast cancer, and sex hormone metabolism. *Ann. N. Y. Acad. Sci.* 595:281–290.

Adlercreutz, H.; Hämäläinen, E.; Gorbach, S.R.; Goldin, B.R.; Woods, M.N.; Dwyer, J.T. 1989. Diet and plasma androgens in postmenopausal vegetarian and omnivorous women and postmenopausal women with breast cancer. *Am. J. Clin. Nutr.* 49:433–442.

Adlercreutz, H.; Höckerstedt, K.; Bannwart, C.; Bloigu, S.; Hämäläinen, E.; Fotsis, T.; Ollus, A. 1987. Effect of dietary components, including lignans and phytoestrogens, on enterohepatic circulation and liver metabolism of estrogens and on sex hormone binding globulin (SHBG). *J. Steroid Biochem.* 27:1135–1144.

Adlercreutz, H.; Höckerstedt, K.; Bannwart, C.; Hämäläinen, E.; Fotsis, T.; Bloigu, S. 1988. Association between dietary fiber, urinary excretion of lignans and isoflavonic phytoestrogens, and plasma non-protein bound sex hormones in relation to breast cancer. *Prog. Cancer Res. Therap.* 35:409–412.

Alberts, D.S.; Einspahr, J.; Rees-McGee, S.; Ramanujam, P.; Buller, M.K.; Clark, L.; Ritenbaugh, C.; Atwood, J.; Pethigal, P.; Earnest, D.; Villar, H.; Phelps, J.; Lipkin, M.; Wargovich, M.; Meyskens, F.L., Jr. 1990. Effects of dietary wheat bran fiber on rectal epithelial cell proliferation in patients with resection for colon cancer. *J. Natl. Cancer Inst.* 82:1280–1285.

Allinger, U.G.; Johansson, G.K.; Gustafsson, J.-A.; Rafter, J.J. 1989. Shift from a mixed to a lactovegetarian diet: influence on acidic lipids in fecal water—a potential risk factor for colon cancer. *Am. J. Clin. Nutr.* 50:992–996.

Bingham, S.A. 1990. Mechanisms and experimental and epidemiological evidence relating dietary fibre (non-starch polysaccharides) and starch to protection against large bowel cancer. *Proc. Nutr. Soc.* 49:153–171.

Brisson, J.; Verreault, R.; Morrison, A.S.; Tennina, S.; Meyer, F. 1989. Diet, mammographic features of breast tissue, and breast cancer risk. *Am. J. Epidemiol.* 130:14–24.

Burkitt, D.P. 1971. Epidemiology of cancer of the colon and rectum. *Cancer* 28:3–13.

Burkitt, D.P. 1973a. Epidemiology of large bowel disease: the role of fibre. *Proc. Nutr. Soc.* 32:145–149.

Burkitt, D.P. 1973b. Some diseases characteristic of modern Western civilization. *Br. Med. J.* 1:274–278.

Byers, T. 1988. Diet and cancer: any progress in the interim? *Cancer* 62:1713–1724.

Calvert, R.J.; Reicks, M. 1988. Alterations in colonic thymidine kinase enzyme activity induced by consumption of various dietary fibers. *Proc. Soc. Exp. Biol. Med.* 189:45–51.

Cohen, L.A.; Kendall, M.E.; Zang, E.; Meschter, C.; Rose, D.P. 1991. Modulation of *N*–nitrosomethylurea–induced mammary tumor promotion by dietary fiber and fat. *J. Natl. Cancer Inst.* 83:496–501.

DeCosse, J.J.; Miller, H.H.; Lesser, M.L. 1989. Effect of wheat fiber and vitamins C and E on rectal polyps in patients with familial adenomatous polyposis. *J. Natl. Cancer Inst.* 81:1290–1297.

Doll, R.; Peto, R. 1981. The causes of cancer: quantitative estimates of avoidable risks of cancer in the United States today. *J. Natl. Cancer Inst.* 66:1191–1308.

*This bibliography contains all reference citations that are either in the text or the appendix table or both.

Freudenheim, J.L.; Graham, S.; Marshall, J.R.; Haughey, B.P.; Wilkinson G. 1990a. A case–control study of diet and rectal cancer in western New York. *Am. J. Epidemiol.* 131:612–624.

Freudenheim, J.L.; Graham, S.; Horvath, P.J.; Marshall, J.R.; Haughey, B.P.; Wilkinson, G. 1990b. Risks associated with source of fiber and fiber components in cancer of the colon and rectum. *Cancer Res.* 50:3295–3300.

Friedman, E.; Lightdale, C.; Winawer, S. 1988. Effects of psyllium fiber and short-chain organic acids derived from fiber breakdown on colonic epithelial cells from high-risk patients. *Cancer Lett.* 43:121–124.

Gerhardsson de Verdier, M.; Hagman, U.; Steineck, G.; Rieger, A.; Norell, S.E. 1990. Diet, body mass and colorectal cancer: a case–referent study in Stockholm. *Int. J. Cancer* 46:832–838.

Ghadirian, P.; Simard, A.; Baillargeon, J.; Maisonneuve, P.; Boyle, P. 1991. Nutritional factors and pancreatic cancer in the francophone community in Montreal, Canada. *Int. J. Cancer* 47:1–6.

Graham, S.; Marshall, J.; Haughey, B.; Mittelman, A.; Swanson, M.; Zielezny, M.; Byers, T.; Wilkinson, G.; West, D. 1988. Dietary epidemiology of cancer of the colon in western New York. *Am. J. Epidemiol.* 128:490–503.

Heilbrun, L.K.; Nomura, A.; Hankin, J.H.; Stemmermann, G.N. 1989. Diet and colorectal cancer with special reference to fiber intake. *Int. J. Cancer* 44:1–6.

Higginson, J.; Oettlé, A.G. 1960. Cancer incidence in the Bantu and "Cape Colored" races of South Africa: report of a cancer survey in the Transvaal (1953–55). *J. Natl. Cancer Inst.* 24:589–671.

Hoff, G.; Moen, I.E.; Trygg, K.; Frφlich, W.; Sauar, J.; Vatn, M.; Gjone, E.; Larsen, S. 1986. Epidemiology of polyps in the rectum and sigmoid colon: evaluation of nutritional factors. *Scand. J. Gastroenterol.* 21:199–204.

Howe, G.R.; Hirohata, T.; Hislop, T.G.; Iscovich, J.M.; Yuan, J.-M.; Katsouyanni, K.; Lubin, F.; Marubini, E.; Modan, B.; Rohan, T.; Toniolo, P.; Shunzhang, Y. 1990a. Dietary factors and risk of breast cancer: combined analysis of 12 case–control studies. *J. Natl. Cancer Inst.* 82:561–569.

Howe, G.R.; Jain, M.; Miller, A.B. 1990b. Dietary factors and risks of pancreatic cancer: results of a Canadian population-based case–control study. *Int. J. Cancer* 45:604–608.

Jacobs, L.R. 1988. Fiber and colon cancer. *Gastroenterol. Clin. North Am.* 17:747–760.

Katsouyanni, K.; Willett, W.; Trichopoulos, D.; Boyle, P.; Trichopoulou, A.; Vasilaros, S.; Papadiamantis, J.; MacMahon, B. 1988. Risk of breast cancer among Greek women in relation to nutrient intake. *Cancer* 61:181–185.

Klurfeld, D.M.; Davidson, L.M.; Kritchevsky, D. 1991. Additive inhibition of colonic carcinogenesis by wheat bran and energy restriction. *FASEB J.* 5:A1285.

Kolonel, L.N.; Hankin, J.H.; Yoshizawa, C.N. 1987. Vitamin A and prostate cancer in elderly men: enhancement of risk. *Cancer Res.* 47:2982–2985.

Kolonel, L.N.; Yoshizawa, C.N.; Hankin, J.H. 1988. Diet and prostatic cancer: a case–control study in Hawaii. *Am. J. Epidemiol.* 127:999–1012.

Koo, L.C. 1988. Dietary habits and lung cancer risk among Chinese females in Hong Kong who never smoked. *Nutr. Cancer* 11:155–172.

Kritchevsky, D. 1983. Fiber, steroids, and cancer. *Cancer Res.* 43 (Suppl.):2491s–2495s.

Kritchevsky, D.; Klurfeld, D.M. 1986. Influence of caloric intake on experimental carcinogenesis: a review. *Adv. Exp. Med. Biol.* 206:55–68.

Lee, H.P.; Gourley, L.; Duffy, S.W.; Estève, J.; Lee, J.; Day, N.E. 1989. Colorectal cancer and diet in an Asian population—a case–control study among Singapore Chinese. *Int. J. Cancer* 43:1007–1016.

Le Marchand, L.; Hankin, J.H.; Kolonel, L.N.; Wilkens, L.R. 1991. Vegetable and fruit consumption in relation to prostate cancer risk in Hawaii: a reevaluation of the effect of dietary beta-carotene. *Am. J. Epidemiol.* 133:215–219.

Li, J.-Y.; Ershow, A.G.; Chen, Z.-J.; Wacholder, S.; Li, G.-Y.; Guo, W.; Li, B.; Blot, W.J. 1989. A case–control study of cancer of the esophagus and gastric cardia in Linxian. *Int. J. Cancer Res.* 43:755–761.

Lyon, J.L.; Mahoney, A.W.; West, D.W.; Gardner, J.W.; Smith, K.R.; Sorenson, A.W.; Stanish, W. 1987. Energy intake: its relationship to colon cancer risk. *J. Natl. Cancer. Inst.* 78:853–861.

Marlett, J.A. 1990. Issues in dietary fiber analysis. *Adv. Exp. Med. Biol.* 270:183–192.

Marlett, J.A.; Chesters, J.G.; Longacre, M.J.; Bogdanske, J.J. 1989. Recovery of soluble dietary fiber is dependent on the method of analysis. *Am. J. Clin. Nutr.* 50:479–485.

Miettinen, T.A.; Tarpila, S. 1989. Serum lipids and cholesterol metabolism during guar gum, plantago ovata and high fibre treatments. *Clin. Chim. Acta* 183:253–262.

National Research Council, Committee on Diet and Health. 1989. *Diet and health: implications for reducing chronic disease risk*. Washington, DC: National Academy Press.

National Research Council, Committee on Diet, Nutrition and Cancer. 1982. *Diet, nutrition and cancer*. Washington, DC: National Academy Press.

Oishi, K.; Okada, K.; Yoshida, O.; Yamabe, H.; Ohno, Y.; Hayes, R.B.; Schroeder, F.H. 1988. A case–control study of prostatic cancer with reference to dietary habits. *Prostate* 12:179–190.

Painter, N.S.; Almeida, A.Z.; Colebourne, K.W. 1972. Unprocessed bran in treatment of diverticular disease of the colon. *Br. Med. J.* 2:137–140.

Paul, A.A.; Southgate, D.A.T. 1978. *McCance and Widdowson's the composition of foods*. New York: Elsevier/North-Holland Biomedical Press.

Pennington, J.A.T. 1976. *Dietary nutrient guide*. Westport, CT: AVI Publishing Company.

Peto, R. 1986. Cancer around the world: evidence for avoidability. In: Hallgren, B.; Levin, O.; Rössner, S.; Vessby, B.; Ingvar, D.H.; Pernow, B.; Pellborn, L.A., eds. *Diet and prevention of coronary heart disease and cancer*. New York: Raven Press. p. 1–16.

Pickle, L.W.; Greene, M.H.; Ziegler, R.G.; Toledo, A.; Hoover, R.; Lynch, H.T.; Fraumeni, J.F., Jr. 1984. Colorectal cancer in rural Nebraska. *Cancer Res.* 44:363–369.

Pilch, S.M., editor. 1987. *Physiological effects and health consequences of dietary fiber*. Prepared for the Center for Food Safety and Applied Nutrition, Food and Drug Administration under Contract No. FDA 223-84-2059 by the Life Sciences Research Office, Federation of American Societies for Experimental Biology. Available from: FASEB Special Publications Office, Bethesda, MD.

Pryor, M.; Slattery, M.L.; Robison, L.M.; Egger, M. 1989. Adolescent diet and breast cancer in Utah. *Cancer Res.* 49:2161–2167.

Pusateri, D.J.; Roth, W.T.; Ross, J.K.; Shultz, T.D. 1990. Dietary and hormonal evaluation of men at different risks for prostate cancer: plasma and fecal hormone–nutrient interrelationships. *Am. J. Clin. Nutr.* 51:371–377.

Reddy, B.; Engle, A.; Katsifis, S.; Simi, B.; Bartram, H.-P.; Perrino, P.; Mahan, C. 1989. Biochemical epidemiology of colon cancer: effect of types of dietary fiber on fecal mutagens, acid, and neutral sterols in healthy subjects. *Cancer Res.* 40:4629–4635.

Rogers, A.E.; Longnecker, M.P. 1988. Biology of disease—dietary and nutritional influences on cancer: a review of epidemiologic and experimental data. *Lab. Invest.* 59:729–759.

Rohan, T.E.; McMichael, A.J.; Baghurst, P.A. 1988. A population-based case–control study of diet and breast cancer in Australia. *Am. J. Epidemiol.* 128:478–489.

Rose, D.P. 1990. Dietary fiber and breast cancer. *Nutr. Cancer* 13:1–8.

Rosen, M.; Nyström, L.; Wall, S. 1988. Diet and cancer mortality in the counties of Sweden. *Am. J. Epidemiol.* 127:42–49.

Ross, J.K.; Pusateri, D.J.; Shultz, T.D. 1990. Dietary and hormonal evaluation of men at different risk for prostate cancer: fiber intake, excretion and composition, with in vitro evidence for an association between steroid hormones and specific fiber components. *Am. J. Clin. Nutr.* 51:365–370.

Severson, R.K.; Nomura, A.M.; Grove, J.S.; Stemmermann, G.N. 1989. A prospective study of demographics, diet, and prostate cancer among men of Japanese ancestry in Hawaii. *Cancer Res.* 49:1857–1860.

Slattery, M.L.; French, T.K.; Egger, M.J.; Lyon, J.L. 1989. Diet and survival of patients with colon cancer in Utah: is there an association? *Int. J. Epidemiol.* 18:792–797.

Slattery, M.L.; Sorenson, A.W.; Mahoney, A.W.; French, T.K.; Kritchevsky, D.; Street, J.C. 1988. Diet and colon cancer: assessment of risk by fiber type and food source. *J. Natl. Cancer Inst.* 80:1474–1480.

Spiller, G.A.; Jenkins, D.J.A. 1986. Dietary fiber supplements, physiological and pharmacological aspects: a workshop report. In: Taylor, T.G.; Jenkins, N.K., eds. *Proceedings of the XIII International Congress of Nutrition.* London: John Libbey. p. 184–185.

Tannenbaum, A. 1945. The dependence of tumor formation on the degree of caloric restriction. *Cancer Res.* 5:609–615.

Trock, B.; Lanza, E.; Greenwald, P. 1990. Dietary fiber, vegetables, and colon cancer: critical review and meta-analyses of the epidemiologic evidence. *J. Natl. Cancer Inst.* 82:650–661.

U.S. Department of Health and Human Services. 1988. *The Surgeon General's report on nutrition and health.* Available from: U.S. Government Printing Office, Washington, DC.

Van't Veer, P.; Kolb, C.M.; Verhoef, P.; Kok, F.J.; Schouten, E.G.; Hermus, R.J.J.; Sturmans, F. 1990. Dietary fiber, beta-carotene and breast cancer: results from a case–control study. *Int. J. Cancer* 45:825–828.

West, D.W.; Slattery, M.L.; Robison, L.M.; Schuman, K.L.; Ford, M.H.; Mahoney, A.W.; Lyon, J.L.; Sorensen, A.W. 1989. Dietary intake and colon cancer: sex- and anatomic site-specific associations. *Am. J. Epidemiol.* 130:883–894.

Willett, W.C.; Stampfer, M.J.; Colditz, G.A.; Rosner, B.A.; Speizer, F.E. 1990. Relation of meat, fat, and fiber intake to the risk of colon cancer in a prospective study among women. *N. Engl. J. Med.* 323:1664–1672.

Wilson, J.D. 1972. Recent studies on the mechanism of action of testosterone. *N. Engl. J. Med.* 287:1284–1291.

Appendix

Criteria for Inclusion of Articles in Appendix Table

Articles in peer-reviewed journals related to the topic of this review were selected primarily on the basis of date and content. In general, papers appearing in 1987 or thereafter were included, provided that they presented original data from studies in humans Certain items tabulated for the sake of completeness may not have been cited in the body of the text if their weight or relevance did not add significantly to development of the author's argument. Reviews have not been listed except as they included new data or useful meta-analyses.

APPENDIX TABLE   Influence of Dietary Fiber on Cancer[1]

		A. Colorectal		
Reference	Study Design	Number and Description of Subjects	Duration	Source and Identity of Test Material
Alberts et al., 1990	Prospective clinical trial of fiber on markers of carcinogenesis NR, SC. Rectal biopsy 1 mo after low-fiber diet, measured thymidine uptake in intact rectal crypt cells and in minced tissue.	17 pts, 54–70 yr, at high risk of recurrent colorectal cancer	8 wk	All Bran® wheat base supplement
Allinger et al., 1989	Dietary intervention study of effect of lactovegetarian diet on fecal bile acids and deoxycholate	26 volunteers (6 ♂, 20 ♀) 26–61 yr	3 mo	Increased intake of fruit and vegetables
DeCosse et al., 1989	PRCT of wheat fiber, and vitamins C and E on number and size of rectal polyps	62 pts with familial adenomatous polyposis who had colectomies and ileo-rectal anastomoses	4 yr	Commercial bran cereal
Freudenheim et al., 1990a	Retrospective CC study	Rectal cancer: cases: 277 ♂, 145 ♀ controls: 277 ♂, 145 ♀	1978–1986	Vegetables, cereals and grains Food-frequency interviews
Freudenhiem et al., 1990b	Reassessment of results of Graham et al. (1988) and Freudenheim et al. (1990a)	Graham et al. (1988): cases: 205 ♂, 223 ♀ controls: 205 ♂, 223 ♀	1975–1986	Vegetables, cereals, grains
Friedman et al., 1988	In vitro study of effect of fiber on deoxycholic acid (DOC)-induced lysis of cultured colonic epithelial cells	Colonic epithelial cells from 18 ♂ and 13 ♀ at high risk of colon cancer		Purified psyllium fiber
Gerhardsson de Verdier, 1990	Population-based case–referent study of diet, body mass, and colorectal cancer	720 ♂ and ♀ cancer pts (452 colon, 268 rectum). 624 controls.	January 1986 –March 1988	Food-frequency questionnaire and analysis for fiber
Graham et al., 1988	Retrospective CC study	Colon cancer population: cases: 205 ♂, 223 ♀ controls: 205 ♂, 223 ♀	1975–1984	Vegetables, cereals, and grains. Food-frequency interviews.

[1]The references cited in this table refer either to the text, this table, or both.

		A. Colorectal		
Dosage	Base Diet	Other Factors Affecting Data Interpretation	Results	Assessment of Study
13.5 g/d	Usual diet	Pilot study, small N, NR, short-term	Overall 22% lower in DNA synthesis and rectal cell proliferation after 2 mo of wheat bran supplementation.	Results appear to confirm a mechanism of action of wheat bran fiber.
DF estimated at 30 g/d	Usual mixed diet before experiment	Uncertainty about biologic mechanisms of DF	Lower concentration of soluble fatty acids and deoxycholic acid in fecal water.	Useful contribution; source of test hypotheses
High-fiber: 22.5 g/d plus 400 mg α-tocopherol and 4 g ascorbic acid/d	Usual diet	Fiber consumption showed downward trend with time, but greater intake prevailed in high-fiber group. Study population was ambulatory.	58 pts assessable in study. Benign large bowel neoplasia was inhibited by grain fiber supplements > 11 g/d; however, the effect was "limited." Prescribed high-fiber supplement seemed to lower polyp size and number.	Useful results in a unique difficult-to-acquire and administer study population. It is not clear whether changes in rectal cell proliferation reflect similar changes in colon.
Low to high: ♂ by quartiles ♀ by tertiles	Usual diet	Some unavoidable error in dietary intake estimates; many CC studies had few cases of rectal cancer.	Increased intakes of vitamin C, carotenoids, and vegetable fiber were protective.	High quality study
Low to high	Usual diet		Colon: ♂—grain fiber, veg fiber = decreased risk; ♀—Grain fiber = decreased risk Rectum: ♂,♀—veg fiber = decreased risk	A reassessment of earlier data. Sex differences exist.
Amount not specified			Increase in percentage of surviving colonies at 10 nM, 0.1mM, 0.5 mM, and 1.0 mMDOC were 5.1, 4.1, 3.8, and 4.6. Propionate was potent colonocyte mitogen.	Relevance to in vivo effects not clear
Low to high by quintiles	Usual diet during 5 yr before cancer dx	Dietary recall up to 5 yr in the past limits accuracy of intake estimates	High fiber intake associated with decreased risk of colon cancer in ♂ and rectal cancer in ♂ and ♀ RR—♂ 0.5; ♀ 1.2 for colon RR—♂ 0.5; ♀ 0.4 for rectum	A carefully conducted study
Low to high by quintiles	Usual diet	Some unavoidable error in dietary intake estimate despite great care in food-frequency interviews	Dietary fiber only equivocally associated with colon cancer risk. Seems to reduce risk for ♀ (For added information see Freudenheim et al., 1990b.)	Carefully conducted study

(continued)

APPENDIX TABLE *(continued)*

Reference	Study Design	Number and Description of Subjects	Duration	Source and Identity of Test Material
Heilbrun et al., 1989	Cohort and CC study	Cohort—8006 American Japanese ♂. Cancer cases during > 16 yr follow-up: 102 colon, 60 rectal. Cancer-free control: 361♂.	1965–1985	Vegetables, cereals, grains from usual diet
Lee et al., 1989	Hospital-based CC study of colorectal cancer	Singapore Chinese Cases: Colon—77♂; 55♀. Rectum—44 ♂; 27♀. Controls: 239 ♂; 187 ♀.	1985–1987	Vegetables
Reddy et al., 1989	Prospective dietary intervention trial in healthy volunteers to determine effects of different DFs on fecal mutagens, acid and neutral sterols. Randomized, crossover design, each subject tested for 5 wk on each of 3 DF supplements.	19 healthy volunteers who exhibited high levels of fecal mutagens	7 mo (Approximately)	Wheat bran, oat fiber, cellulose
Rosen et al., 1988	Swedish correlational study of colon cancer mortality and food acquisition for households in different regions	N/A		Fiber calculated from food expenditure
Slattery et al., 1988	Population-based CC study of dietary fiber in relation to colon cancer	Cases: 112 ♂, 119 ♀ Controls: 185 ♂, 206 ♀	1979–1983	Dietary fruits, vegetables, grains, estimated by food-frequency questionnaire
Slattery et al., 1989	Correlation analysis of 2 population-based CC studies. Dietary intakes were estimated 2–5 yr before cancer dx.	411 colon cancer pts	Cancers dx 1976–1871	Dietary fiber
Trock et al., 1990	Review and appraisal of all epidemiological studies of colorectal cancer and fiber, vegetables, grains, or fruit published from 1970 through 1988. Meta-analysis of 16 CC studies. Total covered: 37 observational and 23 CC.	N/A	Span of studies about 18 yr	Fiber from all fiber-containing foods

Dosage	Base Diet	Other Factors Affecting Data Interpretation	Results	Assessment of Study
Cancer cases: 11.5–12.1 g/d Controls: 11.6 g/d	Usual diet	Only one 24-hr dietary-recall interview to estimate fiber and nutrient intakes	When fat intake < 61 g/d, colon cancer risk drops as fiber increases—$p = 0.042$. No significant association between fiber intake and risk of rectal cancer	Preliminary results
Low to high by tertiles of intake	Usual diet	Uncertainties of actual dietary intakes	Cruciferous vegetables protect against colon and rectal cancer. High meat to vegetable ratio increases risk of colon cancer; no consistent trend for fat and fiber.	Apparent lack of fat and fiber influence needs further study.
10 g/d as dietary supplement. Normal diets in control periods	Self-selected, high-fat, low-fiber		Effects on fecal secondary bile acids and mutagenic activity: wheat bran—decrease cellulose—decrease oat fiber—no effect	Type of fiber appears important in determining effects.
Usual Diet		Gross uncertainties of actual dietary intakes; time mismatch between survey of food purchases and mortality data	Inverse relationship between consumption of dietary fiber, crisp bread and colon cancer mortality in ♂ and ♀ $r = 0.62$	Data suggest protective effect of dietary fiber but statistical power is weak
Low to high by quartiles	Usual diet	Small N to support the various parameters analyzed; uncertainty of dietary intake	♂ and ♀ intake of fruits, vegetables inversely related to colon cancer risk. Grains not protective. DF and NDF: no consistent relationship; mannose, galactose protective in ascending colon in ♂; galactose and uronic acid protective in ascending colon in ♀.	Useful study
Low to high by quartiles	Usual diet, precancer dx	Dietary recall 2–5 yr in the past limits accuracy of intake estimates	Highest quartile of fiber intake associated with decreased survival compared with lowest quartile of intake	Limited statistical power
High and low levels of consumption	Usual diets		A majority of studies showed protective effect associated with fiber-rich foods. When highest and lowest quintile of intake were compared the estimated combined ORs were: 0.57 for fiber-rich diets 0.48 for vegetable consumption.	A useful analysis

(*continued*)

APPENDIX TABLE *(continued)*

Reference	Study Design	Number and Description of Subjects	Duration	Source and Identity of Test Material
West et al., 1989	CC study of diet and colon cancer	Cases: 112 ♂, 119 ♀ Control: 185 ♂, 206 ♀	1979–1983	Dietary fruits, vegetables, estimated on food-frequency questionnaire and analysis for crude fiber, NDF, and sugar fractions
Willett et al., 1990	Prospective cohort study of relationships between intakes of meat, fat, and fiber and colon cancer	Cohort 88,751 ♀, 34–59 yr By 1986, incident cases of colon cancer = 150	1980–1986	Dietary questionnaire and estimation of fiber content

	B. Breast			
Katsouyanni et al., 1988	CC study of diet and breast cancer	120 cases controls: 120 non-cancer pts	1983–1984	Dietary intake estimates from food frequency questionnaire
Pryor et al., 1989	Population-based CC study of adolescent diet and breast cancer.	172 cases 190 controls 20–54 yr	1980–1983	Dietary intakes estimates from food-frequency interviews
Rohan et al., 1988	Population-based CC study of diet and breast cancer	Cases: 451; 20–74 yr Controls: 451 no hx breast cancer, age-matched	1982–1984	Dietary intakes estimated from self-administered food-frequency questionnaire and food composition tables
Van't Veer et al., 1990	Population-based CC study of dietary fiber, β-carotene, and breast cancer	133 cases, 25–44 yr 238 controls, 55–64 yr	1985–1987	Dietary intakes estimated from dietary history interviews

	C. Pancreas			
Ghadirian et al., 1991	Population-based CC study of diet and pancreatic cancer in French-speaking Canadians	Cases: 179 (97 ♂, 82 ♀) Controls: 239, age- and sex-matched	1984–1988	Dietary intakes estimated from interviewer-administered food-frequency questionnaire. Fiber estimated as total and crude

Dosage	Base Diet	Other Factors Affecting Data Interpretation	Results	Assessment of Study
Low to high by quartiles	Usual diet 1–2 yr before cancer dx	Dietary recall limits accuracy of intake estimates	Fiber (or crude fiber) was protective in ♀ (OR—0.5). ♂ risk estimates for fibers = 0.3 and cruciferous vegetables = 0.3.	Data support the fiber hypothesis
Low to high by quintiles	Usual diet, pre-cancer dx	Dietary recall limits accuracy of intake estimates	Low intake of fiber from fruits was associated with increased risk of colon cancer, but not statistically independent of meat intake.	A carefully conducted study

B. Breast

Dosage	Base Diet	Other Factors Affecting Data Interpretation	Results	Assessment of Study
ND	Usual precancer dx diet	Uncertainty of actual dietary intakes	No evidence of a protective effect of dietary fiber, but Vitamin A protective. No ↑ risk from dietary fat.	Apparent lack of fiber effect needs validation.
ND	Adolescent diet as estimated by diet interview	Possible biased estimate from low response rate, recall bias, and lack of precision in dietary instrument	Postmenopause: high-fiber intake related to ↑ ORs, but grain fiber related to ↓ risk in pre- and postmenopause subjects	Level of risk unclear, nutrient source may be important.
ND	Usual pre-dx diet	Uncertainty of actual dietary intakes. Dietary energy, protein, fat, carbohydrate (including fiber), and vitamin A were study foci.	Risk decreased nonuniformly at upper 3 quintiles of fiber intake; statistically nonsignificant	Extensive study that suggests a protective effect of fiber
ND	Usual diet during 12 mo preceding dx	Uncertainty of actual dietary intakes	Fiber intake lower in cases than controls. β-carotene similar in both groups. OR for highest quartile intake of cereal products: 0.42; OR for fiber intake = 0.55, but trend NS	Results suggest a diet rich in vegetable products may lower risk of breast cancer.

C. Pancreas

Dosage	Base Diet	Other Factors Affecting Data Interpretation	Results	Assessment of Study
ND	1- and 10-yr pre-dx diet estimate	Uncertainty of actual dietary intakes despite extra care in administering food-frequency questionnaire	No significant effect of estimated fiber intake on risk	Fiber was not a primary study focus.

(continued)

APPENDIX TABLE *(continued)*

Reference	Study Design	Number and Description of Subjects	Duration	Source and Identity of Test Material
Howe et al., 1990b	Population-based CC study of diet and pancreatic cancer	Cases: 249 (141 ♂, 108 ♀) 35–79 yr Controls: 505, age- and sex-matched	1983–1986	Total fiber from fruit, vegetables, and cereals. Dietary intakes estimated from interviewer-administered food-frequency question- naire. Fiber estimat- ed from food tables.

D. Prostate

Reference	Study Design	Number and Description of Subjects	Duration	Source and Identity of Test Material
Le Marchand et al., 1991	Further analysis of a 1987 CC study of vitamin A and prostate cancer (Kolonel et al., 1987)	Cases: 452 multi- ethnic ♂	1977–1983	Quantitative hx of food frequency and portion size
Oishi et al., 1988	CC study of prostatic cancer and diet	Cases: 100, 50–79 yr Age-matched controls: 100 BPH 100 hospital pts with no prostatic pathology	1981–1984	Food consumption and portion size interview
Severson et al., 1989	Prospective cohort study of demographics, diet, and prostate cancer	7999 Japanese- American ♂. Incident cases: 74	1965–1986	Food-frequency questionnaire plus 24-hr diet recall at interview

E. Other

Reference	Study Design	Number and Description of Subjects	Duration	Source and Identity of Test Material
Koo, 1988	Retrospective CC study of diet and lung cancer in non-smoking Hong Kong Chinese women	Cases: 88 ♀, mean age 57.8 yr District-matched con- trols: 137 All subjects never smoked tobacco.	1981–1983	Dietary interview of food consumption patterns
Li et al., 1989	Population-based CC study of diet, other risk factors, and can- cers of esophagus, cardia, in Linxian, China	1244 cases (758 ♂, 468 ♀), 35–64 yr Age- and sex-matched controls (789 ♂, 525 ♀)	1984–1985	Interviewer admin- istered food- frequency question- naire

ABBREVIATIONS:

BPH—benign prostatic hypertrophy	N/A—not applicable	OR—odds ratio
CC—case control	ND—not described	PRCT—prospective, randomized, controlled trial
DF—dietary fiber	NDF—neutral detergent fiber	pt—patient
dx—diagnosis	NR—nonrandom	RR—relative risk
FA—fatty acid	NS—nonsignificant	SC—self-controlled
hx—history		

Dosage	Base Diet	Other Factors Affecting Data Interpretation	Results	Assessment of Study
ND	Usual diet 1–2 yr before interview	Uncertainties related to actual dietary intakes and validity of information from proxies	Fiber—highest quartile of intake RR = 0.42 p < 0.0004. Positive association with total caloric intake.	Study carefully conducted; supports the need for added investigation

D. Prostate

	Usual pre-dx diet	Limitations in dietary data	No association of yellow-orange fruits and vegetables, tomatoes, dark green veg., and cruciferous veg., with risk of prostate cancer except in ♂ > 70.9 yr; papaya increased OR to 2.5 p < 0.0001	Useful study leading to test hypotheses
	Usual diet 5 yr before interview	Limitation in accuracy of dietary intake estimates	Estimated fiber intake was not correlated with risk of prostate cancer.	Fiber was 1 of 7 dietary component categories analyzed.
ND	Usual diet at time of interview	Limitation in dietary data. 23 foods or food-component categories analyzed	RRs: tofu 0.35 fruit 1.31 seaweed 1.74 rice 0.38	More research needed to sort out diet-prostate cancer relationships

E. Other

	Usual diet 1 yr before cancer dx	Limitations in dietary data and number of patients	Adjusted RR: 2.4 and 2.8 for lowest tertile of intake of fresh fruit and fresh fish, respectively. Protective effects of vegetables, carrots, tofu, fresh fruit, and fresh fish mostly applied to adenocarcinoma or large cell tumors. Only fresh fruit affected risk of squamous and small cell tumors.	Fruit may contain a protective factor other than fiber.
	Usual diet in the late 1950s and the late 1970s	Limitations in dietary data	ORs: wheat 2.0, corn 1.5, millet 0.7, fresh veg. 1.5, dried veg. 0.8, fruit 1.0	Slight increased risk for fiber-rich foods. Cause of high incidence of esophageal cancer in Linxian was not identified.

Dietary Fiber and Cancer: An Update

David Kritchevsky, Ph.D.

Howe et al. (1992) have published a meta-analysis reviewing data on dietary fiber intake and risks of colorectal cancer. Data from 13 case–control studies were combined for analysis. Original data records for 5287 cases and 10470 controls were combined and relative risks and confidence levels were estimated for intakes of fiber, vitamin C and β-carotene using logistic regression analysis. All but one study showed that there was an inverse relationship between increasing intake of fiber and risk of colorectal cancer compared to the lowest quintile of fiber intake, increasing fiber intake gave relative risks of 0.79, 0.69, 0.63 and 0.53 ($p < 0.0001$). The inverse association was true regardless of cancer site, gender or age of the subject. Only a weak inverse association was found for intakes of vitamin C or β-carotene. The authors conclude that risk of colorectal cancer in Americans could be reduced by 31 percent if fiber intake from food sources were increased by 13 g/d.

Dwyer and Ausman (1992) have reviewed the subject of fiber and its protective effects and enumerated a number of questions which remain to be answered. Among the unanswered questions are most effective type of fiber, dose-response, the "more-fiber–less-fat" relationship and mechanism(s) of action. In subsequent publications both authors (Ausman, 1993; Dwyer, 1993) address the evidence regarding the role of dietary fiber in carcinogenesis and comment on the overall inconsistency of the data and need for delineation of mechanisms of action.

Giovannucci et al. (1992) examined the relationship between diet and risk of colorectal adenoma in men. Studying quintiles of intake they found significant positive associations with total fat ($p = 0.003$), saturated fat ($p = 0.006$), monounsaturated fat ($p = 0.04$), no relationship of protein or cholesterol and a significant negative trend for total carbohydrate intake ($p < 0.001$). Dietary fiber was inversely associated with risk of adenoma ($p < 0.0001$) as were all sources of fiber, namely, vegetables, fruits and grains. The data were derived from the Health Professionals Follow-Up Study in which the authors compared 170 cases with 7284 controls.

Sandler et al. (1993) also investigated the relationships between diet and risk of colorectal adenomas. In women, carbohydrate intake was inversely related to adenoma risk ($p = 0.002$). Intake of fruits per se or fiber derived from fruits or vegetables was also inversely related to risk of adenoma ($p = 0.028$ for fruit, 0.012 for fiber). The risks in men were similar in direction and magnitude but did not reach statistical significance. The case–control study included 236 cases (105 men, 131 women) and 409 controls (165 men, 244 women).

The adenoma study also showed a strong positive relation between dietary fat and adenomas in women ($p = 0.004$) whereas the analysis by Howe did not include fat. Thus we still must resolve the question of fiber being effective because high-fiber diets are usually low-fat diets. In a third diet–adenoma study (Neugut et al., 1993) incident and recurrent polyps were compared. There were 286 patients (162 men, 124 women) in the incident group and they were compared with 480 controls (210 men, 270 women). In the recurrence study 186 patients (130 men, 56 women were compared with 330 controls (187 men, 143 women).

Increased caloric intake increased risk for incidence and recurrence in both sexes. Otherwise consistent relationships were only found in the female probands. Measuring quintiles of intake, positive trends between incident polyps and diet were seen for intake of saturated fat ($p = 0.07$) and ratio of red meat to chicken and fish ($p = 0.06$). A significant negative relationship was found between incident polyps and vitamin A intake ($p = 0.02$). The p value for the trend between incidence of polyps and dietary fiber was >0.2.

In the case of recurrent polyps, only total fiber intake yielded a significant negative trend ($p = 0.01$). Trends for positive relationships with total ($p = 0.09$) and saturated fat ($p = 0.15$) and negative relationships with intake of carbohydrates ($p = 0.10$) and vitamin A ($p = 0.12$) did not reach significance.

The relationship of polyp occurrence and recurrence to diet seems to be a particularly appropriate area of study. The discrepancies among the data in the three cited papers emphasize the need for further study but even in the face of the differences (in gender, for instance) the results are exciting and promising.

Willett et al. (1992) in an 8-year follow-up of the Nurses Health Study reported that they found no evidence for an adverse effect of dietary fat or beneficial effect of dietary fiber on incidence of breast cancer in their cohort of 84494 women.

Bibliography

Ausman, L.M. 1993. Fiber and colon cancer: Does the current evidence justify a preventive policy? *Nutr. Rev.* 51: 57–63

Dwyer, J. 1993. Dietary fiber and colorectal cancer risk. *Nutr. Rev.* 51:147–155.

Dwyer, J.T. and Ausman, L.M. 1992. Fiber: Unanswered questions. *J. Natl. Cancer Inst.* 84:1851–1853.

Giovannucci, E.; Stampfer, M.J.; Colditz, G.; Rimm, E.B. and Willett, W.C. 1992. Relationship of diet to risk of colorectal adenoma in men. *J. Natl. Cancer Inst.* 84:91–98.

Howe, G.R.; Benito, E.; Castalleto, R.; Corneé, J.; Esteve, J.; Gallagher, R.P.; Iscovich, J.M.; Deng-ao, J.; Kaoks, R.; Kune, G.A.; Kune, S.; L'Abbé, K.A.; Lee, H.P.; Lee, M.; Miller, A.B.; Peters, R.K.; Potter, J.D.; Riboli, E.; Slattery, M.L.; Trichopoulos, D.; Tuyns, A.; Tzonou, A.; Whittermore, A.S.; WuWilliams, A.H. and Shu, Z. 1992. Dietary intake of fiber and decreased risk of cancers of the colon and rectum: Evidence from combined analysis of 13 case–control studies. *J. Natl. Cancer Inst.* 84:1887–1896.

Neugut, A.I.; Garbowski, G.C.; Lee, W.C.; Murray, T.; Nieves, J.W.; Forde, K.A.; Treat, M.R.; Waye, J.D and Fenoglio-Preiser, C. 1993. Dietary risk factors for the incidence and recurrence of colorectal adenomatous polyps. A case–control study. *Arch. Int. Med.* 118:91–95.

Sandler, R.S.; Lyles, C.M.; Perpins, L.A.; McAuliffe, C.A.; Woosley, J.T. and Kupper, L.L. 1993. Diet and risk of colorectal adenomas: Macronutrients, cholesterol and fiber. *J. Natl. Cancer Inst.* 85:884–891.

Willett, W.C.; Hunter, D.J.; Stampfer, M.J.; Colditz, G.; Manson, J.E.; Spiegelman, D.; Rosner, B.; Hennekens, C.H. and Speizer, F.E. 1992. Dietary fat and fiber in relations to risk of breast cancer. An. 8-year follow-up. *J. Am. Med. Assoc.* 268:2037–2044.

Chapter 2

Vitamin A and Cancer

A. Catharine Ross, Ph.D.

I. Introduction

The possibility of a relationship between vitamin A and cancer first became apparent shortly after vitamin A was recognized as a distinct, new nutritional entity in 1913 (McCollum and Davis). In the 1920s, Mori (1922) and Wolbach and Howe (1925) reported that vitamin A deficiency was associated with a change from normal epithelial morphology to a xerotic, squamous, keratinized epithelium in various tissues including the mucosal linings of the trachea, larynx, and bronchi. Since metaplastic change is often the precursor of malignant transformation, it was reasonable to propose that vitamin A functions in the maintenance of normal tissue morphology and control of cellular growth. Experiments conducted from the mid-1950s to the present have provided strong evidence that natural vitamin A (retinol and its fatty acid esters) and synthetic analogues of retinol, collectively known as retinoids, can regulate cellular differentiation in a variety of experimental systems [see ref. Roberts and Sporn (1984) for review]. Many of the retinoids are potent inhibitors of neoplastic change initiated by chemical carcinogens or other transformants (Roberts and Sporn, 1984), and several of the retinoids have gained importance as therapeutic agents in certain proliferative diseases, mainly of the skin (Bollag, 1983).

A. Diet and Cancer

The magnitude of the relationship between environmental risk factors and the development of human cancers is still unknown. In 1981, Doll and Peto (1981) estimated that some 80–90 percent of human cancers may be attributable to environmental factors, and that the etiology of about 35 percent (range 10–70 percent) of human cancers may be related to dietary factors. Estimates made by other researchers have been similar (United States Department of Health and Human Services [USDHHS], 1988). Given the hypothesized role of vitamin A in growth control and cellular differentiation, the relationship of vitamin A as a nutrient to cancer incidence and the relationship of vitamin A or its analogues to cancer treatment have become a subject of great interest to biologists, clinicians, and the public.

Several major reports on nutrition and health, summarized below, have reviewed the scientific literature through the late 1980s on which our current understanding of the potential relationships of vitamin A and human cancer is based. These reports form the benchmarks from which this update and review are based. Between 1988 and the present, over 50 new reports have been published on the relationship of vitamin A in the diet, or vitamin A status as determined by serological measures, to indices of cancer risk. The major objective of this chapter will be to assess our current knowledge based on the benchmark references and on these additional human studies and basic experiments.

B. Vitamin A: Nomenclature and Exposure

In this review, the term vitamin A will be used in the nutritional sense to describe both dietary retinol and the portion of those dietary carotenoids which, through metabolism, give rise to retinol. Thus, dietary vitamin A comprises *retinol and retinyl esters* which are obtained exclusively from foods of animal origin or from vitamin supplements and the *carotenoids with provitamin A activity* that are obtained mainly from foods of plant origin (leafy green and yellow-orange vegetables) or, to a more limited extent, from milk, eggs, or other tissues of animals which have absorbed dietary carotenoids. Of the over 500 carotenoids that have been identified chemically, only about 50 have any vitamin A activity (Bendich and Olson, 1989). In the common leafy green and yellow-orange vegetables, the predominant provitamin A activity is due to a hydrocarbon carotene, beta (β)-carotene, which makes up 75–85 percent of the total carotenoid in these foods (Bendich and Valez, 1987; Micozzi, 1989; Vitamin Nutrition Information Service [VNIS], 1987). Other members of the carotenoid family such as the oxygenated carotenoids (e.g., lutein, epoxycarotenoids) and other hydrocarbon carotenoids (e.g., lycopene) may be absorbed and are found in the circulation but cannot be converted to retinol and thus do not have provitamin A activity (Micozzi, 1989). It is nearly always desirable to distinguish the individual chemical forms of retinoids or carotenoids; however, this information is not always available or has not been distinguished in published reports. In these cases, the general terms vitamin A, retinoids, provitamin A, or carotenoids will be used.

In the typical U.S. diet, preformed vitamin A constitutes approximately two-thirds to three-quarters of the total vitamin A; the remaining portion is derived from carotenoids with provitamin A activity (National Research Council [NRC], 1989a,b; Ziegler, 1991). In other parts of the world, carotenoids typically provide 80–90 percent of dietary vitamin A (see Underwood in ref. VNIS, 1987).

Few of the studies on diet and cancer published prior to the mid-1980s were intentionally designed to discriminate between the retinol and carotene components of total dietary vitamin A. However, when the results of dietary questionnaires pointed towards the protective effects of foods which are major sources of β-carotene, a potential relationship between dietary or plasma carotene(s) and cancer rates emerged. In 1981, Peto and colleagues (1981) reviewed the literature available at that time and formulated the provocative question "Can dietary beta-carotene materially reduce cancer rates?" Since then, there has been a gradual evolution toward experiments designed to discriminate between the potential capabilities of preformed vitamin A vs. provitamin A to modulate human cancer risks. Thus, one goal of this review will be to evaluate the strength of evidence that retinol or β-carotene is independently associated with the risk of human cancer.

II. Status of Scientific Opinion: The Benchmark Documents

Both the Surgeon General's Report on Nutrition and Health (USDHHS, 1988) and the National Research Council Report on Diet and Health (NRC, 1989a) have considered in detail the information available through 1987 on the relationship of specific nutrients and nutritional status to the development of various types of cancer. Cancers, described as populations of cells that have acquired the ability to multiply and spread without the usual biological restraints (NRC, 1989a), may form in nearly all tissues of the body. Collectively, cancers of all sites are the second leading cause of death in the U.S. (USDHHS, 1988); in 1984, cancer accounted for 22 percent of all deaths in the U.S. (USDHHS, 1988). The distribution of cancers within the population and their etiological determinants differ according to individual cancer sites. Most cancers are classified by organ site, while some are classified histologically (NRC, 1989a). Most cancers occur with greater frequency as people age and thus cancer, like several other degenerative diseases, is largely a disease of aging. Cancers which are common in the U.S. and associated with dietary factors include: cancers of the gastrointestinal, digestive tract (esophageal, stomach, pancreatic, and colorectal cancers), cancers associated with the reproductive organs (breast, endometrial, and ovarian cancers in women and prostate cancer in men) and lung, liver, and bladder cancer (NRC, 1989a).

A. Vitamin A and Cancer: Conclusions of the Benchmark Reports

There is substantive agreement, with some difference in emphasis, between the Surgeon General's Report (USDHHS, 1988) and the report of the National Research Council (NRC, 1989c) regarding the evidence relating vitamin A and cancer, as is summarized below. Most of the studies of diet and human cancer have been observational, epidemiological investigations (see further below). Such studies have the ability to weigh associations and correlations but cannot demonstrate a cause-and-effect relationship. Thus, these studies have either provided suggestive evidence of varying strength for a relationship or have not provided evidence of a statistically significant association.

Both the Surgeon General's Report (USDHHS, 1988) and the NRC report (1989a) concluded that the consumption of *foods* which are high in β-carotene may protect against some epithelial cancers, and both concurred that the evidence is strongest in the case of cancer of the lung. The Surgeon General's Report (USDHHS, 1988) found the evidence relating the consumption of foods high in vitamin A and carotenoids to protection against lung cancer to be strongly suggestive, while the NRC report reached a similar conclusion regarding foods rich in β-carotene that was stated somewhat more guardedly. The evidence upon which these reports were based regarding preformed vitamin A was, indeed, inconsistent. The weight of the evidence did not support a significant, positive association between the amount of preformed vitamin A in the diet or the levels of retinol in blood and reduced cancer rates.

B. Significant Recent Developments

Since the early 1980s, the concept of retinol and β-carotene as distinct entities and distinct exposures in experimental studies has gained recognition and importance (NRC, 1989a; Ziegler, 1991). In these benchmark reports, retinol and β-carotene were discussed as distinct exposures which can be evaluated independently as risk factors in epidemiological and experimental studies. Since the conduct of the studies that were reviewed in 1987–88, there has been considerable progress in understanding the fundamental metabolism and functions of retinol and its metabolites. There has also been substantial improvement in the food composition database regarding carotenoids (Lachance, 1988; Micozzi, 1989; Ziegler, 1991) which has been critical for analysis of the separate effects of dietary provitamin A or non-provitamin A carotenoids. These recent developments will be commented upon briefly before reviewing the new human studies on vitamin A and site-specific cancers.

1. Vitamin A: Metabolism

The general features of the metabolism of retinol and carotene have been described previously (Goodman, 1984a; NRC, 1989d; Peto et al., 1981; USDHHS, 1988; VNIS, 1987) and will be discussed only briefly here. Dietary retinol is absorbed relatively efficiently into the intestinal mucosa where it is esterified with long-chain fatty acids and incorporated into the chylomicron for transport from the intestine to the circulation. Two mechanisms for retinol esterification in the intestine have been proposed (Blomhoff et al., 1990; Ong et al., 1987), and recent evidence from biochemical studies has pointed to an important role of one of the intracellular retinol-binding proteins in the esterification of intestinal retinol (Ong et al., 1987). After secretion from the intestine and movement to the circulation, the majority of chylomicrons containing newly absorbed retinyl esters are rapidly taken up by hepatocytes, most likely via a newly described receptor (Herz et al., 1990). It has also been demonstrated recently that a smaller portion of chylomicron vitamin A is taken up by other organs (Hussain et al., 1989); this means of distribution of vitamin A may have relevance for differentiation in non-hepatic tissues. In liver, newly absorbed vitamin A undergoes a series of metabolic steps leading to deposition of vitamin A (as retinyl esters) in hepatic stellate cells (Blomhoff et al., 1990). When retinol is mobilized from the liver to the circulation, it is secreted in association with a specific transport protein, retinol-binding protein (RBP) (Goodman, 1984b).

Numerous reviews have emphasized that the concentration of retinol and RBP in plasma is under tight homeostatic regulation and does not vary measurably with an individual's vitamin A status, except in extremes of vitamin A deficiency. The concentration of retinol and RBP does vary with age and gender (Pilch, 1985), in diseases of the liver and kidneys (Goodman, 1984b) and with the use of certain hormones such as are found in oral contraceptives (Goodman, 1984b; Pilch, 1985). When retinol intake was varied through the use of vitamin A supplements, small but significant increases in serum retinol and RBP were observed (Wald et al., 1985). The administration of certain synthetic retinoids has been observed to rapidly lower the plasma retinol concentration of animals whose vitamin A nutritional status was normal (Formelli et al., 1987), suggesting interference with a normal, regulatory step in vitamin A transport.

The efficiency with which dietary β-carotene is utilized is more variable. Carotenoids in foods require sufficient bile salts and fat for effective digestion and emulsification prior to uptake into the intestine (Underwood, 1984). Despite the seeming ability of one β-carotene molecule to generate two molecules of retinol, the nutritional value is actually much lower (6 μg of β-carotene is nutritionally equivalent to 1 μg of retinol). The efficiency of carotene absorption decreases somewhat as intake increases (Brubacher and Weiser, 1985). Likewise, there is evidence that the cleavage of β-carotene to retinol in the intestinal mucosa becomes less efficient as intake increases (Underwood, 1984). A portion of β-carotene is cleaved and converted in the mucosa to retinol which then follows the same pathways of transport and metabolism as preformed dietary retinol. Human beings also absorb an appreciable amount of unmodified carotenoids, including β-carotene and other carotenoids which lack vitamin A activity. Like retinyl esters, these carotenoids are also transported from the intestine to blood in the chylomicron and are thought to be rapidly cleared into tissues.

In contrast to retinol, the plasma concentration of carotenoids is sensitive to dietary intake. In individuals on a typical diet, only about 15–30 percent of plasma total carotenoid is β-carotene; this plasma pool represents some 1 percent of total body carotenoid (Bendich and Olson, 1989). Most carotenoids circulate in association with low-density lipoproteins (LDL), which may help to explain the observed association between concentrations of plasma carotenes and lipids (e.g., cholesterol). It is also likely that tissue uptake of carotenoids is determined by the interaction of LDL with tissue lipoprotein receptors. A substantial portion of total body carotene is stored in adipose tissue, with lesser amounts in liver and other tissues (Bendich and Olson, 1989). Recent analysis of human serum and adipose tissue has shown that lutein, cryptoxanthin, lycopene, α- and β-carotene are present in both (Parker, 1989).

When supplemental β-carotene was administered in amounts (50 mg/d) far exceeding usual dietary intake (≈ ca. 1.5 mg/d [Lachance, 1988]), the plasma concentration of β-carotene increased 10-fold (Nierenberg et al., 1991). There was, however, no change in plasma retinol (Nierenberg et al., 1991).

The factors other than diet that determine plasma β-carotene levels are becoming better understood. In a correlation study, Nierenberg et al. (1989) found that plasma β-carotene concentrations were greater in women than men and were inversely related to cigarette smoking and an index of body fatness. The effect of smoking on plasma β-carotene concentration was seen across four intervals of dietary β-carotene (Nierenberg et al., 1989).

2. Vitamin A: Functions

Studies over a number of years have implicated a metabolite of retinol, retinoic acid, in the regulation of cellular differentiation. A most exciting and important breakthrough in understanding the mechanism of action of vitamin A began in 1987 with the discovery of nuclear receptor proteins that bind retinoic acid (Giguere et al., 1987; Petkovich et al., 1987). These retinoic acid receptors (RAR), which are highly similar in structure to the receptors that mediate steroid hormone effects, have been described in a number of tissues and are thought to have important regulatory roles during embryogenesis and in maintaining the differentiated state of more mature cells [see ref. (Ross, 1991; Wolf, 1990) for reviews]. Only a very few of the genes that are regulated by the RARs have been identified. As further data become available, a much improved understanding of the relationship between vitamin A (as retinoic acid) and cancer is likely to follow rapidly. There is a low but measurable concentration of retinoic acid in plasma (DeLeenheer et al., 1982); however, it is generally thought that it is the intracellular generation of retinoic acid [through oxidation of retinol (Napoli and Race, 1987)] that is related to maintenance of the normal phenotype and function of cells.

A very recent finding strongly implicates one form of RAR (RAR-α) and, by extension, retinoic acid with one type of cancer, acute promyelogenous leukemia. It was noticed that the position of a breakpoint on human chromosome 17 that is specifically associated with acute promyelogenous leukemia maps is in the same region of the chromosome as the RAR-α. Recent reports (Chang et al., 1991; Chen et al., 1991) by several groups have provided evidence that the RAR-α gene is frequently disrupted by this chromosomal break and translocation to chromosome 15 in patients with acute promyelogenous leukemia. Aberrant transcription of the RAR-α gene leading to a dysfunction of retinoic acid in cell regulation is thus implicated in the development of this form of leukemia. It is very interesting that treatments with vitamin A or other retinoids in pharmacologic quantities have had some success in producing remissions of leukemia (see Castaigne et al., 1990).

It is possible that carotenoids play their putative role as anti-cancer agents after conversion into retinol or in a fundamentally different way from retinol. Beta-carotene has been shown in chemical studies to have antioxidant properties (Burton, 1989) which are not shared by retinol (Bendich and Valez, 1987). The eleven conjugated double bonds of β-carotene enable it to efficiently quench singlet oxygen or free radicals generated through chemical or photochemical reactions, thereby breaking chains of oxidative reactions (Bendich and Valez, 1987; Burton, 1989). Although this property has led to the frequent categorization of β-carotene as an antioxidant vitamin, it is important to keep in mind that the evidence for this role under physiological circumstances is quite limited (Bendich and Olson, 1989) and that there are other potential means by which this molecule could exert biological activity. For instance, β-carotene may modulate membrane properties important to cell–cell signaling or possibly serve as an intracellular precursor to retinoic acid (Napoli and Race, 1988). It seems likely that the physiologically important concentrations of both retinol and β-carotene are those within cells and that plasma concentrations, although accessible, may have a limited relationship to intracellular events.

3. Vitamin A: Pharmacodynamics

Differences in the pharmacodynamics of carotenoids versus retinoids were highlighted in an earlier review by Peto et al. (1981), and some of these differences have already been mentioned above. Evidence from animal studies has indicated that the rate of utilization of retinol varies with vitamin A intake. Following the initial report by Lewis et al. (1981), which indicated that retinol recycles between liver and other tissues before it is irreversibly degraded, recent work has confirmed and quantified the extent of retinol recirculation (Green et al., 1987; Lewis et al., 1990). In contrast, there is no evidence for a similar reutilization of RBP. The availability of exogenous retinoic acid can reduce the irreversible degradation of retinol (Keilson, 1979). While there is as yet no direct evidence for such recycling of retinol in man, it is most likely that a similar basic process exists. Thus, while plasma retinol concentrations are nearly invariant over a range of liver retinol reserves, the *flux* through the plasma compartment and between tissues is related to some aspects of vitamin A status.

The dynamics of β-carotene transport and utilization are less well known. Major unanswered questions concern the local metabolism of carotenoids within human tissues and the resolution of whether β-carotene or other carotenoids have physiological roles outside of those associated with vitamin A. Regarding local metabolism, Napoli and Race (1988) have demonstrated that rodent tissues in vitro are capable of converting β-carotene to retinoic acid, presumably with retinaldehyde as an intermediate, but by-passing formation of retinol. If this pathway also functions in vivo then there may be two, distinct, intracellular precursors of retinoic acid, retinol, and β-carotene, and the production of retinoic acid from these precursors may be regulated separately.

4. Dietary Assessment of Vitamin A

The interpretation of many of the studies which have reported a linkage between consumption of carotene-rich foods and cancer rates has been limited by weakness in the food composition databases with regard to the carotenoid composition and content of specific foods. Additionally, some food-frequency questionnaires have not adequately probed the consumption of foods rich in provitamin A carotenoids versus carotenoids without provitamin A activity. Recent improvements in analytical methods have been important in strengthening the food composition database. As noted by Ziegler (1991), the older, approved spectrophotometric method did not resolve β-carotene from several chemically similar carotenoids. Newer HPLC methods have provided the necessary resolution. Using HPLC, all the green, leafy vegetables were found to contain the same profile of carotenoids but at varying concentrations (Micozzi, 1989). The α- and β-carotene contents of these vegetables equalled only 9–18 percent of total carotenoids while the majority were oxygenated carotenoids (Micozzi, 1989). The yellow-orange vegetables, in contrast, contained predominantly α- and β-carotene (Micozzi, 1989).

Considerable uncertainty exists regarding the bioavailable content of carotenoids because of their inherent instability to light, oxygen, and heat during storage, cooking, or other culinary processes (Lachance, 1988). Nonetheless, improvements in the database constitute an important step towards developing valid tests of whether fruits and vegetables, or β-carotene per se, confer protection against cancer. Lachance (1988) has used information on both the β-carotene content of various vegetables and fruits in the U.S. diet and their per capita disappearance to estimate the major dietary contributors of β-carotene. According to these estimates, just five food items contribute nearly 85 percent of the β-carotene in the average diet. These include carrots, sweet potatoes/yams, tomatoes, melons, and spinach. Notably also, a number of green vegetables and most fruits have a low content of β-carotene (Lachance, 1988).

III. Vitamin A and Human Cancer

A. Types of Studies: Methodological Considerations

Most of the studies conducted before and since 1987 have been epidemiological, observational studies of the case–control design. A number of recent reviews have addressed the types of designs used in epidemiological research and the strengths and limitations of each (Boone et al., 1990; DeWys et al., 1986; Mettlin, 1988; Vogel and McPherson, 1989). Correlational studies can be used to identify ecological associations between a potential risk factor and disease. Case–control studies involve retrospective identification of persons with particular disease characteristics and comparison of that individual's diet or other habits with those of one or more individuals without the disease who have been matched for potentially confounding characteristics (usually gender, age, and other characteristics thought to influence the variables under study). Controls may be hospital controls, that is patients in the same setting but with disease unrelated to the one under investigation, or they may be community (population) controls chosen from the same general population as the cases. Results are usually expressed as the relative risk (ratio of cases to controls) or an odds ratio (ratio of risks). Trends are examined by testing the significance of the dose–response gradient across categories of an exposure (e.g., tertiles of vitamin A intake) for relative risk.

As noted by Mettlin (1988), dietary exposures in such retrospective studies are usually measured by questionnaire and interview, requiring recall of dietary habits across extended intervals, thus exposures are observed *post hoc*. In the experiments to be reviewed, the primary data in nearly all studies have been information on *food items* or *groups of foods* from which secondary data on nutrient composition have sometimes been derived.

Prospective studies provide a higher level of epidemiological evidence and seek to correlate nutrient intake and disease occurrence. The success of such studies depends on their ability to study a range of intakes (Vogel and McPherson, 1989); therefore, a study population with dietary heterogeneity best serves this type of design.

Intervention trials or clinical trials are truly experimental, providing an opportunity to compare treatment and control groups. Such studies are usually preceded by significant results in case–control or prospective studies and by pilot or feasibility work to determine the size of the study necessary for statistically meaningful results and, perhaps, operational logistics. Although intervention trials could involve true dietary modification, those that have been conducted recently have examined the effects of supplemental nutrients on disease outcome. The process by which potential chemopreventative agents, including β-carotene and certain retinoids, have been identified and moved towards clinical trials has been reviewed recently by DeWys et al. (1986) and by Boone et al. (1990).

B. Vitamin A and Cancer: By Site

As noted in both the summaries of the Surgeon General's Report (USDHHS, 1988) and the National Research Council's report, *Diet and Health* (NRC, 1989a), the strongest evidence for a protective effect of vitamin A, principally in the form of β-carotene, has been found previously for cancer of the lung. Seven studies since 1987 that address dietary or plasma vitamin A and lung cancer will be reviewed first. Carotenoids and/or vitamin A have also been postulated to protect against epithelial cancers at sites other than the lung. New studies have been reported which have addressed the protective effect of diets including vitamin A, carotenoids, and β-carotene on cancers of the mouth and pharynx, esophagus, stomach, pancreas, and colon or rectum. These will be considered together as cancers of the gastrointestinal-digestive tract. Other studies have addressed cancers with a hormonal relationship, namely, cancers of the breast, ovary, endometrium and cervix in women, and cancer of the prostate in men. Finally, studies of cancers of the bladder and skin will be considered.

All of the human epidemiological studies considered in this text have been summarized by organ site in the Appendix Table.

1. Lung Cancer

Lung cancer is the leading cause of cancer mortality among men in the U.S. and most technologically advanced countries and is approaching equality with the rate of breast cancer for women (NRC, 1989a). The most important causal factor for both men and women is cigarette smoking; certain occupational exposures also contribute to lung cancers in men (NRC, 1989a). The strongest evidence for a role of vitamin A in the prevention of human cancers has come from epidemiological investigations which have correlated the consumption of foods rich in preformed vitamin A or provitamin A and the risk of lung cancer (USDHHS, 1988). The Surgeon General's Report of 1988 summarized results from 8 case–control studies and 4 prospective studies published between 1978 and 1987 that examined the relationship of foods (leafy green vegetables) or nutrients (total vitamin A, retinol, total carotenoids, or β-carotene) and lung cancer rates (measured as incidence or death). A consistent observation was a greater relative risk of lung cancer, after adjustment for smoking habits in nearly all studies, in individuals whose nutrient level was in the lowest category (lowest half, tertile or quartile) in comparison to those whose nutrient level was in the highest category. Generally, the relative risk (lowest category of intake compared to the highest category of intake) was about 1.7–2.0. Recent reviews by Colditz et al. (1987), Willett (1990), and Ziegler (1991) have also presented summaries and critiques of these data and some of the more recent studies on dietary vitamin A and lung cancer.

Despite the overall consistency of these earlier studies, there were discrepancies which limited the inferences that could be drawn. All were observational studies which, inherently, could not distinguish between associations and causal relationships. The studies varied considerably in the form and quality of interview and dietary data, whether use of vitamin A supplements was considered, in the number of cases examined, in the detail to which smoking habits were examined, and in whether or not disease was classified by histological type. In some studies the dietary data were consistent with a protective effect of foods rich in β-carotene, while in others the protective relationship was also seen with dietary or supplemental retinol or with the use of certain vegetables (e.g., tomatoes, cruciferous vegetables) that are not good sources of β-carotene. Studies have differed with respect to whether men and women appeared to be equally protected, whether protection was limited to, or more likely for, squamous cell carcinoma versus adenocarcinoma, and in whether or not dietary retinol was also protective. Thus, collectively these studies supported the conclusion that a diet high in leafy green and yellow-orange vegetables and fruits is generally protective against cancers of the lung. It was unlikely, but not disproved, that this protection was due to dietary retinol. The distinct contributions of dietary β-carotene, other carotenoids, or other factors concentrated in carotenoid-rich foods could not be clearly discerned.

Connett et al. (1989) reported results from a case–control study of the relationship between baseline nutrient intake, serum nutrient levels, and cancer mortality among participants in the Multiple Risk Factor Intervention Trial (MRFIT). Of the 156 initially healthy men who subsequently died from cancers, 66 died of lung cancer; all of these were current or past smokers. Controls matched for age, smoking status, and participation variables were chosen from the study survivors. For all cancers, there were no significant differences in serum levels of total carotenoids, β-carotene, retinol, RBP, or α-tocopherol. However, for lung cancer cases, serum total carotenoids were significantly lower in cases than controls. A similar tendency was observed for serum β-carotene levels, but these did not differ significantly from controls. No differences were found for retinol or RBP. Dietary intake of vitamin A, β-carotene, retinol, vitamin E, and cholesterol were calculated from a 24-hour dietary recall taken at baseline. Intake of β-carotene was about 25 percent lower in lung cancer cases, but this difference was not significant. The authors recognized that a single 24-hour dietary recall is generally a poor measure of usual dietary intake. Thus, to the extent that serum carotenoid levels and a 1-day dietary record reflected dietary patterns, this study was consistent with an inverse relationship between carotenoid intake and risk of lung cancer. However, the low serum total carotenoids may also have been related to subtle differences in smoking habits or to dietary differences related to smoking habits.

Bond et al. (1987) conducted a case–control study of 308 former employees of a Texas chemical company who had died of lung cancer between 1940 and 1980 in comparison to matched living or decedent controls. The frequency of consumption of 29 food items was determined by interviews with subjects (for controls) or next-of-kin (for all cases and some of the controls). Standard food portion sizes were assumed, and a vitamin A index and a carotenoid index were calculated. After adjustment for smoking, vitamin supplement use, and education, vitamin A intake was inversely associated with lung cancer risk. The effect was strongest in comparison to the living controls and appeared to be greatest for heavy smokers. Similar odds ratios were found when the dose–response relationship of carotenoid intake and lung cancer was examined. When the frequency of consumption of specific food items was analyzed, there was no association with consumption of squash or sweet potatoes (rich in β-carotene), but there was an inverse association with consumption of carrots and melon (also rich in β-carotene) and with tomatoes (low in β-carotene) and with consumption of certain low-fat foods. The results of this study were generally in agreement with the previous conclusions that frequent consumption of fruits and vegetables is protective against lung cancer. Due to the long interval between case death and the collection of much of the dietary data by proxy there were obvious concerns about the reliability of the dietary information and the potential for misclassification. In a validation study conducted 3–5 months later in a subset of respondents, there was less than 50 percent agreement with the original response category for the frequency of use of four food items which would contribute significantly to the vitamin A or carotenoid indices.

A large case–control study of lung cancer incidence in a high-risk region of southern Louisiana was reported by Fontham et al. (1988). Twelve hundred fifty-three lung cancer cases were compared to 1274 hospital controls. The monthly frequency of consumption of 59 food items prior to onset of illness was determined by questionnaire, and cancer rates were analyzed by race, gender and histological type. The consumption of fruits and vegetables was lower in cases than in controls. For carotene intake, there was an inverse relationship between relative risk and tertiles of intake in cases of squamous cell and small-cell carcinomas, but the trend was not significant. In contrast, the inverse gradient for vitamin C was highly significant. Because intakes of carotene and vitamin C were strongly correlated (r = 0.64), it was not surprising that adjustment for vitamin C eliminated the effect of carotene. However, the opposite adjustment left the effect of vitamin C intact. Although most studies have not supported a relationship of vitamin C and lung cancer (NRC, 1989a), the authors pointed out that vitamin C intake in this population is generally low so that effects of higher intakes may have been more readily discerned. Overall, the results were most consistent with a strong protective effect for fruits, a weaker effect for vegetables, and only a modest indication that carotenoids were protective. Retinol showed little association except in cases of adenocarcinoma for which there was a significant inverse relationship, especially among black men and women whose diets contained more preformed retinol from organ meats (livers).

Koo (1988) reported results of a case–control study of lung cancer among women in Hong Kong who had never actively smoked. Eighty-eight cases of lung cancer, by histological type, were compared with 137 population controls (Koo, 1988; Koo et al., 1987). Because of the difficulty in quantifying the intake of Chinese foods from mixed dishes, women were queried only about their frequency of use of certain foods. In this study, more frequent consumption of fresh fruit or fresh fish conferred protection against lung cancer. There were inverse trends between tertiles of intake of both β-carotene and retinol for all cases combined but these were not statistically significant. However, trends approached statistical significance for both β-carotene and retinol intakes in women with adenocarcinoma or large-cell lung cancer. The strongest inverse trend was found for a composite indicator of a "good diet" (based on frequency of consumption of cruciferous vegetables, fresh leafy green vegetables, carrots, beans/legumes, tofu/soy, fresh fruit, soup, milk, and fresh fish). Thus, the weight of evidence from this unique study supported a protective role of fresh fruits and a diet pattern containing a variety of fresh fruits and vegetables. These effects were observed among individuals in whom tobacco smoking was not a risk factor.

Le Marchand et al. (1989) reported results of a case–control study of lung cancer among men and women in Hawaii. Lung cancer cases (230 men and 102 women) were matched by age and gender to population controls (597 men and 268 women). A diet history was obtained by home interview using a quantitative food-frequency questionnaire designed to probe consumption of foods which provided greater than 85 percent of the intakes of carotene, retinol, vitamin C, and other nutrients. The use of nutrient supplements, tobacco, and alcohol was also queried. Most subjects were interviewed directly but proxy interviews (with next-of-kin, usually the spouse, who had lived with the case subject for at least 5 years) were obtained for 29 percent of the cases and 7 percent of the controls. In this study, total vitamin A (foods plus supplements) was inversely related to lung cancer risk for both sexes. Of total vitamin A, only β-carotene intake was inversely related; there was no relationship for retinol or supplements. The protective effect of total vitamin A, β-carotene, and other carotenoids with vitamin A activity showed consistency across tertiles of intake, with gender, among ethnic groups, and with histological classification. Protection was observed for both men and women who had reported ever smoking. All vegetables, including several not rich in β-carotene, showed a stronger inverse relationship with risk than was found for β-carotene. The results of this study were consistent with a protective effect of carotenoids but pointed more strongly to a beneficial effect of a diet rich in vegetables. As noted by the authors, the constituent(s) most strongly associated with lowering risk may be common to all the food types; components of vegetables other than β-carotene were also implicated by the results of this study.

Jain et al. (1990) reported an analysis of dietary data from men and women in the Toronto area who had a histologically-confirmed diagnosis of lung cancer. The estimated intake of 34 nutrients was assessed from a diet history conducted by a trained interviewer in which the frequency and the usual intake of 81 food items chosen to cover the complete intake of both retinol and β-carotene, and of cholesterol. A detailed smoking history and occupational history were also obtained, and the very strong association of smoking with lung cancer was confirmed by this study. Regarding diet, there was a significant inverse association with vegetable intake but there were no significant relationships with consumption of fruit, total vitamin A from foods, or the intakes of retinol or β-carotene. The study did reveal a significant, inverse, association with cholesterol intake and a strong inverse association with the consumption of nitrate, primarily from certain vegetables (lettuce, broccoli, spinach, and beets), some of which are also rich sources of β-carotene. Thus, this study did not lend additional support to the hypothesis that dietary vitamin A or β-carotene is protective against cancer of the lung and, instead, provided further evidence that constituents of vegetables, other than β-carotene, may be significant in reducing the risk of lung cancer.

A case–control study reported by Dartigues et al. (1990) examined the relationship of dietary intake of preformed vitamin A and β-carotene to risk of lung cancers classified histologically as epidermoid. One hundred forty-three cases of lung cancer admitted to six urban hospitals in southwestern France and 290 hospital controls were selected; of these, 106 cases and 212 controls were matched, interviewed, and complete data were obtained for analyses. Cases and controls were mostly men over the age of 60 who were farmers or blue-collar workers for whom tobacco and alcohol use was stated to be high. The exposure factor used in the analysis was the average vitamin A and β-carotene intake during the 6 months preceding the interview and the average intake over the past 10 years when the interview indicated that diet had changed during the preceding 6 months. The authors considered recall bias to be the most likely source of information bias in this study. The median daily intakes of preformed vitamin A were 600 μg retinol equivalents (RE) in cases and 1020 in controls while the medians for β-carotene were 1510 and 2170 RE, respectively, yielding odds ratios of 4.3 for preformed vitamin A and 4.1 for β-carotene. However, the trend with increasing consumption of either form of vitamin A was not significant. The results of this study are consistent with a protective effect of β-carotene on the risk of developing epithelial lung cancer and also suggest that a higher intake of preformed vitamin A may also be protective. The authors commented that consumption of preformed vitamin A from dairy products is relatively high in this population as compared to some of the populations that have taken part in U.S. studies of diet and lung cancer.

In a prospective study, Paganini-Hill et al. (1987) followed a cohort of over 10,000 residents of a California retirement community for 5 years during which 643 new cancers were diagnosed. Of these, 56 were cancers of the lung. At baseline, information was obtained on the frequency of consumption of 59 food items that were subsequently used to construct a quantitative index of vitamin A and β-carotene intake. Information was also obtained on vitamin supplement use, smoking habits, and personal habits. The results for 56 lung cancers were analyzed according to tertiles of intake for dietary vitamin A, dietary β-carotene, supplemental vitamin A, and total vitamin A. No significant differences or trends in the age-adjusted incidence rates were observed by level of nutrient intake for all cancers combined or for lung cancer specifically. The authors noted that this population is generally well-fed so that even those in the lowest tertile did not have an absolutely low nutrient intake.

This study (Paganini-Hill et al., 1987) also illustrated some of the significant factors that may confound interpretation of the vitamin A–cancer relationship. The investigators examined whether vitamin A intake differed substantially with smoking habits in this population. Indeed, current smokers were more likely to be in the lowest tertile for vitamin A intake than either past smokers or those who had never smoked. The investigators also examined whether the report of dietary habits agreed over time. Some participants were asked to complete a second questionnaire; the agreement between reports at baseline and after 5 years was only 50 percent for the intake of β-carotene and 72 percent for the intake of vitamin A from supplements.

Thus, this prospective study, in which information on diet and supplement use was collected in a comparatively thorough and quantitative fashion, did not lend support to the hypothesis that either dietary vitamin A, retinol, or β-carotene is protective against cancer of the lung.

Stähelin et al. (1987) reported results of a prospective study in which plasma nutrients were measured in 1971–73 in a cohort of male employees of Swiss pharmaceutical firms and follow-up was continued until 1980. Of 268 deaths, 37 were attributed to lung cancer. Plasma β-carotene levels, without adjustment for smoking, were significantly lower for all cases including lung cancers separately. No dietary data were provided. The emphasis of this report was not on vitamin A or carotenoids, and analysis of the β-carotene data by smoking status was not presented in sufficient detail for evaluation. Since plasma nutrient concentrations were measured near the time of blood collection, nutrient losses during sample storage were not a major concern for this study.

Kune et al. (1989) reported that the serum concentrations of retinol and β-carotene were significantly lower in 72 men consecutively diagnosed for lung cancer at a Melbourne, Australia, hospital than for 73 consecutively admitted hospital controls. Neither the extent of cancer (local, regional, or metastatic) nor the type of cancer (squamous, adenocarcinoma, large cell or small cell) significantly influenced these results.

In a study of similar design conducted in Louisiana, LeGardeur et al. (1990) examined the serum levels of vitamin A, β-carotene, RBP, vitamin E and vitamin C in 59 cases (57 men and 2 women of which 51 percent were black and 49 percent white) with newly diagnosed, histologically or cytologically confirmed, primary lung cancer. Cases were compared to both hospital and community controls. In comparison to the hospital controls (only 11 percent of whom had never smoked) the lung cancer cases had significantly lower levels of carotenoids, vitamin E, vitamin C, and cholesterol, but differences in serum vitamin A were not significant ($p = 0.07$). On average, the hospital controls also had lower levels of each serum nutrient, except cholesterol, than the community controls, although the only significant difference was for vitamin C. With the designs of these studies, it could not be determined whether the lower concentrations of serum retinol (Kune et al., 1989) and carotene (Kune et al., 1989; Le Gardeur et al., 1990) reflect manifestations of cancer or may be risk factors predisposing to disease.

Knekt et al. (1990) reported the results of a prospective serological study which examined the association between serum retinol, RBP and β-carotene levels and the subsequent incidence of cancer in a large cohort (consisting of 25 smaller cohorts which made up the Finnish Mobile Clinic Health Examination Survey carried out in 1968–72). Information on smoking habits, occupation and parity was obtained, height and weight were determined and a blood sample was drawn for storage of serum (–20°C). Of 36,265 men and women, ages 15–99, who had no prior history of cancer at baseline, 766 cancer cases (all sites) developed over an 8-year follow-up period.

At baseline, the mean age for cases and controls was identical (57 yr). Each case was then matched with two controls by age, sex, and municipality. Of cases, 39.7 percent were smokers at baseline as compared to 28.9 percent of controls. For 453 male cases and matched controls, mean serum retinol concentrations equalled 645 μg/L for cases and 667 μg/L for controls; this difference was statistically significant, as were differences for RBP

(58.6 and 60.2 mg/L) and for β-carotene (72.3 and 84.1 μg/L). For females, the comparable values showed the same pattern but did not differ as greatly and were not statistically significant. When data were adjusted for smoking, there was a significant, inverse relationship between relative cancer risk for men and the concentrations of serum retinol, RBP, and β-carotene. Differences for women were not significant. When case–control differences were computed for men according to cancer, site differences were highly significant for lung cancer (p < 0.005) and for "cancers related to smoking" (defined as cancers of the lip, oral cavity, pharynx, esophagus, respiratory organs and urinary bladder) (p < 0.001). No other site-specific differences were significant. Similarly, for RBP there were significant case–control differences for cancer of the lung, urinary organs, and cancers related to smoking, while for β-carotene differences were significant for cancer of the lung and for cancers related to smoking. Low β-carotene at baseline was also significantly related to increased risk of prostate cancer in men and of breast cancer in women. The associations observed in this study were generally greater during the first 2 years of follow-up, suggesting that the lower values in cases may reflect the existence of occult, preclinical disease at baseline.

Concern has been raised previously about the validity of vitamin A, and particularly β-carotene, assays on serum which has been stored for years; however, it appears that, at least, all sera were treated comparably in this study. Thus, this study, which is notable for its large case number, provides evidence that serum β-carotene, and to a lesser extent retinol, is inversely associated with cancer risk, particularly with smoking-related cancers.

In summary, the results of six (Bond et al., 1987; Connett et al., 1989; Dartigues et al., 1990; Fontham et al., 1988; Koo, 1988; Le Marchand et al., 1989) of the eight recent studies on lung cancer that included dietary information are generally consistent with the earlier literature. Most of the studies have provided evidence, in the form of a statistically significant association or a non-significant tendency, that consumption of carotene-rich foods is associated with some protection against cancer of the lung. Three of the studies (Bond et al., 1987; Koo, 1988; Le Marchand et al., 1989) also found evidence consistent with a protective effect of retinol, while three studies did not (Connett et al., 1989; Fontham et al., 1988; Paganini-Hill et al., 1987). Thus, while the majority of previous and recent studies have not pointed to a protective effect of a high intake of retinol, the strength of this inference has been weakened somewhat by two of the recent studies. *The most consistent finding among all studies was the protective quality of diets in which fruits and vegetables are regularly consumed.* Upon further analysis by nutrient content, the evidence supports a role(s) for a variety of nutrients including carotene, vitamin A in some studies, vitamin C in some studies, and, most likely, other constituents that are also concentrated in leafy green, cruciferous and yellow-orange vegetables and fresh fruits. Thus, the question of a specific protective effect for β-carotene in the usual diet in prevention of lung cancer is still open.

The interpretation of the serological studies is complicated by the use of stored sera in some investigations and uncertainty as to whether differences in serum nutrient levels are related to diet, other health-related habits (e.g., smoking), metabolic differences that precede cancer, or other factors. The relationship of serum β-carotene to smoking status is a strong one and may mediate the differences between cases and controls observed in these studies.

The Surgeon General's Report (USDHHS, 1988) has listed eight ongoing, clinical prevention trials in a variety of populations which have been designed to critically test the ability of *supplemental* β-carotene to protect against cancers of the lung. The results of these trials should become available within the next few years.

2. Head and Neck (Oral/Pharyngeal, Laryngeal, and Esophageal) Cancers

Oral/pharyngeal cancers (cancers of the head and neck) are strongly associated with the use of tobacco and alcohol (McLaughlin et al., 1988). Recent case–control studies have addressed whether dietary factors including vitamin A and carotenoids influence risk of oral/pharyngeal cancer, and a short-term intervention trial has tested the ability of supplemental β-carotene or β-carotene plus retinol to prevent progression of oral leukoplakia. A clinical trial of 13-*cis*-retinoic acid in chemoprevention has been reported recently.

McLaughlin et al. (1988) conducted a large case–control study in four areas of the U.S. in which 871 cases of oral cancer were matched with 979 population controls. This report examined only the white members of a study population (83 percent of total cases) that also included non-white and Hispanic cases. The frequency of consumption of 61 food items was determined and standard portion sizes were assumed to construct indices of nutrient intake. Supplement use was not included. The results of this study showed an inverse relationship between the intake of fruit and the risk of oral and pharyngeal cancers. Results were consistent for men and women. Individuals in the highest quartile for intake had about half the relative risk of those in the lowest quartile. However, the authors noted that the vitamin C, carotene, or fiber contents of fruits did not appear to fully account for this relationship because these nutrients in vegetables did not provide similar protection.

Franco et al. (1989) reported results from a case–control study conducted in Brazil of 232 men and women with newly diagnosed cancers of the oral cavity compared to hospital controls. An interview-questionnaire was used to ascertain frequency of consumption of broad groups of foods including carotene-rich foods (carrots, pumpkins, and papaya) as well as citrus fruits and green vegetables. Significant reductions in risk were associated with more frequent consumption of carotene-rich foods and citrus fruits. After adjustment for smoking and alcohol use, the association with carotene-rich foods was marginally significant, and that with citrus fruits was statistically significant. There was no association with the intake of green vegetables. Thus, both the studies of McLaughlin et al. (1988) and Franco et al. (1989) are consistent with a protective effect of fruits which may be related, in part, to their content of carotenoids. However, it seems most likely that other constituents or a combination of constituents contributed to this protective effect.

In 1988, Stich et al. (1988) reported results of a 6-month intervention trial in which supplemental β-carotene or vitamin A was provided to Indian men with well-developed oral leukoplakia. These men were from a population that habitually chews betel nut (areca) and has a high rate of alcohol use. Thirty-five men were supplemented with β-carotene (180 mg/wk), 60 with an equal dose of β-carotene plus vitamin A (100,000 IU/wk), and 35 with a placebo capsule. The habitual use of betel nut continued during the study. No adverse reactions due to treatment were reported. However, the development of skin yellowing in the β-carotene-supplemented men prevented the trial from remaining double-blind. The appearance and size of leukoplakia and the percent of micronucleated cells were evaluated after 3 and 6 months.

By 6 months, there was significant reduction in appearance and size of oral leukoplakia in the group supplemented with both β-carotene and vitamin A and a marginal reduction in those supplemented with β-carotene alone. The percent of micronucleated cells, an indicator of the genotoxic activity of areca constituents, was reduced very significantly after 3 months with either supplement. This trial supported the therapeutic efficacy of supplemental β-carotene and vitamin A in the regression of oral leukoplakia, even during continued exposure to genotoxic agents.

Recently, de Vries and Snow (1990) have compared the serum vitamin A, vitamin E, and β-carotene levels in 71 patients with a single primary head and neck tumor to 15 patients with a recurrence (second primary tumor). No other information regarding the two groups of patients was provided. The results of serum analysis revealed that both serum vitamin A and vitamin E, but not serum β-carotene, levels were significantly lower in the single tumor group than in the group with second primary tumors. The authors commented that there were no differences in standard measures of nutritional status and suggested that levels of circulating vitamins A and E may be protective against recurrence of epithelial tumors of the head and neck.

In a study of 22 patients with laryngeal cancer in Poland, Drozdz et al. (1989) found serum retinol and RBP to be lower in cancer patients than in either controls or patients with nonmalignant laryngeal disease. As with several other studies of serum nutrients in patients with diagnosed cancer, it is unclear whether low serum retinol levels were a manifestation of disease or were a pre-existing factor related to cancer risk.

Despite the successes of surgery and radiotherapy in cancers of the head and neck, the failure rate is still high due mainly to the development of secondary primary tumors which are thought to have been in the premalignant state at the time of the first tumor. Thus, treatments that prevent or delay the development of these second primary tumors are of interest. A recent study of Hong et al. (1990) showed that daily administration of *high* levels of 13-*cis*-retinoic acid to disease-free patients after primary treatment for squamous carcinomas of the larynx, pharynx, and oral cavity resulted in a significantly lower rate of new second primary tumors in a 12-month period.

Previous epidemiological and case–control studies have demonstrated a direct association between consumption of alcoholic beverages and esophageal cancer (NRC, 1989a). It is likely that smoking acts synergistically with alcohol in this disease (NRC, 1989a). There are substantial international differences in rate (NRC, 1989a). In the U.S., the rate of esophageal cancer is greater among blacks than whites (NRC, 1989a). According to a recent review by Hargreaves et al. (1989), blacks have a poorer nutritional status with respect to a number of nutrients including vitamins A and C. Previous correlational studies have implicated diets low in fresh fruits, vegetables, vitamins A and C, or high in pickled or moldy foods in the etiology of esophageal cancer (NRC, 1989a).

The relationship between dietary factors and esophageal cancer has been addressed in four recent studies. Brown et al. (1988) studied 207 cases and 422 controls among men in a coastal region of South Carolina which is known to have an elevated rate of esophageal cancer. The cases were further divided into an incidence series (identified through referral and hospital admissions and matched to 2 patient controls) and a mortality series (consisting of men who had died of primary esophageal cancer within a 4-year period) which were evaluated separately. The use of alcohol and tobacco and the frequency of intake of 65 selected foods were determined. As may be expected, this study identified alcohol and tobacco use as strong risk factors for esophageal cancer. Increased risk was also associated with a diet low in fresh fruits, particularly citrus fruits and juices. There was no association with fruits high in β-carotene, thus these data were not supportive of an effect of total vitamin A or β-carotene but did suggest that vitamin C may have had protective value.

Li et al. (1989) conducted a case–control study in Linxian, China in which 1244 new cases of esophageal or gastric cancer were matched with community controls. The diet evaluation in this study was difficult to compare to typical studies, but it appeared that consumption of fresh vegetables was associated with an increased risk of esophageal cancer in this population.

Graham et al. (1990) conducted a case–control study in western New York in which 743 cases were identified from hospital records from 1975 to 1986. Of these, usable interviews were obtained from 178 cases (136 men and 42 women) regarding their usual diet 1 year before the start of symptoms; community controls for these cases were matched for age, gender, and neighborhood. In addition to confirming the strong associations of alcohol intake and smoking with esophageal cancer, the results of this study indicated an inverse association between esophageal cancer and intakes of vitamin A (essentially β-carotene) from vegetable sources, with a statistically significant trend for quartiles of intake. Conversely, preformed retinol was associated with esophageal cancer in a direct manner, and this association remained significant after adjustment for smoking and alcohol intake.

The relationship of diet to risk of esophageal cancer was also investigated in a case–control study by Tuyns et al. (1987a) in Calvados, France, a region with a high rate for this type of cancer. The investigators recruited 743 cases (704 males and 39 females) and 1975 age-matched population controls (922 men and 1053 women); however, most of the analysis used only the male controls. A diet-history questionnaire concerning weekly intake of 40 food items was administered by dieticians, and portion sizes were estimated to calculate nutrient values. On average, cases consumed significantly more calories, less protein of animal origin, more carbohydrate and less polyunsaturated fat than controls. The relative risk of esophageal cancer was not significantly associated with the intake of total vitamin A; however, analysis of the sources of vitamin A revealed a sharp contrast between β-carotene which decreased risk (OR = 0.53 for the highest quartile) and retinol which increased the relative risk (OR = 3.09 for the highest quartile of intake). The high relative risk observed for retinol intake was shown to be due to a higher intakes of organ meats and butter by cases than by controls and was not observed for retinol obtained from other foods (eggs, cheese, and dairy products). A conclusion drawn by the investigators from these results was that "… the role of food items is as important as that of individual nutrients, if not more so."

In summary, the results of these recent studies have been equivocal in implicating dietary intakes of carotene or retinol, or serum levels, as factors associated with esophageal cancer. Some investigations have provided no evidence of significant relationships, while other studies have suggested a protective role for β-carotene but a direct association with high intakes of preformed retinol.

3. Digestive Cancer

The rate of stomach cancer in the U.S. has decreased greatly both in incidence and mortality during the past 40 years and is now among the lowest in the world (NRC, 1989b). Previous correlational and case–control studies have provided evidence for an association between consumption of dried, salted, or pickled foods and gastric cancer (NRC, 1989a). In the past 3 years, results of three case–control studies relevant to the effects of vitamin A or carotenoids have been reported.

Kono et al. (1988) compared 139 cases of newly diagnosed stomach cancer to both hospital and community controls. The frequency of consumption of foods in fairly broad categories was determined by questionnaire. Compared to hospital controls, cases showed no significant difference or trend with consumption of raw vegetables or green-yellow vegetables or fruits other than mandarin oranges. Compared to the general population controls, there was a significant decrease in relative risk only at the highest frequency of fruit consumption. Thus, this study did not support a role for vitamin A or β-carotene in protection against cancer of the stomach.

You et al. (1988) reported a large case–control study of rural Chinese men and women in which 564 cases were compared to 1131 population controls. Information was collected about 85 food items consumed prior to onset of disease. The odds ratio for stomach cancer decreased with increasing consumption of vegetables and fruits, reaching 0.4 for the highest quartile. Retinol intake showed little or no association with stomach cancer, but there was a trend for carotene across quartiles of intake after adjustment for non-dietary variables. This study generally supported the protective effect of a vegetable-rich diet. The authors noted that intakes of carotene and vitamin C were highly correlated (r = 0.6) so that the separate contributions of these nutrients could not be distinguished.

Coggon et al. (1989) conducted a mail-interview study among 95 cases of stomach cancer in England in comparison to population controls. A low intake of "salad vegetables" (mostly lettuce and tomatoes) and a high intake of salt were positively associated with stomach cancer.

The serological study reported by Stähelin et al. (1987), described above under lung cancer, provided evidence that individuals with a low plasma level of vitamins A, C, E, and β-carotene were at greater risk of subsequently developing stomach or large bowel cancers.

Collectively, the data on diet and stomach cancer do not indicate a strong protective effect for vitamin A or β-carotene. The studies are, however, consistent with modest beneficial effects of a diet high in vegetables and fruits.

4. Colorectal Cancer

International comparisons have shown a strong association between colorectal cancer and cancers of the breast, endometrium, ovary, and prostate (NRC, 1989a). An association with dietary fat has been demonstrated in some of the case–control and correlational studies (NRC, 1989a). A few previous investigations have shown a relationship between the intake of vitamin A or consumption of certain vegetables (NRC, 1989a; Vogel and McPherson, 1989). The dietary epidemiology of colon cancer has recently been reviewed by Vogel and McPherson (1989) who concluded that "the laboratory and epidemiologic studies to date do not provide supporting evidence for the association of vitamin A-active foods with the risk of colon cancer." Thus, overall, intake of vitamin A and β-carotene does not seem to be closely associated with risk of colorectal cancer (Rogers and Longnecker, 1988; Vogel and McPherson, 1989).

Kune et al. (1987) reported the results of a comparison of 715 cases of colon or rectal cancer and community or hospital controls in Melbourne, Australia. Both food-frequency and food-portion data were collected for 300 foods so that a quantitative assessment of nutrient intake could be made. The relative risk of colorectal cancer was about half in individuals with a diet high in fiber, vegetables, cruciferous vegetables, and vitamin C. Both the reduction in relative risk and the trend by quartiles of intake were significant in a univariate model for both men and women and for both colon and rectal cancers. There was no association of relative risk with retinol intake, but there was an inverse tendency with the use of vitamin A supplements. In a multivariate model, dietary β-carotene had no separate association with the risk of colorectal cancer. This study, which is notable for the quality of dietary information and use of multiple controls, provided evidence that a diet high in fiber and vegetables, including but not limited to those rich in β-carotene, was protective against cancers of the colon and rectum.

La Vecchia et al. (1988) compared 575 cases of colon or rectal cancer in northern Italy with hospital controls. The frequency of nutrient intake was determined from a questionnaire regarding weekly consumption of 29 food items selected to include major sources of retinol and carotenoids. The frequency of intake of green vegetables, tomatoes, and melons was inversely associated with both colon and rectal cancers, and trends across tertiles of intake were significant. Individuals in the highest tertile of carotenoid intake had a relative risk of about 0.6 compared with those in the lowest tertile. No association was found for retinol. The strongest indicator of cancer risk, however, was a combined score based on a high consumption of pasta/rice and beef and a low consumption of green vegetables and coffee.

Tuyns et al. (1987b) also conducted a large case–control study of colorectal cancer among men and women in two cities in Belgium. Eight hundred eighteen cases were compared to over 2800 population controls. The investigators used a diet history method and food photographs to construct a quantitative measure of retinol and carotenoid intake. Retinol intake was positively associated with colon and rectal cancers, and the trend with quartile of intake was significant. For β-carotene, however, there was no significant trend.

West et al. (1989) examined the relationship of colon cancer in men and women in Utah to dietary intake of macronutrients, dietary fiber, and vitamin A, β-carotene, vitamin C, and cruciferous vegetables. The 4-year study included 231 white male and female cases, ages 40–79 yr, with histologically-confirmed primary colon cancer and 391 population controls matched for age, sex, and address. Questionnaires were administered in respondents' homes by trained interviewers on the average frequency of consumption of 99 foods selected to account for all sources of dietary fiber and over 90 percent of all foods eaten by Utah residents. Quantities consumed were evaluated by use of food models. Nutrient values were calculated and grouped by quartiles for males and females separately.

A high body–mass index was associated with increased risk of colon cancer for both men and women, and dietary fiber was protective in both sexes after adjustment for body mass and energy consumption. Intakes of vitamins A and C did not alter colon cancer risk after adjustment for age, body–mass index, crude fiber, and energy intake. However, there was a significant inverse association with the intake of β-carotene for both males and females (adjusted OR of 0.4 and 0.5, respectively, in the highest quartile of intake). A high intake of cruciferous vegetables was also significantly related to reduced risk of colon cancer for men, but not for women. Thus, this study which is notable for quantitative dietary data supports the hypothesis that β-carotene, but not vitamin A, protects against cancer of the colon.

In the prospective study of Californians living in a retirement community by Paganini-Hill et al. (1987), described above under lung cancer, 110 cases of colon cancer were also studied. As was the case for cancer of the lung, there was no association in either men or women between the level of nutrient intake (either for dietary retinol or β-carotene, or supplemental or total vitamin A) and the rate of colon cancer.

A serological study of French men and women undergoing hospital therapy for cancers of the digestive tract was reported by Charpiot et al. (1989). Little information was provided regarding the patient population or specific types of digestive tract cancers except that hepatocellular carcinomas were excluded, the characteristics of the control group were not described, and no dietary information was collected. The concentrations of retinol, RBP, transthyretin, and α-tocopherol were determined for 50 age-matched, cancer–control pairs. Although each comparison revealed a statistically significant decrease in the cancer group, the simultaneous reduction in serum concentrations of RBP and TTR was interpreted by the authors as an indicator of general malnutrition in the group with cancers of the digestive tract. Thus, this study did not support any preexisting relationship between serum nutrient levels and the subsequent development of digestive tract cancer. In a serological study in Poland, Ostrowski et al. (1987) also found that serum retinol levels were significantly lower in patients with advanced colorectal cancer or metastases. These authors also suggested that these low levels were likely to be a consequence rather than a precursor of the neoplastic process.

Freudenheim et al. (1990a) designed a case–control study in western New York to investigate the relationship of diet to risk of rectal cancer. A series of incident cases (277 Caucasian males and 145 females greater than 40 yr with pathologically confirmed adenocarcinoma of the rectum) were compared to controls matched on age, sex and neighborhood. Detailed interviews by a trained examiner were designed primarily to obtain information on the frequency and approximate quantity of consumption of 129 food items. From these data, indices of intake for energy, fiber, and 15 nutrients were determined.

For males, the risk of rectal cancer increased significantly with increasing intake of total energy, fat, and carbohydrate energy. For females, these relationships were less pronounced but followed the same pattern. For males, there was an increased risk of rectal cancer with increasing intake of preformed vitamin A. However, this relationship was no longer significant after adjustment for either calorie or fat intake. The unadjusted data showed a significant protective effect of carotenoids in males and this trend became stronger after control for calorie or fat intake. Generally, the risk at the highest tertile of carotenoid intake was about half that for the lowest tertile for each level of calorie or fat intake. For females, for whom there were fewer case–control pairs, the tendency for increased risk of rectal cancer with higher retinol consumption and decreased risk with higher carotenoid consumption was also apparent but of lesser magnitude. The data also suggested an inverse association of intakes of vitamin C, and vegetable fiber with risk of rectal cancer, but there was no evidence of protection by vitamin E. The carotenoids, vitamin C and vegetable fiber were highly correlated in food items (r = 0.64 to 0.76 for the male controls). Foods associated with decreased rectal cancer risk included broccoli, celery, lettuce, carrots, green peppers, cucumber, and tomatoes. In all, the results of this study are consistent with protection by diets lower in fat and higher in vegetable fiber, vitamin C, and carotenoids.

Graham et al. (1988) used methodology similar to that in the study by Freudenheim et al. (1990a) to investigate the relationship of total fats, calories, and obesity to risk of colon cancer in the western New York area. Four hundred twenty-eight cases and 428 matched neighborhood controls were interviewed to obtain data on the intake of individual vegetables, some of which are rich in carotene. Although no significant relationship was found for carotene, vitamin C, and cruciferous vegetables, there were significant reductions in risk for high intakes of tomatoes, peppers, carrots, onions, and celery. Thus, whereas some specific foods were implicated in protection by this study, the overall conclusion regarding a protective effect of β-carotene was, nevertheless, negative.

In summary, several of these recent studies examined a relatively large number of cases and controls, and the quality of dietary information, when obtained, was generally high. While the study of La Vecchia et al. (1988) and particularly those of West et al. (1989) and Freudenheim et al. (1990a) provided some indication for a protective effect of carotenoids, the strongest and most consistent effect was from diets that are high in fiber and vegetables. There was no evidence for any protective effect of dietary retinol. Two clinical intervention trials of the effects of β-carotene on colorectal cancer are currently underway (USDHHS, 1991).

5. Pancreatic Cancer

The rate of pancreatic cancer in the U.S. has increased over the past 20–30 years, is greater in men than in women, and is somewhat greater for blacks than for whites (NRC, 1989a). Only cigarette smoking has been established as a major risk factor (NRC, 1989a).

Most of the previous investigations of the association of fruit and vegetable consumption with pancreatic cancer have reported inverse associations (Rogers and Longnecker, 1988). Since 1988, four studies have addressed the relationship of vitamin A to pancreatic cancer.

Falk et al. (1988) conducted a 5-year, hospital-based, case–control study in a high-risk region of southern Louisiana. Three hundred sixty-three cases were compared to over 1200 controls. A food-frequency questionnaire was used to collect information about 59 food items; standard portions were assumed to determine intakes of vitamin A, retinol, and β-carotene. Due to the rapid deterioration of patients with pancreatic cancer, more than half of the cases were unavailable for direct interview, in which case dietary information was collected from next of kin. Consumption of fruits was inversely associated with risk of pancreatic cancer, while consumption of vegetables showed a slight, negative association. For β-carotene intake there was no significant association, while for total vitamin A and for retinol, there was a significant *positive* association at the highest tertile of intake for men but not for women.

The relationship between diet and pancreatic cancer was studied by Farrow and Davis (1990) in a case–control study of married men, aged 20–74 yr, in and around Seattle, Washington. One hundred forty-eight men with newly diagnosed pancreatic cancer were enrolled over a 4-year period. Population controls (n = 188) were matched to cases by 5-year age groups. Information on dietary intake was collected through telephone interviews with wives, even if husbands were available for interview, who subsequently completed a self-administered, semi-quantitative, food-frequency questionnaire concerning intake 3 years prior to diagnosis of foods that represent 96 percent of vitamin A intake, 97 percent of vitamin C intake, and 95 percent of fat intake. In this study, cases tended to have less education than controls, and almost half were current smokers, compared with less than one-fourth of controls. This study found no association between pancreatic cancer risk and the intake of fat or vitamins A or C, although a high intake of protein was implicated as a risk factor.

Burney et al. (1989) have conducted a serological study of 22 cases of pancreatic cancer and 44 controls in western Maryland. Blood was collected in 1974 and stored; cases were collected between 1975 and 1986. These investigators reported no association between subsequent development of cancer of the pancreas and the serum concentration of retinol, β-carotene, total carotenoids, RBP or selenium.

A prospective study of fatal pancreatic cancer in California Seventh-Day Adventists was conducted by Mills et al. (1988). Following enrollment in 1976 and completion of a lifestyle questionnaire which included food frequency, there were 40 deaths from pancreatic cancer during 6 years of follow-up. Lower risk was associated with the frequent consumption of vegetarian protein products, beans, lentils and peas, and dried fruits. However, the use of some other items including cooked green vegetables, green salad, tomatoes, and fresh fruit was not associated with risk of pancreatic cancer. A strength of this study was its prospective nature, including the collection of dietary data well before the onset of disease. However, the lifestyle questionnaire was largely a household questionnaire so that, for some participants, it was filled out by proxy. This study supported the general conclusion that frequent consumption of some vegetables was protective, but it did not lend support to the hypothesis that a diet high in retinol or carotenoids is beneficial.

Thus, none of the dietary studies nor the serological study revealed a consistent or strong association between dietary β-carotene and cancer of the pancreas. The positive relationship between dietary retinol and risk of pancreatic cancer in the Louisiana study may have been due to the more frequent consumption of organ meats by men in this region.

6. Liver Cancer

In Western countries, liver cancer is rare (NRC, 1989a). Limited epidemiological evidence has linked alcohol to primary liver cancer. In Africa and parts of Asia, liver cancer is linked to hepatitis B infection and to use of aflatoxin-contaminated foods (NRC, 1989a). No new studies have directly addressed diet and liver cancer.

The study by Kanematsu et al. (1989) examined the associations of serum retinol and liver retinol and of liver retinol and cellular retinol-binding protein (CRBP) in 26 Japanese patients with hepatocellular carcinoma. Serum retinol concentrations were low in these patients. In comparison to normal tissue, carcinomas contained equal concentrations of CRBP, but their retinol content was about one-fifth as great, perhaps reflecting a lower number of vitamin A-storing cells in the cancerous tissue. This study helped to eliminate loss of CRBP as a likely factor in the dedifferentiation of cancerous liver cells. Beta-carotene concentrations have been reported to be lower in cancerous tissue than in adjacent normal tissue at several sites (Palan et al., 1989), but it is unknown whether these differences represent an etiological factor or a consequence of disease.

7. Breast Cancer

Breast cancer is a common cause of death among U.S. women, especially Caucasians, is closely correlated with hormonal activity, and in some cases has a genetic predisposition (NRC, 1989a). Nutrients or foods which are considered to be risk factors for breast cancer include fats (NRC, 1989a), total calories, and alcoholic beverages (NRC, 1989a; USDHHS, 1988). Previous studies that have examined a relationship of dietary vitamin A to risk of breast cancer have generally found an inverse association (Rogers and Longnecker, 1988). Serological studies, however, did not show a relationship (Rogers and Longnecker, 1988). Vitamin A and synthetic retinoids have shown strong potential in the chemoprevention of chemically-induced mammary tumors in rodents (Moon, 1989; Moon and Mehta, 1990) and are under clinical study for women at risk of recurrence of breast cancer (Mehta et al., 1991).

Howe et al. (1990) published a review and reanalysis of original data from 12 previously-published, case–control studies conducted in the U.S., Canada, and other countries. Although investigation of the relationship of dietary fat to breast cancer was a major aim of this analysis, information on the intake of vitamin A, β-carotene, retinol, and vitamin C was also available for most of the studies. In all, over 4400 cases and 6000 controls were compared. For postmenopausal women, there was an inverse association between risk and intake of total vitamin A, β-carotene, and vitamin C, but not of retinol. None of these were significant for cases of premenopausal breast cancer. The effects were strongest and statistically significant only for vitamin C. These data are important because of the large experience that these studies represent. It would be desirable to determine whether the effects of β-carotene and vitamin C are independent.

Marubini et al. (1988) investigated 214 cases of breast cancer in Milan, Italy in comparison to hospital controls. Blood was drawn on the first day in the hospital, and a dietary questionnaire with 69 food items was used to calculate an index of dietary retinol and β-carotene. This study reported no association of either dietary retinol or dietary β-carotene and risk of breast cancer. Likewise, plasma β-carotene concentration was not associated with breast cancer. However, a significant direct association between plasma retinol and risk of breast cancer was reported. Because of the well-known effect of disease on plasma nutrient levels, concern may be raised regarding the significance of the plasma data. However, usually disease is associated with decreased plasma nutrient levels and the use of hospital controls should, in principle, have controlled for non-specific effects of illness. Thus, this study provided no evidence for a protective effect of either dietary vitamin A, plasma retinol, or β-carotene on the risk of breast cancer in pre- or postmenopausal women.

Van't Veer et al. (1990) conducted a case–control study in The Netherlands of 133 Caucasian women with newly diagnosed breast cancer in comparison to population controls. Interviews were conducted by trained dieticians using a questionnaire that included 236 foods; portion sizes were also estimated to provide a quantitative assessment of nutrient intake. The levels of consumption of dietary fiber, cereal products and total vegetable products were associated with a somewhat lower risk of breast cancer although the trend was significant only for cereals. There was a significant correlation between dietary β-carotene intake and plasma levels of β-carotene and carotenoids, thus providing a form of validation for the dietary data. For β-carotene consumption, the relative risk of breast cancer did not differ significantly from 1 except at the highest quartile of intake (relative risk = 0.63). The trend across quartiles, however, was not significant. Although the results generally supported a protective effect of a diet rich in vegetable products, the data did not indicate that β-carotene content was likely to be responsible.

A case–control study conducted in south Australia by Rohan et al. (1988) investigated the effect of diet on breast cancer in 451 cases and an equal number of community controls. A self-administered, food-frequency questionnaire was used to establish quintiles of intake for retinol and β-carotene. For retinol, there was no association with risk of breast cancer for either pre- or postmenopausal women. For β-carotene, the relative risk for all cases for each of the upper 2 quintiles of intake was 0.76 and the linear trend was significant. When pre- and postmenopausal women were considered separately, the trends were no longer significant. Overall, this study provided modest support for a protective role of dietary β-carotene, but not of retinol, in reducing the risk of breast cancer.

This same group of investigators (Rohan et al., 1990) also conducted a case–control study of the effect of diet on benign proliferative epithelial disorders (BPED) in the same population group. Three hundred eighty-three cases with a biopsy indicating BPED were compared to 192 controls whose biopsy did not show proliferation and to 383 community controls matched on the basis of age and socioeconomic grading. An interviewer-administered questionnaire was used to collect sociodemographic and medical information, and a self-administered, quantitative food-frequency questionnaire was used to ascertain total daily intake of energy and selected nutrients.

For retinol intake, there was a significant trend (inverse relationship) with risk of BPED when cases were compared to community controls but not to biopsy controls. The same pattern was observed for β-carotene intake, as well as for dietary fiber. These authors suggested that these discrepancies in outcome may have been due to the problem of "overmatching" of cases and community controls, i.e., that one or more of the characteristics used for matching may have been a crude proxy for dietary habits (Rohan et al., 1990). Trends between relative risk of BPED and quintile of intake of total and saturated fat, after adjustment for energy intake, were not statistically significant when cases were compared to either control group. Thus, this study did not support a role for fat intake in the etiology of breast cancer but provided some suggestion of an inverse association with the intake of retinol, β-carotene, and fiber.

Ewertz and Gill (1990) conducted a large case–control study among Danish women, aged less than 70 yr, which was principally designed to assess the relationship between dietary fat and breast cancer risk. Diet information was collected by a self-administered, semi-quantitative, food-frequency questionnaire that was mailed 1 year after diagnosis of breast cancer to avoid the period of adjuvant chemotherapy. This questionnaire included

21 food items which covered about 80 percent of the consumption of fat and β-carotene and questions about use of supplements, coffee, tea, sugar, and artificial sweeteners. While there was a highly significant trend for increased risk with increasing intake of fat, the results did not support a relationship between consumption of β-carotene from vegetable or non-vegetable sources and breast cancer risk.

Brisson et al. (1989) conducted a case–control study of 290 women with newly diagnosed breast cancer and 645 population controls. This study differed in design from most case–control studies in that the cases were used to establish mammographic characteristics associated with breast cancer. The mammographic characteristics of the control group were then determined, and this group was divided into women with high-risk or low-risk mammographic characteristics for breast cancer. The dietary component of the study was then conducted on the subgroups of the control women. This experimental design assured that diet was not confounded by disease. A greater extent of high-risk mammographic features was found in women with a high intake of saturated fat, while increasing carotenoid or fiber intake was significantly associated with a reduction in high-risk mammographic features. Retinol had little effect. The authors suggested that an elevation of dietary saturated fat and a reduction of carotenoids and fiber may increase breast cancer risk through effects on breast tissue morphology.

Hislop et al. (1990) reported results of a study of women in Vancouver, Canada, ages 40–59, with benign breast disease classified by two standard histological criteria into proliferative lesions associated with a high risk of breast cancer and lesions causing no increased risk. Dietary data were obtained from a self-administered questionnaire and consisted of the usual frequency of intake during the past year of 39 food items selected for their fat, provitamin A, and vitamin A content. From over 7000 women who initially took part in a breast-screening project, there were 124 and 274 case–control pairs in the increased risk group and no increased risk group using one criterion (proliferative lesions showing moderate or severe epithelial hyperplasia regardless of atypia classified as at increased breast cancer risk), and somewhat fewer cases and controls in the increased-risk group when a second, more stringent, histological criterion (ductal and lobular hyperplastic lesions with severe atypia classified as at-increased-risk) was applied.

Using criterion 1, a significantly greater number of women classified as at-increased-risk of breast cancer were non-users of vitamin A supplements, although quantitative measures of use were not examined. Consumption of green vegetables was marginally significant, but intakes of yellow vegetables, carrots, and fruit or animal sources of vitamin A were not. Using criterion 2, neither the use of vitamin A supplements nor intake of any of the foods rich in vitamin A or β-carotene was associated with a significant difference in risk. Thus, the results of this study only weakly support the hypothesis that vitamin A is protective against breast changes associated with increased cancer risk.

Katsouyanni et al. (1988) compared 120 women with newly diagnosed breast cancer to 120 patients admitted for trauma or orthopedic conditions in an Athens, Greece hospital. Interviews were conducted in the hospital to determine the typical use of 120 food items. Cases reported significantly less frequent consumption of total vitamin A, with a relative risk ratio of 0.46 after adjustment for potentially confounding factors. When analyzed by retinol and β-carotene content, the inverse associations were similar, but the significance of each was less than for total vitamin A. Overall, this study provided support for a protective role of foods containing dietary vitamin A.

In a 2-year study of women in northern Italy with histologically diagnosed breast adenocarcinoma who were free of local or distant metastases, Toniolo et al. (1989) used a semi-quantitative, food-frequency questionnaire to collect data on intake of 70 food items from which the daily intake of β-carotene, retinol, vitamin C, vitamin E, and fat were calculated. Data were analyzed for 251 cases and 499 age-matched population controls. The intake of β-carotene was slightly higher among cases than controls while that of retinol was slightly lower, but these differences were not significant. There were no apparent differences in intake of vitamins C and E. Although this study supported the concept that a low fat intake is protective against breast cancer, it provided no evidence in support of either β-carotene or vitamin A, or of intake of vegetables or fruits, as protective factors.

A 1-year, case–control study was conducted by Potischman et al. (1990) in women in western New York who were being evaluated for a breast mass but who had no previous history of cancer. Prior to biopsy, a fasting blood sample was collected and a self-administered dietary questionnaire of 30 food items (selected to account for 90 percent of vitamin A) intake was completed. Women were classified according to their pathology report into those with breast cancer (n = 83), controls (n = 113, including 34 without biopsy), and those with high-risk atypical hyperplasia (n = 40) who were excluded from the study. Cancer cases were somewhat older than controls (mean ages 58 and 50 yr, respectively). The mean dietary intakes of total vitamin A and vitamin A from vegetable sources were not significantly different. The plasma levels of retinol were identical between cases and controls. However, the plasma levels of β-carotene and lycopene, but not α-carotene, were significantly lower in cases than controls. The trend with quartile of plasma nutrients was significant for β-carotene both before and after adjustment for plasma lipid concentration and, on further analysis, was restricted to postmenopausal cases. There was no correlation between dietary vitamin A calculated from vegetable sources and plasma β-carotene (r = −0.02), but the food-frequency instrument used in this study was acknowledged to be relatively weak. In all, the study did not point to a relationship between dietary vitamin A or β-carotene and breast cancer but did suggest a possible relationship between plasma β-carotene and this disease.

In a retrospective serological study, Basu et al. (1989) found no statistically significant differences in the concentrations of serum vitamin A, β-carotene, vitamin E, or selenium in 30 women with advanced breast cancer whose stored sera were compared to sera from 30 women with benign breast disease and 30 healthy, age-matched controls. Although the mean values for vitamin A and RBP were somewhat lower in women with breast cancer than in the control group, they were also lower in the group with benign breast disease; only in the case of serum RBP were differences significant between the women with breast cancer and the healthy controls. This report lacked information on the year of the study, the time since sample collection, characteristics of the study population excepting age, and it did not address dietary intake. The authors concluded that the somewhat lower values for serum vitamin A may well have been a consequence of disease in general rather than breast cancer per se.

In the prospective dietary study of Paganini-Hill et al. (1987), described above, 123 cases of breast cancer occurred in women in a California retirement community. The consumption of dietary vitamin A or β-carotene as well as supplemental vitamin A was determined by a quantitative food frequency questionnaire. As was the case for lung and colon cancers, there was no evidence that more frequent use of any of these forms of vitamin A resulted in protection from breast cancer.

The prospective serological study of Knekt et al. (1990) in Finnish men and women (see under Lung Cancer) provided evidence for an association of low serum β-carotene, but not retinol, and subsequent risk of breast cancer. Of cancers at all sites, this was the only statistically significant association for females.

In summary, the results of several dietary studies on vitamin A and human breast cancer are inconclusive. None of the recent or previous reports provided strong evidence of an inverse association, some studies were consistent with a very modest beneficial effect, while in others no measurable protection was afforded. None of the ongoing clinical trials listed in the Surgeon General's report (USDHHS, 1988) has been designed to address the effects of vitamin A on breast cancer.

8. Cervical/Ovarian Cancer

In the U.S., ovarian cancer is the major cause of death from cancer of the reproductive tract in women. No clear dietary association has been reported (NRC, 1989a). In an earlier study, a very small direct association was seen between vitamin A intake and the risk of ovarian cancer. Two recent case–control studies have examined dietary factors associated with ovarian cancer.

Slattery et al. (1989) compared 85 cases with first primary ovarian cancer to 492 population controls in Utah. Information was obtained by interview on the frequency and quantity of consumption of 183 common food items. This study did not find evidence of association between calories, protein, or fat and risk of ovarian cancer. For intake of vitamins A and C there was a slight but non-significant inverse association with risk. For β-carotene, the inverse association was statistically significant. Women in the highest tertile of β-carotene intake consumed about twice as much β-carotene and had half the risk of ovarian cancer as compared to women in the lowest tertile of β-carotene intake.

In a case–control study in China (Shu et al., 1989), 172 cases were compared to 172 community controls. Information was obtained on the consumption of 63 common foods. This study identified calories and fat from animal sources as positive risk factors. There was no association between risk of ovarian cancer and either vitamin A or carotene in foods. There was no evidence that frequent consumption of dark green, yellow-orange vegetables, or cruciferous vegetables conferred protection from ovarian cancer.

In summary, no consistent pattern regarding a protective effect of either retinol or β-carotene has emerged from the few dietary studies that have examined ovarian cancer. The collection of dietary data in the study of Slattery et al. (1989) was especially thorough, and the results of this study suggested a modest, beneficial effect of β-carotene-rich foods.

The relationship of diet to cervical cancer was not addressed in the benchmark references (NRC, 1989a; USDHHS, 1988). Cervical cancer is, like lung cancer, primarily a squamous cell epithelial tumor. Its prevalence is greater among women of low socioeconomic status and thus may be related to poor nutrition (Ziegler, 1991). Epidemiological evidence for the role of vitamins in the etiology of cervical neoplasia was reviewed by Schneider and Shah (1989). Of six case–control studies including dietary analysis that were reported previously, two found no association between vitamin A and cervical cancer risk, while four reported a significant relationship between low β-carotene intake and risk (Schneider and Shah, 1989). Five case–control studies and one prospective clinical trial have been published recently.

A case–control study by Brock et al. (1988) in Australia compared the plasma β-carotene concentrations and quantitative nutrient intakes for 117 cases with cervical carcinoma in situ and 196 community controls. These authors reported no significant association between dietary retinol or β-carotene and risk of cervical carcinoma in situ. There was also no relationship with plasma retinol. However, the plasma concentration of β-carotene was significantly lower for cases than for controls. Since plasma β-carotene is thought to reflect dietary intake, the lack of association with dietary β-carotene in the face of a significant difference in plasma β-carotene was puzzling. Although it is possible that the lower plasma β-carotene concentrations were related to incipient disease, the authors commented that carcinoma in situ is an early form of cancer that is not known to be associated with changes in appetite and metabolism that could affect blood nutrient concentrations.

Verreault et al. (1989) compared 189 women in Seattle with a diagnosis of cervical cancer to 227 community controls. Dietary habits during the year preceding diagnosis were determined by a telephone interview–questionnaire. Although cases and controls were matched for age, the case group tended to have somewhat less education, more smokers, and a history of more sexual activity. Regarding diet, retinol intake showed no relationship to risk of cervical cancer. Frequent consumption of dark green, leafy vegetables was related to a lower risk. After adjustment for energy intake and known risk factors including smoking, the inverse relationship between dietary β-carotene and risk of cervical cancer remained, but it was not statistically significant. An inverse relationship was also found for fruit juice; this association remained significant after adjustment. The results of this study were consistent with a protective effect of β-carotene, but the effect was not strong. The stronger association seen with fruit juice might suggest that the vitamin C in foods that are also rich in β-carotene was responsible for some of the protective effect.

De Vet and colleagues (1991) have recently reported the results of a randomized, blind, multi-center clinical trial of the efficacy of supplemental β-carotene to retard progression or cause regression of cervical dysplasia, a condition thought to be a precursor to cervical cancer. Two hundred eighty-one women, ages 20–65, with a recent diagnosis of cervical dysplasia were stratified by age, location, and degree of dysplasia; 137 were assigned to receive 10 mg of β-carotene daily for 3 months. Habitual dietary intake was determined by a mid-study questionnaire. There was insufficient progression of dysplasia to be analyzed. Regarding regression, there were no statistically significant differences between the experimental and the control groups. The authors considered that the time of study may have been too short, or that the typical Dutch diet may be sufficient in β-carotene to mask a small effect of additional β-carotene. By comparison, it may be recalled that while histologic improvement in oral leukoplakia (reduction in cells with micronuclei) was observed after 3 months of β-carotene supplementation at a dose of 180 mg per week, regression was evident only after 6 months (Stich et al., 1988); thus, both the time of treatment and the dose of β-carotene may have been too little for differences in cervical dysplasia to become manifest.

A case–control study of invasive cervical cancer among women in five geographically diverse areas of the U.S. was reported recently (Ziegler, 1991; Ziegler et al., 1990). Data were reported for white women with whom an interview could be obtained (271 cases equalling 73 percent of white, non-Hispanic cases and 502 controls equalling 74 percent of identified controls). Diet was assessed by asking about the usual frequency of consumption of 75 food items that included the major sources of carotenoids, vitamin A, vitamin C, and folate in the diets of U.S. women. The weekly frequency of consumption was derived for each food item; typical portions were assumed. Ten cases and 4 controls were excluded due to incomplete data for 6 or more food items. Cervical cancer diagnoses (histological classification and stage) were based on hospital records: of 261 cases, 218 were squamous cancers, 14 adenosquamous cancers, and 29 adenocarcinomas.

Analysis of the relative risks of invasive squamous cell cervical cancer, by either quartiles or quintiles of intake of carotenoids, vitamin A, vitamin C, or folate, did not reveal significant trends. Similar results were found for both crude relative risks and after adjustment for factors related to cervical cancer risk. Analysis by food groups (including vegetables and fruit, dark green vegetables, and dark yellow-orange vegetables) also did not reveal significant trends, nor were there trends with the use of multivitamin supplements nor with specific vitamins including vitamin A in supplements. Thus, the findings of this study of U.S. women did not implicate consumption of vitamin A or other antioxidant vitamins as protective for invasive squamous cell cervical carcinoma. The authors noted that their results differ from those of other investigations with comparable cases and controls in which intake of at least one micronutrient was lower in women with cervical disease (dysplasia, carcinoma, or invasive cervical cancer) and that the results are not readily explained by bias in subject selection, inadequate power, or lack of control of confounding factors.

Palan et al. (1988) reported that the serum β-carotene concentrations, but not those of retinol, were significantly lower in women with newly diagnosed mild or moderate dysplasia, severe dysplasia or carcinoma in situ, or cancer of the cervix than in disease-free controls. There was a stepwise, progressive decline in β-carotene concentration with increased severity of disease. As with other studies of this type, it is unclear whether the low serum β-carotene concentrations are a manifestation of disease or reflect risk factors related to disease. The authors commented that patients with cervical dysplasia are asymptomatic, and the low plasma β-carotene levels may reflect differences in dietary intake, as shown in earlier work.

Cuzick et al. (1990) reported results of a case–control study of London women, aged 16–40 yr, with histologically classified cervical intraepithelial neoplasia and community controls. Blood was collected from 86 percent of the cases and 68 percent of the randomly selected controls; serum was analyzed for vitamins A and E. No dietary information was reported. There were no significant differences for vitamin A in either the means, odds ratios, or trends with quintile of serum vitamin A. Significant trends were observed for vitamin E for both classifications of neoplasia examined, with higher levels of vitamin E being protective. Thus, this study did not reveal any relationship between serum vitamin A and cervical neoplasia, even in women with diagnosed disease at the time of blood sampling.

Overall, the results of the recent studies of diet and cervical cancer provide very little, if any, support for a protective role of β-carotene-rich foods. The results of the short-term intervention trial (de Vet et al., 1991) did not support a therapeutic effect for supplemental β-carotene in cervical dysplasia. The results of serological studies may be of etiologic significance, but they could also reflect occult disease; further long-term prospective studies would be needed to address these data.

9. Prostate Cancer

Cancer of the prostate is common in the U.S.. The incidence increases with age after about 45 yr of age (NRC, 1989a). The rate for black men is greater than for white men and is increasing (Hargreaves, 1989; NRC, 1989a). Male hormones and sexual activity appear to contribute to risk (NRC, 1989a). A number of dietary studies have identified fats and vitamin A as probable risk factors (NRC, 1989a). For prostate cancer, particularly in older men, some of the previous studies had identified retinol as a *positive* risk factor. Some studies had suggested a protective effect for dietary β-carotene (NRC, 1989a; Rogers and Longnecker, 1988).

Hsing et al. (1990a) reported a case–control serological study with 103 men in western Maryland who developed prostate cancer, in comparison to matched community controls. This study examined serum nutrient concentrations after a long period of blood storage which is likely to have led to deterioration of some nutrients. For serum retinol, there was a small downward shift in the distribution for cases (mean 61 μg/dL) versus controls (mean 64 μg/dL). There was a tendency for greater risk of prostate cancer to be associated with a lower serum retinol. For β-carotene, the opposite tendency was observed. In all, this study provided little support for reduced risk in men with either a high concentration of serum retinol or β-carotene.

A study conducted in the Netherlands by Hayes et al. (1988) examined both plasma retinol and β-carotene levels in 94 cases of clinical prostate cancer in comparison to 130 men with benign prostatic hyperplasia (BPH) and 130 hospital controls. Men with prostate cancer had lower mean retinol concentrations and lower mean β-carotene and α-tocopherol concentrations than the controls. Some of this difference may have been related to disease because plasma nutrient levels tended to rise slightly after surgical treatment. At face value, the results indicated that a low plasma retinol concentration was associated with increased risk of prostate cancer.

Two publications (Ohno et al., 1988; Oishi et al., 1988) have reported on a group of 100 men with newly diagnosed prostate cancer in Japan who were compared to 100 men with benign prostatic disease and 100 hospital controls. Beta-carotene intake was significantly lower in prostate cancer patients than in either men with BPH or hospital controls. When β-carotene intake was examined by quartiles for all ages, the relative risk of prostate cancer in the lowest quartile for intake was about three times greater than that in the upper quartile; this difference was highly significant. When effects were examined by age, a diet high in β-carotene appeared to confer protection in older men (≥70 yr) but not in younger men. Thus, the results of this study indicated a modest protective effect of dietary β-carotene for cancer of the prostate.

Mettlin et al. (1989) examined the dietary habits of 371 men with newly diagnosed prostate cancer in comparison to hospital controls. A food-frequency checklist was completed shortly before hospital admission and standard food portions were assumed. For men < 68 yr, the relative risk was lower in men who consumed more β-carotene. However, for older men this difference was not apparent. For the entire study, the evidence was consistent with some reduction of risk of prostate cancer with higher consumption of β-carotene.

Ross et al. (1987) conducted a case–control study of black men and white men in a region of southern California with a high rate of prostate cancer among blacks. One hundred forty-two cases were matched with population controls. Among dietary variables, a high intake of fat was a risk factor for both black men and white men. There was no significant or consistent association of dietary vitamin A or β-carotene with prostate cancer.

Kolonel et al. (1988) compared 452 men with prostate cancer in Hawaii with 899 population controls. Data were analyzed by age and ethnic group. Collection of dietary data in this study was very thorough so that a quantitative assessment of nutrient intake could be calculated. This study found a *positive* association between the intake of total vitamin A, carotenoids, and β-carotene and prostate cancer in older men (≥70 yr), but not in younger men. The overall trend was significant. For dietary retinol, however, there was no significant relationship with prostate cancer. It is of interest that the same diet methodology had been used previously in this population in a study of lung cancer (Le Marchand et al., 1989) and an inverse relationship had been observed between total vitamin A or β-carotene intake and cancer of the lung.

A re-evaluation of these data on diet and prostate cancer were reported in 1991 (Le Marchand et al.). Data were further analyzed by food groups rich in β-carotene. Le Marchand et al. (1991) concluded that the greater β-carotene intake in controls versus cases was due to more frequent consumption of papaya. However, there was no association between risk of prostate cancer and consumption of other β-carotene-rich foods. Thus, they concluded that the intake of β-carotene, lycopene, lutein, or other phytochemicals was *not* associated with prostate cancer risk.

A prospective study was reported by Reichman et al. (1990) of a cohort of 2440 men who participated in the NHANES I Epidemiologic Follow-up Study. Eighty-four cases of prostate cancer developed during a 10-year period. Data for initial serum vitamin A concentration was compared between cases and the remaining group. For the entire population, serum vitamin A level was itself positively correlated with education, serum cholesterol, alcohol consumption and, to a lesser extent, with body–mass index. A significant difference was found between the mean serum vitamin A concentration for cases (59 μg/dL) versus non-cases (65 μg/dL). When considered by quartiles of serum vitamin A, there were significantly fewer cases whose initial vitamin A level had been high. While it is possible that some of the men who developed clinically-recognized cancer had incipient disease at the time of the initial blood sampling, the authors did not think this was likely to have confounded the results because there was no relationship between the time interval between blood sampling and diagnosis and the initial serum vitamin A level. Thus, this study indicated that a low serum retinol concentration could be a risk factor for cancer of the prostate.

Another prospective study was reported by Hsing et al. (1990b) of a cohort of over 17,500 white males who were part of the Lutheran Brotherhood Study. During a 20-year period, 149 died of prostate cancer. Information on the frequency of consumption of 35 food items, grouped in 9 food groups, was collected in 1966. However, a number of potentially important sources of vitamin A (such as liver, cheese, butter, broccoli, spinach, and cantaloupe) were not included in the questionnaire. This study found no significant association between frequency of intake of any of the 9 food groups (including vegetables, cruciferous vegetables, and fruits) and the relative risk of prostate cancer. When analyzed by retinol and β-carotene content, risk was *directly* related to the intake of total vitamin A, retinol, and β-carotene for men < 75 yr, while risk *decreased* significantly with total vitamin A and β-carotene for older men. Thus, this study suggested that there may be age-specific differences in diet–risk relationships for prostate cancer. However, other authors have noted that there is no biological hypothesis regarding differences between age groups for this disease (Mettlin et al., 1989).

A third prospective study was reported by Severson et al. (1989) for a cohort of nearly 8000 men of Japanese ancestry living in Hawaii. One hundred seventy-four cases of prostate cancer were compared to the remaining non-case controls. A 24-hour dietary recall interview with food models was used to collect dietary data. The emphasis of this study was on food items typical of the Japanese versus Western diet and there was no analysis of vitamin A or β-carotene per se. The risk of prostate cancer appeared to be lower in men who consumed more rice and tofu, and there was a marginal, positive relationship between cancer risk and consumption of butter and eggs. Thus, the relationship of prostate cancer to some aspects of the diet was strengthened by this study, but the results provided little direct information concerning vitamin A.

In the prospective study of Paganini-Hill et al. (1987), 93 cases of prostate cancer developed. As was the case for the other cancer sites examined in this study, there was no relationship between intake of total vitamin A, carotenoids, retinol, or β-carotene and subsequent development of prostate cancer.

In contrast, the prospective serological study of Finnish men and women by Knekt et al. (1990) (see Lung Cancer) provided evidence of an association of low baseline serum β-carotene, but not retinol, with the development of prostate cancer during an 8-year follow-up period.

In all, the data relating vitamin A and carotene consumption, or plasma nutrient levels, to risk of prostate cancer continue to be inconsistent. Some of the previous investigations and some of the more recent studies have found a protective effect for retinol or carotenoids, while others have found no effect or even a positive association.

10. Bladder Cancer

Bladder cancer is more common in the U.S. than in many other parts of the world and is more frequent in men than in women (NRC, 1989a). Bladder cancer is associated with cigarette smoking and certain occupational hazards (NRC, 1989a). A few previous dietary studies have suggested either a protective effect of vitamin A and β-carotene or no effect (NRC, 1989a). Synthetic retinoids have been effective in the prevention of experimental bladder cancer in animals (NRC, 1989a), and one of these retinoids, etretinate, has shown efficacy in clinical trials of prevention of recurrent superficial bladder cancer (reviewed in Lippman and Meyskens, 1988). Four recent epidemiological studies have reported on the relationship of diet or serological measurements and bladder cancer.

La Vecchia et al. (1989) reported a case–control study of 163 histologically confirmed cases of bladder cancer vs. 181 hospital controls in northern Italy. A questionnaire was used to determine the frequency of consumption, before illness, of foods selected to include major sources of retinoids and carotenoids. This study reported that the intake of green vegetables and carrots was significantly lower for cases, as was intake of total carotenoids and total vitamin A. For retinol intake, there was no significant difference.

In the prospective study of Paganini-Hill et al. (1987), no relationship between dietary intake of total vitamin A, retinol, carotenoids, or β-carotene was found for 59 men and women who subsequently developed cancer of the bladder. However, it is of interest that these authors subsequently analyzed their data, for all cancer sites combined, by histological type into five categories: adenocarcinomas, transitional cell, epithelial cell, squamous cell, and all others (Paganini-Hill et al., 1987). Data were then analyzed by tertile of dietary vitamin A or β-carotene intake and by supplement use. For tumors with transitional cell histology, but not for any other classification, there was a significant, inverse trend for β-carotene intake and a near-significant inverse trend for vitamin A intake. There was no significant trend for supplements. The 53 transitional cell cancers included 45 bladder cancers. Thus, this follow-up analysis of all cancer sites may be interpreted as suggesting a beneficial effect of carotene intake on the risk of certain types of bladder cancer.

In a prospective serological study conducted in western Maryland, serum concentrations of retinol, RBP, β-carotene, and lycopene were compared for 35 cases of bladder cancer versus matched controls. There were no significant differences between bladder cancer cases and population controls for any of these measurements (Helzlsouer et al., 1989).

A study of the relationship of urothelial cancer to dietary habits and vitamin supplement use among men and women in Stockholm, Sweden was reported by Steineck et al. (1990). Data were analyzed for 323 cases less than 74 yr who had histologically or cytologically confirmed urothelial cancer and/or squamous cell cancer of the lower urinary tract (renal pelvis, ureter, urinary bladder and urethra, of which 305 cases were of bladder cancer) and for 392 population controls. Dietary information was obtained of 56 food items chosen primarily to cover the major contributors of carotene, retinol, vitamin C, and fried foods in the Swedish diet. Information about smoking habits and the frequency of use of supplements mainly containing vitamins A, B, and C was also obtained. This study reported a strong inverse association between use of supplements mainly containing vitamin A and the risk of urothelial cancer; however, this conclusion was based on use of such supplements by none of the cases and only eight of the controls. Additionally, nearly all the subjects exposed to vitamin A supplements were also exposed to vitamin C supplements. Regarding dietary vitamins, there were no significant associations with β-carotene, retinol, or vitamin C intake and risk of urothelial cancer.

In summary, the number of human studies regarding diet and bladder cancer is still quite small, and consistent effects for dietary vitamin A or carotenoids have not yet emerged.

11. Skin Cancer

Skin cancer was not considered specifically in the benchmark reports. Synthetic retinoids have become a major form of chemotherapy for a number of previously intractable dermatological disorders (Bollag, 1983; Lippman and Meyskens, 1988), and high-dose β-carotene has been used successfully for a number of years in the treatment of the photosensitive disease, erythropoietic protoporphyria (Matthews-Roth, 1989). In animal models of chemically-induced photosensitization, both high-dose β-carotene and a structurally-similar carotenoid without provitamin A activity were effective, pointing to a mechanism not involving retinol (Mathews-Roth, 1989). Since 1987, a case–control study and a major clinical trial have addressed the ability of vitamin A or β-carotene from the diet, or supplemental β-carotene, to prevent cancer of the skin.

A case–control study of malignant melanoma was conducted by Stryker et al. (1990) among patients at a Massachusetts dermatology clinic. Two hundred four cases were compared to 248 controls with other dermatological conditions. A semiquantitative food-frequency questionnaire was used and plasma was collected at the first visit for analysis of retinol, β-carotene, α-carotene, lycopene and α-tocopherol. For plasma α- or β-carotene, there were no appreciable differences between cases and controls. The intake of preformed vitamin A was similar in both groups. Controls had a tendency to consume more β-carotene, but there were no significant associations with specific β-carotene-rich foods. Thus, the overall result of this study was that neither diet nor blood levels of retinol nor carotenoids were associated with risk of malignant melanoma.

The results of a major, prospective, clinical trial on the efficacy of supplemental β-carotene to prevent basal-cell and squamous-cell cancers of the skin was reported by Greenberg and colleagues (1990). The authors noted that patients who have recently had a non-melanoma skin cancer are at high risk for another skin cancer and thus this group seemed well-suited for a clinical prevention trial. Over 1800 patients at four medical centers who had a recent non-melanoma skin cancer were randomly assigned to either the treatment group (50 mg β-carotene/d by capsule) or the control group (placebo capsule). These groups were well matched at the study's outset. All subjects underwent an annual dermatological examination and plasma was analyzed at enrollment and annually thereafter for retinol and β-carotene. A limited dietary questionnaire was administered at intervals throughout the study. The primary end point was the first occurrence of a new basal-cell or squamous-cell skin cancer. Nearly all lesions were confirmed histologically.

After 5 years, the study was halted and results were thoroughly analyzed. The risk of a new skin cancer in the β-carotene-supplemented group and the placebo group was essentially identical. Subgroup analysis indicated that β-carotene did not lower the risk of skin cancer for patients who smoked or for those whose plasma β-carotene concentration was low at enrollment. Compliance appeared to have been good. It is noteworthy that the plasma β-carotene concentration was 8-fold greater in the β-carotene-supplemented group than in the placebo group. Since not all subjects completed 5 years of treatment, it was important to analyze whether protection could be observed in those treated with β-carotene for longer times. The results showed no evidence that efficacy increased with the length of β-carotene treatment. Thus, this carefully designed and conducted study did not provide evidence that supplemental β-carotene protects against recurring cancers of the skin.

It has been commented that the latency for skin cancer is long such that the efficacy of supplemental β-carotene in preventing primary skin cancers still should be subjected to long-term follow-up (Manson et al., 1991).

IV. Summary and Conclusions

A. Vitamin A: Normal Metabolism and Physiology

It is now recognized that vitamin A functions in multiple physiological processes. Outside of its critical function in vision, retinol or one of its metabolites is required for normal cell differentiation, growth, and reproduction. It is possible that the role of vitamin A in each of these processes is associated with more than one type of biochemical, regulatory event. As more has been learned about the processes in which retinol functions, the physiological function(s) of retinol or its metabolite, retinoic acid, appear to be more like those of the hormones that govern a wide variety of biological processes and which frequently interact to maintain homeostasis. The recent recognition of nuclear receptors for retinoic acid, described in Section II. C., has further strengthened the analogy between vitamin A and the steroid hormones. Despite this improved understanding, it is still unknown exactly how retinol or related retinoids regulate differentiation, or whether any of these processes is related directly to preventing the type of unregulated cell growth that characterizes cancer.

B. Basis of the Association Between Vitamin A and Cancer

An important question to be addressed in any diet–cancer relationship is whether cancer risk is associated with a specific *nutrient* (e.g., retinol, β-carotene, carotenoids, or other nutrients), with a particular *food*(s), or with some combination of factors. The recent human studies on vitamin A and cancer summarized above support most strongly an inverse relationship between cancer risk and the frequent intake of certain foods. The most consistent protective effect was seen with diets high in vegetables and/or fruits. Significant differences or tendencies consistent with a beneficial effect of such diets were seen in studies of cancer of several sites: the lung (Bond et al., 1987; Connett et al., 1989; Dartigues et al., 1990; Fontham et al., 1988; Jain et al., 1990; Koo, 1988; Le Marchand et al., 1989), mouth and pharynx (Franco et al., 1989; McLaughlin et al., 1988), esophagus (Brown et al., 1988; Graham et al., 1990), stomach (You et al., 1988), colon/rectum (Freudenheim et al., 1989, 1990; Kune et al., 1987; La Vecchia et al., 1988; Tuyns et al., 1987b; West et al., 1989), pancreas (Falk et al., 1988; Mills et al., 1988), breast (Brisson et al., 1989; Howe et al., 1990; Katsouyani et al., 1988; Rohan et al., 1989, 1990; Van't Veer et al., 1990), ovaries (Slattery et al., 1989), cervix (Verreault et al., 1989), prostate (Mettlin et al., 1989; Ohno et al., 1988; Oishi et al., 1988), and bladder (La Vecchia et al., 1989).

As stated by Micozzi (1989), "People consume (and epidemiological studies inquire about) foods, culturally processed in different ways, as opposed to nutrients." The primary data in all of the dietary studies above were the frequency of use or the quantity of intake of *food items or groups of foods*. Thereafter, data on the consumption of *nutrients* such as retinol or β-carotene were derived by calculation. These data on nutrient intake thus rest on various assumptions about quantities of foods actually consumed as well as their nutrient content. A protective effect of β-carotene or retinol could be inferred from some studies but not from others. If the association between the intake of foods rich in β-carotene or retinol and cancer risk was consistently strong and if correlations with other nutrients were not apparent, then it would be possible to argue that the beneficial effect of these foods is highly likely (though still not proven) to be due to their contents of vitamin A.

In a number of the studies cited above, cancer risk was associated with consumption of certain provitamin A-rich foods but not with others, or the protective effect of fruits and vegetables did not appear to be closely related to their provitamin A content. Possible explanations for these results include:

1) that effects are *due to other factors* which are found in some provitamin A-rich foods;

2) that the effects are largely due to vitamin A but vary with its food source, i.e., that there are significant *interactions* with other factors in foods;

3) that effects of provitamin A are seen primarily in *combination*(s) with other factors that are found in some but not all vitamin A-rich foods; or

4) that some of the data on nutrient content may be inaccurate and unreliable.

In any case, a protective effect of provitamin A (β-carotene) has been observed less consistently than that of a diet high in fruits and vegetables. It therefore seems prudent to conclude that the weight of evidence supports a beneficial effect of *foods or food combinations* more strongly than it supports any specific benefit from dietary β-carotene or retinol. This conclusion is similar to that reached recently by other reviewers who have examined the evidence relating vitamin A to lung cancer (Colditz et al., 1987; Willett, 1990) or to cancers more generally (Freudenheim and Graham, 1989; Ziegler, 1991). For both the previous studies and those since 1987, a protective effect of foods rich in β-carotene has been most clearly demonstrated for cancer of the lung.

The problems of interpreting epidemiological, dietary studies have been considered in detail by other reviewers (Mettlin, 1988; Micozzi, 1989; Vogel and McPherson, 1989; Ziegler, 1991). Due to the high correlation of certain nutrients within foods or food groups, it is sometimes difficult to disassociate the effects of one nutrient from another. For example, two of the studies described above (Fontham et al., 1988; You et al., 1988) reported a correlation coefficient for intakes of carotene and vitamin C of ≥0.6. The results of some studies were more suggestive of a beneficial effect of vitamin C-rich foods than of β-carotene-rich foods. It would seem reasonable that, depending on which nutrients are more limited in a population's diet, effects might appear stronger for one nutrient than for another, even though both nutrients have beneficial effects. It would be helpful if questionnaires were designed to probe more extensively into the use of foods which are rich in β-carotene but lacking in vitamin C versus those foods with a high content of vitamin C but little β-carotene.

As was pointed out recently by Ziegler (1991) and Willett (1990), constituents of fruits and vegetables other than β-carotene might be important in the prevention of cancer. Some of the questionnaires used in the recent studies inquired about food items that could help to distinguish between effects of β-carotene and those of other carotenoids, while other questionnaires lacked this discrimination. The importance of other carotenoids and non-carotenoid constituents of fruits and vegetables has not been adequately explored. For example, the fiber component of fruits and vegetables has been implicated as beneficial in prevention of cancers of the colon and rectum (Freudenheim et al., 1990b). In one study in which the food content of nitrate was examined, this food constituent showed a significant inverse relationship with lung cancer (Jain et al., 1990). Nitrate is primarily found in certain vegetables, some of which are also rich sources of β-carotene, so confounding of the effects of these food constituents could also be possible.

C. Evidence for an Optimal Intake of Vitamin A

Most observational studies have examined the relationship of cancer risk to the *levels of intake* of preformed or provitamin A in the habitual diet, sometimes including supplements as a separate category. Thus, most of our current information is based on usual frequency of intake or, in fewer studies, on a quantitative assessment of the usual dietary intake.

The RDA (NRC, 1989b) for vitamin A (as preformed and provitamin A combined) is 800–1000 Retinol Equivalents (1 RE = 1 µg of retinol). As noted above, the nutritional equivalent of 1 µg of retinol is 6 µg of food carotenoids. In the typical U.S. diet, approximately two-thirds to three-quarters of total vitamin A is preformed, with the remainder supplied by carotenoids with provitamin A activity (NRC, 1989a,b; Ziegler, 1991). The usual intake of β-carotene in the U.S. diet is approximately 1.5 mg/d (Lachance, 1988). A rather similar figure of 2–3 mg/d for Dutch women was reported by de Vet et al. (1991). Lachance (1988) has estimated that, if the current dietary goals of the USDA/HHS which advocate increased consumption of carotene-rich foods were met, the intake of β-carotene would rise to nearly 6 mg/d. Generally, differences between the highest and lowest intakes of β-carotene in most cancer studies did not differ by much more than a factor of 2 to 3.

By comparison, only a few intervention trials have tested the ability of supranormal supplements of vitamin A (retinol and/or β-carotene) to affect precancerous conditions or cancer risk [cervical dysplasia (de Vet et al., 1991), skin cancer (Greenberg et al., 1990) or oral leukoplakia (Stich et al., 1988)]. Only in the case of oral leukoplakia, for which supplements equalled 180 mg/wk of β-carotene and 100,000 IU/wk of vitamin A, was a positive effect reported. If the rather small differences of 2–4 mg of dietary β-carotene described above are truly protective, then it seems that beneficial effects of supplemental β-carotene should also be seen when results of the ongoing clinical trials are analyzed.

D. Evidence for a Protective Effect of Vitamin A

The magnitude of the data supporting a protective effect of dietary vitamin A has been discussed in part in Section VI. B. For preformed retinol, the majority of studies did not find evidence of a protective role. In a few studies, a higher intake of retinol did appear to be associated with decreased risk, but for other studies there was evidence suggestive of a *positive* association with cancer risk. Positive associations have been observed most frequently for cancer of the prostate but also occasionally in studies of colorectal, pancreatic, or breast cancer. In some of the case–control or prospective studies, higher levels of plasma retinol appeared to be related inversely to cancer risk, but the influence of existing or incipient disease on plasma retinol concentration, or analytical differences due to sample storage, could not be ruled out. In all, there is little convincing evidence of a benefit due to higher dietary intake of preformed vitamin A.

Generally, the data are stronger for an inverse association of dietary β-carotene with cancer risk. However, even this association is not highly convincing. For instance, for studies of lung cancer for which the inverse association with β-carotene is most consistent, the relative risk between the groups with the highest and lowest intakes of β-carotene was usually no greater than 2. Confounding by other covariates in carotenoid-rich foods (VI. B.), or by other non-dietary habits such as smoking (see VI. J. below) could significantly influence this small difference in risk. Some of the weakness in demonstrating an association may be due to the quality of the dietary data, which has differed considerably among studies. A number of studies have used food questionnaires of limited scope, have of necessity used proxy interviews, and have assumed standard portion sizes. The limitations in food composition databases, particularly for carotenoids, have been noted above.

In retrospective studies, subjects (or surrogates) must recall food intake patterns from the past. In one study of a generally well-educated population, the agreement between a baseline dietary report and re-interview 5 years later was only 50 percent for β-carotene and 72 percent for vitamin A supplements (Paganini-Hill et al., 1987), while another found <50 percent agreement for β-carotene after a shorter interval (Bond et al., 1987).

In some of the studies in which serum nutrient levels were measured, a low retinol or β-carotene concentration was a positive risk factor for cancer, while other studies did not find this association. The strength of the inferences that can be drawn from serological studies is highly dependent upon each study's experimental design. In a number of the case–control studies conducted before 1987 and in some of those noted above, blood or plasma had been collected at baseline and stored until clinical cases accrued. Carotenoids are known to be sensitive to oxygen and light, and their instability during long-term storage has been noted before [see ref. (Colditz et al., 1987; Willett, 1990; Ziegler, 1991) for discussion]. There is also evidence that retinol and β-carotene concentrations are lower during illness (Drozdz et al., 1989; Kanematsu et al., 1989) so that, in prospective studies having a relatively short follow-up, it is possible that results are biased by preclinical disease. For these reasons, the data from the serological studies conducted to date would seem to be generally less reliable than those from dietary studies.

E. Optimal Level of Consumption

It is unknown at what level of consumption of fruits and vegetables there would be no further benefit regarding cancer risk. As noted by Lachance (1988), adoption of the current USDA/HHS dietary goals would increase the average intake of β-carotene by a factor of 2- to 4-fold. A substantial increase in the consumption of fruits and leafy green or yellow-orange vegetables containing provitamin A, balanced calorically by decreased use of fat-rich foods, is achievable and would be expected to increase significantly the consumption of carotenoids and fiber as well as to reduce intake of total fat and saturated fat. Such an overall dietary change would be predicted to reduce the risk not only of cancer but also of cardiovascular disease and diseases related to obesity.

F. Time Course of Beneficial Effects

It is also unknown how long the benefits of dietary change might persist. However, based on knowledge of epithelial tissues, some speculation is possible. Most epithelial cells are replaced at a regular, relatively rapid, rate. Abnormalities of epithelial morphology and function due to vitamin A deficiency are usually reversed readily after a dietary source of vitamin A is restored. In vitro, the effects of retinol or retinoic acid on cells can often be observed within days or hours. Thus, it is possible that beneficial effects might commence quickly after a change in diet is implemented. On the other hand, studies of induced cancers in laboratory animals have pointed out the need for continuous exposure to vitamin A (or, in most studies, related retinoids) to establish and maintain protection (Moon, 1989; Moon and Mehta, 1990). These data, and knowledge of the latent nature of many cancers, suggest that benefits are likely to accrue slowly from long-term, sustained changes in dietary pattern.

The dynamics of β-carotene are less well known. The types of animal studies which have proved very valuable in understanding vitamin A metabolism are difficult and complicated because most rodents and small mammals absorb carotenoids poorly and store little carotenoid in tissues (Moon, 1989). In humans on a vitamin A-adequate diet, there is considerable storage of vitamin A in the liver as well as β-carotene in adipose tissue and other fatty tissues. Following supplementation with β-carotene, plasma β-carotene concentrations have been observed to increase in less than 2 weeks (Ringer et al., 1991) with a magnitude of change proportional to the β-carotene dose. Based on limited data on tissue carotenoids in humans, there appears to be substantial inter-individual variability in carotenoid storage (Parker, 1989). The relationship of tissue carotenoid level to dietary intake has not been adequately explored.

With respect to cancer, it is not clear at what point during development of disease retinoids or β-carotene would be most likely to exert protective functions. As noted above, there is considerable evidence from carcinogenesis studies in animals that administration of pharmacologic levels of retinoids is effective primarily after tumor initiation (Moon, 1989; Moon and Mehta, 1990). In these studies, protection has depended on continuous retinoid administration (Moon, 1989).

Therefore, from the knowledge at hand, it seems most likely that beneficial effects of dietary modification would begin almost immediately at the cellular level, but that clinical evidence of benefit would be discernable only later for slowly progressing diseases such as cancer. Chronic dietary change would be expected to have greater benefit than intermittent change.

G. Populations to Which Scientific Evidence Can Be Generalized

The retrospective studies reviewed above have been conducted in many parts of the world with populations whose basic dietary habits differ considerably. There is no evidence that geographical or ethnic differences are important. Within studies that have included men and women, a range of ages, or different ethnic groups, there generally has been consistency. There may be some differences between pre- and postmenopausal women with regard to dietary risk factors for breast cancer, and some of the studies on prostate cancer have raised a question about age-related differences for this type of cancer. Otherwise, it seems most likely that the results of the studies conducted to date may be generalized to the adult population at large.

H. Dietary Interactions

There is no substantial evidence that any other components of the diet would interfere directly with a potentially beneficial effect of vitamin A. Experimental studies have shown the efficiency of absorption of β-carotene to be dependent on dietary fat; however, the fat content of nearly all normal human diets is sufficient for optimal β-carotene absorption (Underwood, in VNIS, 1987). The efficiency of carotene absorption varies considerably, and it is possible that carotene bioavailability from some food sources is poor. This has been taken into account as far as possible when the nutritive value of carotenoids has been determined. It is conceivable and even likely that the magnitude of the protective effects that have been seen in cancer studies also depends on the presence or absence of other food components. If nutrients that covary with β-carotene also have protective or deleterious effects, the magnitude of the effects attributed to β-carotene might be an over- or underestimation of its true efficacy.

I. Significant Food Sources of Vitamin A

This subject has been discussed in part in the Introduction and in Section II. C. Lachance (1988) has published recent information on the β-carotene content and the usual per capita use of foods which contribute substantial carotenoids. Five food items were found to contribute 85 percent of the β-carotene in the average U.S. diet. These include carrots

(256 mg per capita per year), sweet potatoes/yams (122 mg per capita per year), tomatoes (86 mg per capita per year), melons (62 mg per capita per year) and spinach (35 mg per capita per year). Other foods that contribute at least 10 mg per capita per year are lettuce, sweet corn, cabbage/sauerkraut, and broccoli.

Foods rich in preformed vitamin A include beef, calf or chicken livers, kidney, dairy products, and, to a lesser extent, meats and eggs. Vitamin and mineral supplements also generally contain preformed vitamin A in the form of retinyl esters.

J. Other Types of Dietary or Lifestyle Interactions

Other dietary or health factors, or habits, may significantly influence the effects of dietary retinol or β-carotene on cancer risk, or may have a more powerful effect on cancer risk than either vitamin A or β-carotene. Cigarette smoking, as is now well known, is the strongest, independent risk factor for cancer of the lung. Smoking has also been implicated in cancers of the pancreas and bladder. Numerous studies cited above included smokers. Therefore, the ability of the investigators to adequately match cases and controls and to adjust for smoking habits was critical for the proper interpretation of these data. Differences in the characteristics of smokers and non-smokers have been noted in various studies. Fehily et al. (1984) found that smokers were lighter and of lower body–mass index and had lower intakes of vitamins, minerals, and dietary fiber than non-smokers or former smokers. The intake of vitamin A or foods rich in β-carotene has been reported to be highly associated with smoking status, being lower for current smokers than for past- or never-smokers (Ross, 1991; Shibata et al., 1989). Cigarette smoking has also been shown to be inversely related to plasma β-carotene levels in a number of studies (Nierenberg et al., 1989; Palan et al., 1989; Russell-Briefel et al., 1985; Stryker et al., 1988). Smokers had lower plasma β-carotene levels in a dose-dependent manner across a 9-fold range of dietary β-carotene intakes (Nierenberg et al., 1989). Heavy smoking and alcohol intake are also highly correlated (Colditz et al., 1987). These data make clear that tight control of smoking is critical for reliable analysis of dietary studies yet, as discussed by others (Ziegler, 1991), it is not always clear from published work how adjustments for smoking were made and whether these truly controlled for smoking-related behaviors.

Certainly in the case of lung cancer, the relative risk due to cigarette smoking is far greater than the relative risks that have been associated with diets low in vitamin A (Ziegler, 1991). The relationship between diet and lung cancer is modest in comparison to the deleterious effect of cigarette smoking (Willett, 1990).

Alcohol consumption is known to decrease the absorption of many nutrients. Although the studies above did not directly address the interaction of alcohol and vitamin A consumption, alcohol has been shown to be positively related to cancers of the pancreas, esophagus, and other sites. The beneficial effects of diets high in fruits and vegetables, or the use of supplemental β-carotene, would be expected to be antagonized by frequent use of alcohol.

Other health behaviors may influence the outcome of research studies. For example, plasma β-carotene concentration has been reported to be lower in women using oral contraceptives (Palan et al., 1989) while retinol concentrations are increased (Palan et al., 1989; Pilch, 1985). The influence of these behaviors on the outcome of nutritional or epidemiological studies would need to be adequately controlled.

K. Safety Concerns

There is no apparent cause for concern about reasonable levels of intake such as could be obtained from the diet. As noted above, the USDA/HHS dietary goals call for increased consumption of fruits and vegetables which would, on average, increase β-carotene intake by about 4-fold.

Toxicity has not been evident for β-carotene (NRC, 1989b), even at high doses used in clinical supplementation trials (de Vet et al., 1991; Greenberg et al., 1990; Stich et al., 1988) and in patients treated for years for photosensitive skin disorders (Matthews-Roth, 1989). In the case of high supplemental doses such as those used in the clinical trial of oral leukoplakia of Stich et al. (Stich et al., 1988) or the skin cancer trial of Greenberg et al. (1990), the accumulation of β-carotene in plasma and skin may cause yellowing. Though cosmetically unacceptable to some, this condition is not associated with known toxicity.

There is good reason for concern, however, about toxicity due to chronic overconsumption of preformed vitamin A. Hypervitaminosis A has been reported following self-medication with vitamin A (Smith and Goodman, 1976) and in explorers subsisting on liver and other tissues with a very high vitamin A content (see Lippman and Meyskens, 1988). Symptoms of acute toxicity (nausea, vomiting, or headache) have been reported in a few studies when normal children in populations with low vitamin A status have been supplemented with vitamin A in single doses of 30–60 mg (Florentino et al., 1990; NRC, 1989b).

Toxicity has also been observed in clinical situations in which pharmacologic doses of retinol or retinoids have been used for chemoprevention or chemotherapy (Yob and Pochi, 1987). Side effects and toxic manifestations have involved a number of organ systems including the skin, eyes, liver, joints, bones, and muscles (Yob and Pochi, 1987). For example, toxicity was associated with the highest doses of 13-*cis*-retinoic acid (100 mg/m² body surface area/d) in a recent prevention trial in patients with previous cancers of the head and neck (Hong et al., 1990). A recent study of adults with advanced acute promyelocytic leukemia who were treated with a high dose of all-*trans*-retinoic acid (45 mg/m² body surface area/d) showed positive therapeutic effects in some patients, but adverse effects of toxicity were also frequently noted (Castaigne et al., 1990). On the other hand, some investigators have reported that administration of high doses of vitamin A for chemotherapy has not been associated with unacceptable side effects. High-dose retinol (approximately 30 times the RDA) has been used chronically to treat children with myelogenous leukemia without apparent, serious toxicity (Lie et al., 1988). Similarly, in a clinical trial of compliance and safety of high dose vitamin A as adjuvant therapy in lung cancer, nearly all patients tolerated doses of ~100 mg/d for over a year without signs of serious liver damage (Pastorino et al., 1991). However, these studies involved careful pre-screening to exclude patients with pre-existing liver disease and, even then, elevations of liver enzymes and of plasma triglycerides were observed during treatment (Pastorino et al., 1991).

Concern is especially great for women of child-bearing age because of the well-known teratogenic effects of high levels of retinol and some of its synthetic analogues (Hall, 1984; NRC, 1989b; Yob and Pochi, 1987). The level of intake causing birth defects, or symptoms of acute toxicity, are well outside those associated with normal dietary practices (NRC, 1989b). Nonetheless, any health message concerning the benefits of vitamin A must be made with great caution because vitamin A supplements almost always contain preformed retinol rather than β-carotene, and the potential for their over-zealous use exists. Currently, approximately one-third of the U.S. adult population consumes vitamin supplements regularly, including vitamin A in doses often meeting or exceeding the RDA (NRC, 1989b).

L. Differences in Efficacy Among Sources of Vitamin A

As commented on above, the bioavailability of carotenoids may vary quantitatively with different food sources. There is evidence that β-carotene supplied in oily solutions is more efficiently converted to retinol, and therefore is of higher potency, than β-carotene in vegetables (NRC, 1989b). Brubacher and Weiser (1985) have estimated that when carotene intake equals 1.5–4.0 mg/d (a normal range), 1 μg of retinol is obtained from 3.33 μg of β-carotene in oily solution or 6 μg of β-carotene in vegetables. Although these data were obtained from animal studies, it seems reasonable that they should also apply to humans. The absorption of retinol or β-carotene, or the conversion of β-carotene to retinol in the intestine, does not appear to vary remarkably between natural foods versus fortified foods such as milk or margarine. There are, however, few experimental studies in this area.

M. Critical Gaps in Knowledge

Progress in understanding the absorption, transport, and tissue metabolism of carotenoids has been slow because the small animal species used effectively as models for studies of retinol metabolism do not absorb carotenoids efficiently. It is known that increasing the consumption of β-carotene or other carotenoids leads to a rapid increase in plasma carotenoid concentrations in humans, but little is known of the cellular consequences of such change. It is possible that the organs which take up carotenoids from plasma are able to convert it to retinol, much as occurs in the intestine, or to retinoic acid which could influence differentiation through nuclear receptors and regulation of gene expression. Although the regulation of intracellular binding-proteins and receptors for retinol and retinoic acid have become an active area of research, very little is known of whether β-carotene, in quantities found in the diet or in supplemental amounts, affects these receptors in any way. A critical area of understanding that is now missing is whether or not β-carotene acts through retinol in the cell, whether the main action of β-carotene is as an antioxidant, or whether it acts primarily through some other process.

The mechanism of transport of retinol and β-carotene into cells is not well understood and constitutes another critical gap in knowledge. It is presently unknown whether the transport protein for retinol (RBP) or the lipoprotein that carries carotenoids (LDL) serves to deliver these molecules to cells in a specific, regulated manner. As vitamin A or β-carotene intake is increased, at what point do these physiological mechanisms become limited or altered?

It is known that the dietary habits of tobacco smokers differ from non-smokers, but further detailed information would be helpful both in interpreting epidemiological studies and providing the most acceptable dietary advice for those who continue to smoke. There is also little information on the extent to which smoking alters the requirement for, or metabolism of, β-carotene, other antioxidant vitamins, or vitamin A. Studies of absorption, turnover, and tissue metabolism would help to fill this gap in knowledge.

While epidemiological studies of the cohort or case–control design have inherent limitations, they have been and are likely to continue to be important means to identify the potential factors in the human diet that protect, or do not protect, against the development of cancer. Studies of this type can be even more informative in the future if use is made of improvements in the food composition/nutrient database and if there are improvements in the questionnaire/interview methods regarding food consumption and personal habits such as smoking. For lung cancer, the evidence supporting a protective role of β-carotene is quite strong at the present time. It does not seem overly optimistic to suggest that the addition of a few large, carefully controlled studies could, if consistent, provide a body of evidence that, collectively, would be compelling. Not withstanding interest in the outcome of clinical trials of β-carotene *supplementation,* there is still a need to evaluate the consequences of *normal dietary patterns* on disease incidence.

There is also a need to evaluate some of the non-vitamin A constituents of fruits and vegetables (e.g., non-provitamin A carotenoids, indoles, and nitrate) to learn whether these are also protective, or whether the protective effects of dietary vitamin A are exerted by themselves or in combination with other food components.

Regarding cancer prevention, most studies to date have had to rely on cancer incidence or mortality as end points. As the processes leading to clinical disease become better understood, it should be possible to use markers of preclinical disease in place of the later end points. The potential for development of biomarkers for cancer chemoprevention studies was recently reviewed (Lippman and Meyskens, 1988) and appears promising. In principle, such markers should also be useful in dietary studies. Occasionally, epidemiological studies have suggested a positive association of high vitamin A intake with increased risk of certain cancers, such as prostate cancer as discussed above. The significance of these observations is unknown but might indicate covariance of vitamin A intake with other risk factors.

N. Summary

The data relating dietary vitamin A and cancer are inconclusive. The strongest evidence supports a protective role of fruits and vegetables in reducing the rates of cancer of various sites, particularly cancers of the lungs, colon/rectum, and breast. For cancer of the lung, it seems most likely that this protective effect is exerted at least in part through the β-carotene contents of these foods. In several studies, the risk of lung cancer was about 2-fold lower in individuals in the highest category of β-carotene intake compared to those in the lowest category of intake. However, the increased risk of lung cancer due to smoking is far stronger than the potentially lower risk associated with diet. Thus, smoking cessation will have a far greater impact on lung cancer rates than can be expected from dietary modification.

For cancers of the colon/rectum and breast, it is possible that the provitamin A component of fruits and vegetables is also protective, but it seems most likely that these foods protect by providing some combination of dietary fiber, provitamin A, vitamin C, reduced fat, or other food constituents.

Based on current knowledge, the dietary goals stated in the Surgeon General's Report and by the USDA/HHS appear to provide excellent directions to a more healthful diet.

V. Bibliography[*]

Basu, T.K.; Hill, G.B.; Ng, D.; Abdi, E.; Temple, N. 1989. Serum vitamins A and E, β-carotene, and selenium in patients with breast cancer. *J. Am. Coll. Nutr.* 8:524–529.

Bendich, A.; Olson, J.A. 1989. Biological actions of carotenoids. *FASEB J.* 3:1927–1932.

Bendich, A.; Velez, R. 1987. The non-vitamin A functions of beta carotene. Report submitted by Hoffman-La Roche. p. 1–55.

Blomhoff, R.; Green, M.H.; Berg, T.; Norum, K.R. 1990. Transport and storage of vitamin A. *Science* 250:399–404.

Bollag, W. 1983. Vitamin A and retinoids: from nutrition to pharmacotherapy in dermatology and oncology. *Lancet* 1:860–863.

Bond, G.G.; Thompson, F.E.; Cook, R.R. 1987. Dietary vitamin A and lung cancer: results of a case–control study among chemical workers. *Nutr. Cancer* 9:109–121.

*This bibliography contains all reference citations that are either in the text or the tables or both.

Boone, C.W.; Kelloff, G.J.; Malone, W.E. 1990. Identification of candidate cancer chemopreventive agents and their evaluation in animal models and human clinical trials: a review. *Cancer Res.* 50:2–9.

Brisson, J.; Verreault, R.; Morrison, A.S.; Tennina, S.; Meyer, F. 1989. Diet, mammographic features of breast tissue, and breast cancer risk. *Am. J. Epidemiol.* 130:14–24.

Brock, K.E.; Berry, G.; Mock, P.A.; MacLennan, R.; Truswell, A.S.; Brinton, L.A. 1988. Nutrients in diet and plasma and risk of in situ cervical cancer. *J. Natl. Cancer Inst.* 80:580–585.

Brown, L.M.; Blot, W.J.; Schuman, S.H.; Smith, V.M.; Ershow, A.G.; Marks, R.D.; Fraumeni, J.F., Jr. 1988. Environmental factors and high risk of esophageal cancer among men in coastal South Carolina. *J. Natl. Cancer Inst.* 80:1620–1625.

Brubacher, G.B.; Weiser, H. 1985. The vitamin A activity of β-carotene. *Int. J. Vitam. Nutr. Res.* 55:5–15.

Burney, P.G.J.; Comstock, G.W.; Morris, J.S. 1989. Serologic precursors of cancer: serum micronutrients and the subsequent risk of pancreatic cancer. *Am. J. Clin. Nutr.* 49:895–900.

Burton, G.W. 1989. Antioxidant action of carotenoids. *J. Nutr.* 119:109–111.

Castaigne, S.; Chomienne, C.; Daniel, M.T.; Ballerini, P.; Berger, R.; Fenaux, P.; Degos, L. 1990. All-*trans* retinoic acid as a differentiation therapy for acute promyelocytic leukemia. I. Clinical results. *Blood* 76:1704–1709.

Chang, K.-S.; Trujillo, J.M.; Ogura, T.; Castiglione, C.M.; Kidd, K.K.; Zhao, S.; Freireich, E.J.; Stass, S.A. 1991. Rearrangement of the retinoic acid receptor gene in acute promyelocytic leukemia. *Leukemia* 5:200–204.

Charpiot, P.; Calaf, R.; Di-Costanzo, J.; Romette, J.; Rotily, M.; Durbec, J.P.; Garcon, D. 1989. Vitamin A, vitamin E, retinol binding protein (RBP), and prealbumin in digestive cancers. *Int. J. Vitam. Nutr. Res.* 59:323–328.

Chen, Z.; Chen, S.-J.; Tong, J.-H.; Zhu, Y.-J.; Huang, M.-E.; Wang, W.-C.; Wu, Y.; Sun, G.-L.; Wang, Z.-Y.; Larsen, C.-J.; Berger, R. 1991. The retinoic acid alpha receptor gene is frequently disrupted in its 5' part in Chinese patients with acute promyelocytic leukemia. *Leukemia* 5:288–292.

Coggan, D.; Barker, D.J.P.; Cole, R.B.; Nelson, M. 1989. Stomach cancer and food storage. *J. Natl. Cancer Inst.* 81:1178–1182.

Colditz, G.A.; Stampfer, M.J.; Willett, W.C. 1987. Diet and lung cancer: a review of the epidemiologic evidence in humans. *Arch. Intern. Med.* 147:157–160.

Connett, J.E.; Kuller, L.H.; Kjelsberg, M.O.; Polk, B.F.; Collins, G.; Rider, A.; Hulley, S.B. 1989. Relationship between carotenoids and cancer: the Multiple Risk Factor Intervention Trial (MRFIT) Study. *Cancer* 64:126–134.

Cuzick, J.; De Stavola, B.L.; Russell, M.J.; Thomas, B.S. 1990. Vitamin A, vitamin E and the risk of cervical intraepithelial neoplasia. *Br. J. Cancer* 62:651–652.

Dartigues, J.-F.; Dabis, F.; Gros, N.; Moise, A.; Bois, G.; Salamon, R.; Dilhuydy, J.-M.; Courty, G. 1990. Dietary vitamin A, beta carotene and risk of epidermoid lung cancer in south-western France. *Eur. J. Epidemiol.* 6:261–265.

De Leenheer, A.P.; Lambert, W.E.; Claeys, I. 1982. All-*trans*-retinoic acid: measurement of reference values in human serum by high performance liquid chromatography. *J. Lipid Res.* 23:1362–1367.

De Vet, H.C.W.; Knipschild, P.G.; Willebrand, D.; Schouten, H.J.A.; Sturmans, F. 1991. The effect of beta-carotene on the regression and progression of cervical dysplasia: a clinical experiment. *J. Clin. Epidemiol.* 44:273–283.

De Vries, N.; Snow, G.B. 1990. Relationships of vitamins A and E and beta-carotene serum levels to head and neck cancer patients with and without second primary tumors. *Eur. Arch. Otorhinolaryngol.* 247:368–370.

DeWys, W.D.; Malone, W.F.; Butrum, R.R.; Sestili, M.A. 1986. Clinical trials of cancer prevention. *Cancer* 58:1954–1962.

Doll, R.; Peto, R. 1981. The causes of cancer: quantitative estimates of avoidable risks of cancer in the United States today. *J. Natl. Cancer Inst.* 66:1191–1308.

Drozdz, M.; Gierek, T.; Jendryczko, A.; Pierkarska, J.; Pilch, J.; Polanska, D. 1989. Zinc, vitamins A and E, and retinol-binding protein in sera of patients with cancer of the larynx. *Neoplasma* 36:357–362.

Ewertz, M.; Gill, C. 1990. Dietary factors and breast-cancer risk in Denmark. *Int. J. Cancer* 46:779–784.

Falk, R.T.; Pickle, L.W.; Fontham, E.T.; Correa, P.; Fraumeni, J.F., Jr. 1988. Life-style risk factors for pancreatic cancer in Louisiana: a case–control study. *Am. J. Epidemiol.* 128:324–336.

Farrow, D.C.; Davis, S. 1990. Diet and the risk of pancreatic cancer in men. *Am. J. Epidemiol.* 132:423–431.

Fehily, A.M.; Phillips, K.M.; Yarnell, J.W.G. 1984. Diet, smoking, social class, and body mass index in the Caerphilly Heart Disease Study. *Am. J. Clin. Nutr.* 40:827–833.

Florentino, R.F.; Tanchoco, C.C.; Ramos, A.C.; Mendoza, T.S.; Natividad, E.P.; Tangco, J.B.M.; Sommer, A. 1990. Tolerance of preschoolers to two dosage strengths of vitamin A preparation. *Am. J. Clin. Nutr.* 52:694–700.

Fontham, E.T.H.; Pickle, L.W.; Haenszel, W.; Correa, P.; Lin, Y.; Falk, R.T. 1988. Dietary vitamins A and C and lung cancer risk in Louisiana. *Cancer* 62:2267–2273.

Formelli, F.; Carsana, R.; Costa, A. 1987. *N*-(4-hydroxyphenyl)retinamide (4-HPR) lowers plasma retinol levels in rats. *Med. Sci. Res.* 15:843–844.

Franco, E.L.; Kowalski, L.P.; Oliveira, B.V.; Curado, M.P.; Pereira, R.N.; Silva, M.E.; Fava, A.S.; Torloni, H. 1989. Risk factors for oral cancer in Brazil: a case–control study. *Int. J. Cancer* 43:992–1000.

Freudenheim, J.L.; Graham, S. 1989. Toward a dietary prevention of cancer. *Epidemiol. Rev.* 11:229–235.

Freudenheim, J.L.; Graham, S.; Marshall, J.R.; Haughey, B.P.; Wilkinson, G. 1990a. A case–control study of diet and rectal cancer in western New York. *Am. J. Epidemiol.* 131:612–624.

Freudenheim, J.L.; Graham, S.; Horvath, P.J.; Marshall, J.R.; Haughey, B.P.; Wilkinson, G. 1990b. Risks associated with source of fiber and fiber components in cancer of the colon and rectum. *Cancer Res.* 50:3295–3300.

Giguere, V.; Ong, E.S.; Segui, P.; Evans, R.M. 1987. Identification of a receptor for the morphogen retinoic acid. *Nature* 330:624–629.

Goodman, D.S. 1984a. Overview of current knowledge of metabolism of vitamin A and carotenoids. *J. Natl. Cancer Inst.* 73:1375–1379.

Goodman, D.S. 1984b. Plasma retinol-binding protein. In: Sporn, M.B.; Roberts, A.B.; Goodman, D.S.; eds. *The retinoids.* Vol. 2. Orlando: Academic Press, Inc. p. 41–88.

Graham, S.; Marshall, J.; Haughey, B.; Brasure, J.; Freudenheim, J.; Zielezny, M.; Wilkinson, G.; Nolan, J. 1990. Nutritional epidemiology of cancer of the esophagus. *Am. J. Epidemiol.* 131:454–467.

Graham, S.; Marshall, J.; Haughey, B.; Mittelman A.; Swanson, M.; Zielezny, M.; Byers, T.; Wilkinson, G.; West, D. 1988. Dietary epidemiology of cancer of the colon in western New York. *Am. J. Epidemiol.* 128:490–503.

Green, M.H.; Green, J.B.; Lewis, K.C. 1987. Variation in retinol utilization rate with vitamin A status in the rat. *J. Nutr.* 117:694–703.

Greenberg, E.R.; Baron, J.A.; Stukel, T.A.; Stevens, M.M.; Mandel, J.S.; Spencer, S.K.; Elias, P.M.; Lowe, N.; Nierenberg, D.W.; Bayrd, G.; Vance, J.C.; Freeman, D.H., Jr.; Clendenning, W.E.; Kwan, T., and the Skin Cancer Prevention Study Group. 1990. A clinical trial of beta carotene to prevent basal-cell and squamous-cell cancers of the skin. *N. Engl. J. Med.* 323:789–795.

Hall, J.G. 1984. Vitamin A teratogenicity. *N. Engl. J. Med.* 311:797–798.

Hargreaves, M.K.; Baquet, C.; Gamshadzahi, A. 1989. Diet, nutritional status, and cancer risk in American blacks. *Nutr. Cancer* 12:1–28.

Hayes, R.B.; Bogdanovicz, J.A.T.; Schroeder, F.H.; de Bruijn, A.; Raatgever, J.W.; van der Maas, P.J.; Oishi, K.; Yoshida, O. 1988. Serum retinol and prostate cancer. *Cancer* 62:2021–2026.

Helzlsouer, K.J.; Comstock, G.W.; Morris, J.S. 1989. Selenium, lycopene, α-tocopherol, β-carotene, retinol, and subsequent bladder cancer. *Cancer Res.* 49:6144–6148.

Herz, J.; Kowal, R.C.; Ho, Y.K.; Brown, M.S.; Goldstein, J.L. 1990. Low density lipoprotein receptor-related protein mediates endocytosis of monoclonal antibodies in cultured cells and rabbit liver. *J. Biol. Chem.* 265:21355–21362.

Hislop, T.G.; Band, P.R.; Deschamps, M.; Ng, V.; Coldman, A.J.; Worth, A.J.; Labo, T. 1990. Diet and histologic types of benign breast disease defined by subsequent risk of breast cancer. *Am. J. Epidemiol.* 131:263–270.

Howe, G.R.; Hirohata, T.; Hislop, T.G.; Iscovich, J.-M.; Yuan, J.-M.; Katsouyanni, K.; Lubin, F.; Marubini, E.; Modan, B.; Rohan, T.; Toniolo, P.; Shunzhang, Y. 1990. Dietary factors and risk of breast cancer: combined analysis of 12 case–control studies. *J. Natl. Cancer Inst.* 82:561–569.

Hsing, A.W.; Comstock, G.W.; Abbey, H.; Polk, F. 1990a. Serologic precursors of cancer: retinol, carotenoids, and tocopherol and risk of prostate cancer. *J. Natl. Cancer Inst.* 82:941–946.

Hsing, A.W.; McLaughlin, J.K.; Schuman, L.M.; Bjelke, E.; Gridley, G.; Wacholder, S.; Chien, H.T.C.; Blot, W.J. 1990b. Diet, tobacco use, and fatal prostate cancer: results from the Lutheran Brotherhood Cohort Study. *Cancer Res.* 50:6836–6840.

Hussain, M.M.; Mahley, R.W.; Boyles, J.K.; Fainaru, M.; Brecht, W.J.; Lindquist, P.A. 1989. Chylomicron-chylomicron remnant clearance by liver and bone marrow in rabbits: factors that modify tissue-specific uptake. *J. Biol. Chem.* 264:9571–9582.

Jain, M.; Burch, J.D.; Howe, G.R.; Risch, H.A.; Miller, A.B. 1990. Dietary factors and risk of lung cancer: results from a case–control study, Toronto, 1981–1985. *Int. J. Cancer* 45:287–293.

Kanematsu, T.; Kawano, T.; Takenaka, K.; Matsumata, T.; Sugimachi, K.; Kuwano, M. 1989. Levels of vitamin A and cellular retinol binding protein in human hepatocellular carcinoma and adjacent normal tissue. *Nutr. Cancer* 12:311–319.

Katsouyanni, K.; Willett, W.; Trichopoulos, D.; Boyle, P.; Trichopoulou, A.; Vasilaros, S.; Papadiamantis, J.; MacMahon, B. 1988. Risk of breast cancer among Greek women in relation to nutrient intake. *Cancer* 61:181–185.

Keilson, B.; Underwood, B.A.; Loerch, J.D. 1979. Effects of retinoic acid on the mobilization of vitamin A from the liver in rats. *J. Nutr.* 109:787–795.

Knekt, P.; Aromaa, A.; Maatela, J.; Aaran, R.-K.; Nikkari, T.; Hakama, M.; Hakulinen, T.; Peto, R.; Teppo, L. 1990. Serum vitamin A and subsequent risk of cancer: cancer incidence follow-up of the Finnish mobile clinic health examination survey. *Am. J. Epidemiol.* 132:857–870.

Kolonel, L.N.; Yoshizawa, C.N.; Hankin, J.H. 1988. Diet and prostatic cancer: a case–control study in Hawaii. *Am. J. Epidemiol.* 127:999–1012.

Kono, S.; Ikeda, M.; Tokudome, S.; Kuratsune, M. 1988. A case–control study of gastric cancer and diet in northern Kyushu, Japan. *Jpn. J. Cancer Res.* 79:1067–1074.

Koo, L.C. 1988. Dietary habits and lung cancer risk among Chinese females in Hong Kong who never smoked. *Nutr. Cancer* 11:155–172.

Koo, L.C.; Ho, J.H.-C.; Saw, D.; Ho, C.-Y. 1987. Measurements of passive smoking and estimates of lung cancer risk among non-smoking Chinese females. *Int. J. Cancer* 39:162–169.

Kune, G.A.; Kune, S.; Watson, L.F.; Pierce, R.; Field, B.; Vitetta, L.; Merenstein, D.; Hayes, A.; Irving, L. 1989. Serum levels of β-carotene, vitamin A, and zinc in male lung cancer cases and controls. *Nutr. Cancer* 12:169–176.

Kune, S.; Kune, G.A.; Watson, L.F. 1987. Case–control study of dietary etiological factors: the Melbourne Colorectal Cancer Study. *Nutr. Cancer* 9:21–42.

Lachance, P. 1988. Dietary intake of carotenes and the carotene gap. *Clin. Nutr.* 7:118–122.

La Vecchia, C.; Negri, E.; Decarli, A.; D'Avanzo, B.; Gallotti, L.; Gentile, A.; Franceschi, S. 1988. A case–control study of diet and colo-rectal cancer in northern Italy. *Int. J. Cancer* 41:492–498.

La Vecchia, C.; Negri, E.; Decarli, A.; D'Avanzo, B.; Liberati, C.; Franceschi, S. 1989. Dietary factors in the risk of bladder cancer. *Nutr. Cancer* 12:93–101.

LeGardeur, B.Y.; Lopez-S, A.; Johnson, W.D. 1990. A case–control study of serum vitamins A, E, and C in lung cancer patients. *Nutr. Cancer* 14:133–140.

Le Marchand, L.; Hankin, J.H.; Kolonel, L.N.; Wilkens, L.R. 1991. Vegetable and fruit consumption in relation to prostate cancer risk in Hawaii: a reevaluation of the effect of dietary beta-carotene. *Am. J. Epidemiol.* 133:215–219.

Le Marchand, L.; Yoshizawa, C.N.; Kolonel, L.N.; Hankin, J.H.; Goodman, M.T. 1989. Vegetable consumption and lung cancer risk: a population-based case–control study in Hawaii. *J. Natl. Cancer Inst.* 81:1158–1164.

Lewis, K.C.; Green, M.H.; Green, J.B.; Zech, L.A. 1990. Retinol metabolism in rats with low vitamin A status: a compartmental model. *J. Lipid Res.* 31:1535–1548.

Lewis, K.C.; Green, M.H.; Underwood, B.A. 1981. Vitamin A turnover in rats as influenced by vitamin A status. *J. Nutr.* 111:1135–1144.

Li, J.-Y.; Ershow, A.G.; Chen, Z.-J.; Wacholder, S.; Li, G.-Y.; Guo, W.; Li, B.; Blot, W.J. 1989. A case–control study of cancer of the esophagus and gastric cardia in Linxian. *Int. J. Cancer Res.* 43:755–761.

Lie, S.O.; Wathne, K.-O.; Petersen, L.B.; Slørdahl, S.H.; Norum, K.R. 1988. High-dose retinol in children with acute myelogenous leukemia in remission. *Eur. J. Haematol.* 40:460–465.

Lippman, S.M.; Meyskens, F.L., Jr. 1988. Vitamin A derivatives in the prevention and treatment of human cancer. *J. Am. Coll. Nutr.* 7:269–284.

Manson, J.E.; Hunter, D.J.; Buring, J.E.; Hennekens, C.H. 1991. [Letter to the editor]. *N. Engl. J. Med.* 324:924.

Marubini, E.; Decarli, A.; Costa, A.; Mazzoleni, C.; Andreoli, C.; Barbieri, A.; Capitelli, E.; Carlucci, M.; Cavallo, F.; Monferroni, N.; Pastorino, U.; Salvini, S. 1988. The relationship of dietary intake and serum levels of retinol and beta-carotene with breast cancer. *Cancer* 61:173–180.

Mathews-Roth, M.M. 1989. β-carotene, canthaxanthin, and phytoene. In: Moon, T.E.; Micozzi, M.S.; eds. *Nutrition and cancer prevention: investigating the role of micronutrients.* New York: Dekker. p. 273–290.

McCollum, E.V.; Davis, M. 1913. The necessity of certain lipins in the diet during growth. *J. Biol. Chem.* 15:167–175.

McLaughlin, J.K.; Gridley, G.; Block, G.; Winn, D.M.; Preston-Martin, S.; Schoenberg, J.B.; Greenberg, R.S.; Stemhagen, A.; Austin, D.F.; Ershow, A.G.; Blot, W.J.; Fraumeni, J.F., Jr. 1988. Dietary factors in oral and pharyngeal cancer. *J. Natl. Cancer Inst.* 80:1237–1243.

Mehta, R.G.; Moon, R.C.; Hawthorne, M.; Formelli, F.; Costa, A. 1991. Distribution of fenretinide in the mammary gland of breast cancer patients. *Eur. J. Cancer* 27:138–141.

Mettlin, C. 1988. Levels of epidemiologic proof in studies of diet and cancer with special reference to dietary fat and vitamin A. In: *Nutrition, growth, and cancer.* New York: Alan. R. Liss, Inc. p. 149–159.

Mettlin, C.; Selenskas, S.; Natarajan, N.; Huben, R. 1989. Beta-carotene and animal fats and their relationship to prostate cancer risk: a case–control study. *Cancer* 64:605–612.

Micozzi, M.S. 1989. Foods, micronutrients, and reduction of human cancer. In: Moon, T.E.; Micozzi, M.S.; eds. *Nutrition and cancer prevention: investigating the role of micronutrients.* New York: Dekker. p. 213–241.

Mills, P.K.; Beeson, W.L.; Abbey, D.E.; Fraser, G.E.; Phillips, R.L. 1988. Dietary habits and past medical history as related to fatal pancreas cancer risk among Adventists. *Cancer* 61:2578–2585.

Moon, R.C. 1989. Comparative aspects of carotenoids and retinoids as chemopreventive agents for cancer. *J. Nutr.* 119:127–134.

Moon, R.C.; Mehta, R.G. 1990. Chemoprevention of mammary cancer by retinoids. *Basic Life Sci.* 52:213–224.

Mori, S. 1922. The changes in the para-ocular glands which follow the administration of diets low in fat-soluble A; with notes of the effect of the same diets on the salivary glands and the mucosa of the larynx and trachea. *John Hopkins Hospital Bulletin* 33:357–359.

Napoli, J.L.; Race, K.R. 1987. The biosynthesis of retinoic acid from retinol by rat tissues in vitro. *Arch. Biochem. Biophys.* 255:95–101.

Napoli, J.L.; Race, K.R. 1988. Biogenesis of retinoic acid from β-carotene: differences between the metabolism of β-carotene and retinal. *J. Biol. Chem.* 263:17372–17377.

National Research Council, Committee on Diet, Nutrition and Cancer. 1989a. Cancer. In: *Diet and health: implications for reducing chronic risk.* Washington, DC: National Academy Press. p. 593–605.

National Research Council, Committee on Diet, Nutrition and Cancer. 1989b. Extent and distribution of chronic disease: an overview. In: *Diet and health: implications for reducing chronic disease risk.* Washington, DC: National Academy Press. p. 99–128.

National Research Council, Committee on Diet, Nutrition and Cancer. 1989c. Fat-soluble vitamins. In: *Diet and health: implications for reducing chronic disease risk.* Washington, DC: National Academy Press. p. 311–323.

National Research Council, Food and Nutrition Board. 1989d. Fat-soluble vitamins. In: *Recommended dietary allowances.* 10th ed. Washington, DC: National Academy Press. p. 78–92.

Nierenberg, D.W.; Bayrd, G.T.; Stukel, T.A. 1991. Lack of effect of chronic administration of oral β-carotene on serum cholesterol and triglyceride concentrations. *Am. J. Clin. Nutr.* 53:652–654.

Nierenberg, D.W.; Stukel, T.A.; Baron, J.A.; Dain, B.J.; Greenberg, E.R.; The Skin Cancer Prevention Study Group 1989. Determinants of plasma levels of beta-carotene and retinol. *Am. J. Epidemiol.* 130:511–521.

Ohno, Y.; Yoshida, O.; Oishi, K.; Okada, K.; Yamabe, H.; Schroeder, F.H. 1988. Dietary β-carotene and cancer of the prostate: a case–control study in Kyoto, Japan. *Cancer Res.* 48:1331–1336.

Oishi, Y.; Okada, K.; Yoshida, O.; Yamabe, H.; Ohno, Y.; Hayes, R.B.; Schroeder, F.H. 1988. A case–control study of prostatic cancer with reference to dietary habits. *Prostate* 12:179–190.

Ong, D.E.; Kakkad, B.; MacDonald, P.N. 1987. Acyl-CoA-independent esterification of retinol bound to cellular retinol-binding protein (type II) by microsomes from rat small intestine. *J. Biol. Chem.* 262:2729–2736.

Ostrowski, J.; Janik, P.; Nowacki, M.; Janczewska, M.; Przybyszewska, M.; Szaniawska, B.; Bartnik, W.; Butruk, E. 1987. Serum retinol level in patients with colorectal premalignant lesions. *Br. J. Cancer* 55:203–205.

Paganini-Hill, A.; Chao, A.; Ross, R.K.; Henderson, B.E. 1987. Vitamin A, β-carotene, and the risk of cancer: a prospective study. *J. Natl. Cancer Inst.* 79:443–448.

Palan, P.R.; Romney, S.L.; Mikhail, M; Basu, J.; Vermund, S.H. 1988. Decreased plasma beta-carotene levels in women with uterine cervical dysplasias and cancer. *J. Natl. Cancer Inst.* 80:454–455.

Palan, P.R.; Romney, S.L.; Vermund, S.H.; Mikhail, M.G.; Basu, J. 1989. Effects of smoking and oral contraceptives on plasma beta-carotene levels in healthy women. *Am. J. Obstet. Gynecol.* 161:881–885.

Parker, R.S. 1989. Carotenoids in human blood and tissues. *J. Nutr.* 119:101–104.

Pastorino, U.; Chiesa, G.; Infante, M.; Soresi, E.; Clerici, M.; Valente, M.; Belloni, P.A.; Ravasi, G. 1991. Safety of high-dose vitamin A: randomized trial on lung cancer chemoprevention. *Oncology* 48:131–137.

Petkovich, M.; Brand, N.J.; Krust, A.; Chambon, P. 1987. A human retinoic acid receptor which belongs to the family of nuclear receptors. *Nature* 330:444–450.

Peto, R.; Doll, R.; Buckley, J.D.; Sporn, M.B. 1981. Can dietary beta-carotene materially reduce human cancer rates? *Nature* 290:201–208.

Pilch, S.M., editor. 1985. *Assessment of the vitamin A nutritional status of the U.S. population based on data collected in the Health and Nutrition Examination Survey.* Prepared for the Food and Drug Administration under Contract No. FDA 223-84-2059 by the Life Sciences Research Office. Available from: Special Publications, Federation of American Societies of Experimental Biology, Bethesda, MD.

Potischman, N.; McCulloch, C.E.; Byers, T.; Nemoto, T.; Stubbe, N.; Milch, R.; Parker, R.; Rasmussen, K.M.; Root, M.; Graham, S.; Campbell, T.C. 1990. Breast cancer and dietary and plasma concentrations of carotenoids and vitamin A. *Am. J. Clin. Nutr.* 52:909–915.

Reichman, M.E.; Hayes, R.B.; Ziegler, R.G.; Schatzkin, A.; Taylor, P.R.; Kahle, L.L.; Fraumeni, J.F., Jr. 1990. Serum vitamin A and subsequent development of prostate cancer in the First National Health and Nutrition Examination Survey Epidemiologic Follow-up Study. *Cancer Res.* 50:2311–2315.

Ringer, T.V.; DeLoof, M.J.; Winterrowd, G.E.; Francom, S.F.; Gaylor, S.K.; Ryan, J.A.; Sanders, M.E.; Hughes, G.S. 1991. Beta-carotene's effects on serum lipoproteins and immunologic indices in humans. *Am. J. Clin. Nutr.* 53:688–694.

Roberts, A.B.; Sporn, M.B. 1984. Cellular biology and biochemistry of the retinoids. In: Sporn, M.B.; Roberts, A.B.; Goodman, D.S.; eds. *The retinoids.* Vol. 2. Orlando, FL: Academic Press, Inc. p. 209–286.

Rogers, A.E.; Longnecker, M.P. 1988. Biology of disease—dietary and nutritional influences on cancer: a review of epidemiologic and experimental data. *Lab. Invest.* 59:729–759.

Rohan, T.E.; Cook, M.G.; Potter, J.D.; McMichael, A.J. 1990. A case–control study of diet and benign proliferative epithelial disorders of the breast. *Cancer Res.* 50:3176–3181.

Rohan, T.E.; McMichael, A.J.; Baghurst, P.A. 1988. A population-based case–control study of diet and breast cancer in Australia. *Am. J. Epidemiol.* 128:478–489.

Ross, A.C. 1991. Vitamin A: current understanding of the mechanisms of action. *Nutr. Today* 26:6–12.

Ross, R.K.; Shimizu, H.; Paganini-Hill, A.; Honda, G.; Henderson, B.E. 1987. Case–control studies of prostate cancer in blacks and whites in southern California. *J. Natl. Cancer Inst.* 78:869–874.

Russell-Briefel, R.; Bates, M.W.; Kuller, L.H. 1985. The relationship of plasma carotenoids to health and biochemical factors in middle-aged men. *Am. J. Epidemiol.* 122:41–44.

Schneider, A.; Shah, K. 1989. The role of vitamins in the etiology of cervical neoplasia: an epidemiological review. *Arch. Gynecol. Obstet.* 246:1–13.

Severson, R.K.; Nomura, A.M.Y.; Grove, J.S.; Stemmermann, G.N. 1989. A prospective study of demographics, diet, and prostate cancer among men of Japanese ancestry in Hawaii. *Cancer Res.* 49:1857–1860.

Shibata, A.; Sasaki, R.; Ito, Y.; Hamajima, N.; Suzuki, S.; Ohtani, M.; Aoki, K. 1989. Serum concentration of beta-carotene and intake frequency of green-yellow vegetables among healthy inhabitants of Japan. *Int. J. Cancer* 44:48–52.

Shu, X.O.; Gao, Y.T.; Yuan, J.M.; Ziegler, R.G.; Brinton, L.A. 1989. Dietary factors and epithelial ovarian cancer. *Br. J. Cancer* 59:92–96.

Slattery, M.L.; Schuman, K.L.; West, D.W.; French, T.K.; Robison, L.M. 1989. Nutrient intake and ovarian cancer. *Am. J. Epidemiol.* 130:497–502.

Smith, F.R.; Goodman, D.S. 1976. Vitamin A transport in human vitamin A toxicity. *N. Engl. J. Med.* 294:805–808.

Stähelin, H.B.; Gey, K.F.; Brubacher, G. 1987. Plasma vitamin C and cancer death: the prospective Basel study. Ann. *N. Y. Acad. Sci.* 498:124–131.

Steineck, G.; Hagman, U.; Gerhardsson, M.; Norell, S.E. 1990. Vitamin A supplements, fried foods, fat and urothelial cancer: a case-referent study in Stockholm in 1985–87. *Int. J. Cancer* 45:1006–1011.

Stich, H.F.; Rosin, M.P.; Hornby, A.P.; Mathew, B.; Sankaranarayanan, R.; Nair, M.K. 1988. Remission of oral leukoplakias and micronuclei in tobacco/betel quid chewers treated with beta-carotene and with beta-carotene plus vitamin A. *Int. J. Cancer* 42:195–199.

Stryker, W.S.; Stampfer, M.J.; Stein, E.A.; Kaplan, L.; Louis, T.A.; Sober, A.; Willett, W.C. 1990. Diet, plasma levels of beta-carotene and alpha-tocopherol, and risk of malignant melanoma. *Am. J. Epidemiol.* 131:597–611.

Toniolo, P.; Riboli, E.; Protta, F.; Charrel, M.; Cappa, A.P.M. 1989. Calorie-providing nutrients and risk of breast cancer. *J. Natl. Cancer Inst.* 81:278–286.

Tuyns, A.J.; Riboli, E.; Doornbos, G.; Péquignot, G. 1987a. Diet and esophageal cancer in Calvados (France). *Nutr. Cancer* 9:81–92.

Tuyns, A.J.; Haelterman, M.; Kaaks, R. 1987b. Colorectal cancer and the intake of nutrients: oligosaccharides are a risk factor, fats are not. A case–control study in Belgium. *Nutr. Cancer* 10:181–196.

Underwood, B.A. 1984. Vitamin A in animal and human nutrition. In: Sporn, M.B.; Roberts, A.B.; Goodman, D.S., eds. *The retinoids.* Vol. 1. Orlando, FL: Academic Press Inc. p. 281–392.

U.S. Department of Health and Human Services. 1988. *The Surgeon General's report on nutrition and health.* Available from: U.S. Government Printing Office, Washington, DC.

U.S. Department of Health and Human Services. 1991. *The Surgeon General's report on nutrition and health.* Available from: U.S. Government Printing Office, Washington, DC.

Van't Veer, P.; Kolb, C.M.; Verhoef, P.; Kok, F.J.; Schouten, E.G.; Hermus, R.J.J.; Sturmans, F. 1990. Dietary fiber, beta-carotene and breast cancer: results from a case–control study. *Int. J. Cancer* 45:825–828.

Verreault, R.; Chu, J.; Mandelson, M.; Shy, K. 1989. A case–control study of diet and invasive cervical cancer. *Int. J. Cancer* 43:1050–1054.

Vitamin Nutrition Information Services. 1987. Presentation summaries, Beta Carotene Health Communicators Conference, April 10–12, Boca Raton, FL. Available from: Vitamin Nutrition Information Services, Nutley, NJ.

Vogel, V.G.; McPherson, R.S. 1989. Dietary epidemiology of colon cancer. *Hematol. Oncol. Clin. North Am.* 3:35–63.

Wald, N.J.; Cuckle, H.S.; Barlow, R.D.; Thompson, P.; Nanchahal, K.; Blow, R.J.; Brown, I.; Harling, C.C.; McCulloch, W.J.; Morgan, J.; Reid, A.R. 1985. The effect of vitamin A supplementation on serum retinol and retinol binding protein levels. *Cancer Lett.* 29:203–213.

West, D.W.; Slattery, M.L.; Robison, L.M.; Schuman, K.L.; Ford, M.H.; Mahoney, A.W.; Lyon, J.L.; Sorensen, A.W. 1989. Dietary intake and colon cancer: sex- and anatomic site-specific associations. *Am. J. Epidemiol.* 130:883–894.

Willett, W.C. 1990. Vitamin A and lung cancer. *Nutr. Rev.* 48:201–211.

Wolbach, S.B.; Howe, P.R. 1925. Tissue changes following deprivation of fat-soluble A vitamin. *J. Exp. Med.* 42:753–777.

Wolf, G. 1990. Recent progress in vitamin A research: nuclear retinoic acid receptors and their interaction with gene elements. *J. Nutr. Biochem.* 1:284–289.

Yob, E.H.; Pochi, P.E. 1987. Side effects and long-term toxicity of synthetic retinoids. *Arch. Dermatol.* 123:1375–1378.

You, W.-C.; Blot, W.J.; Chang, Y.-S.; Ershow, A.G.; Yang, Z.-T.; An, Q.; Henderson, B.; Xu, G.-W.; Fraumeni, J.F., Jr.; Wang. T.-G. 1988. Diet and high risk of stomach cancer in Shandong, China. *Cancer Res.* 48:3518–3523.

Ziegler, R.G. 1991. Vegetables, fruits, and carotenoids and the risk of cancer. *Am. J. Clin. Nutr.* 53:251S–259S.

Ziegler, R.G.; Brinton, L.A.; Hamman, R.F.; Lehman, H.F.; Levine, R.S.; Mallin, K.; Norman, S.A.; Rosenthal, J.F.; Trumble, A.C.; Hoover, R.N. 1990. Diet and the risk of invasive cervical cancer among white women in the United States. *Am. J. Epidemiol.* 132:432–445.

Appendix

Criteria for Inclusion of Articles in Appendix Tables

Articles in peer-reviewed journals related to the topic of this review were selected primarily on the basis of date and content. In general, papers appearing in 1987 or thereafter were included, provided that they presented original data from studies in humans. Certain items tabulated for the sake of completeness may not have been cited in the body of the text if their weight or relevance did not add significantly to development of the author's argument. Reviews have not been listed except as they included new data or useful meta-analyses.

APPENDIX TABLE   Vitamin A, Carotenoids and Cancer (Observational Studies x Site)

		I. Lung Cancer	
Study	Type/Location	Subject Number and Description	Methods
Bond et al., 1987	Nested case–control Texas	308 cases of *lung cancer* who had died between 1940–80 308 control ♂ living 308 control ♂ deceased (dead ≤ 5 yr after matched case). There were 28 overlapping controls for a total of 588. Controls were individually matched with cases for yr of birth (± 5 yr), race, and yr of hire. This cohort came from a larger pool of employees of a chemical plant.	Telephone interviews with subjects or "next of kin" to collect data about occupational history, tobacco use, residential history, and dietary habits 29-item food-frequency questionnaire. Items chosen for high vitamin A content. Reference period was 3–5 yr prior to development of symptoms in cases and 3–5 yr prior to matched case's death for living controls. No reference period described for decedent group. Interviews were completed in 1984. Analyses were adjusted for cigarette smoking, education, and use of vitamin supplements.
Connett et al., 1989	Nested case–control Minnesota	66 cases of lung cancer out of a total 156 cases of cancer deaths. 311 controls matched for age, smoking status, randomization group, date of randomization, and clinical center. Subjects from a pool of 12,866 subjects involved in an intervention trial (MRFIT) for heart disease.	Subject selection was by risk status for CHD: smoking, diastolic BP, serum cholesterol at initial screening. Subjects then seen twice. Bloods collected at second visit and stored at –50°C to –70°C. Matched triads were analyzed within 3 mo of each other. Average duration of sample storage was not reported. The cancer cases (deaths) occurred over a 10-yr period (1973–1983). On the third visit all subjects completed a 24-hr dietary recall. Serum vitamin analysis was by HPLC.
Dartgues et al., 1990	Case–control southwest France	143 cases of epidermoid lung cancer; all histologically confirmed and consecutively admitted. 212 hospitalized controls were admitted to the same hospitals with diagnosis other than cancer; matched for sex, age (± 5 yr), residential area, occupation, smoking habits, and alcohol intake.	All subjects were given a structured interview; each case and matched controls were interviewed by same person. Food-frequency questionnaire consisted of "items likely to be part of the normal diet in southwest France." Subjects asked about frequency of consumption during typical wk. Reference period was the 6-mo period prior to the interview for all subjects.
Fontham et al., 1988	Case–control Louisiana	1253 cases of lung cancer. 1274 controls matched for race, sex, and age (± 5 yr) were all admitted to the same hospitals as cases. There were significantly more non-smokers in the control group (31.6% vs 4.3%).	All subjects were given a questionnaire containing diet and tobacco history, occupational, residential, medical and family health histories. A 59-item food-frequency questionnaire was given with the reference period being before appearance of symptoms. Surrogates were interviewed in both cases (26.7%) and controls (11.5%) where subjects were unable to respond.
Jain et al., 1990	Case–control Toronto, Canada	839 cases of lung cancer; matched pairs of ♂ and ♀ 772 population-based controls; sex-matched to case pairs. Also matched for age (± 4 yr) and borough of residence. <33% refusal by eligible controls. Initial contact of subjects was by mail.	All subjects interviewed to gain data about: SES factors, lifetime residences, occupational history, and detailed smoking history. 81-item food-frequency questionnaire that emphasized vitamin and cholesterol intake. Subjects were asked to approximate portion sizes using reference food models. Data were collected on vitamin and other nutritional supplements. Reference period was 1 yr prior to interview for all subjects. Proxy interviews (primarily spouses) were used for 34% of cases. Time between interview and diagnosis in cases was not reported.

I. Lung Cancer

Results	Comments
Inverse relationship between vitamin A intake and risk of lung cancer. The association was apparent in comparisons with both controls but significant only in "living" control group. There was a stronger effect for subjects with higher carotenoid index indicating a protective effect of vitamin A from plant sources. A negative association between carrots and risk in comparison to living control; a positive association in same comparison between cases and decedent subjects. Cases were reported to have used vitamin supplements more often than either control groups.	Results are presumptive due to lack of biochemistry, extremely long retrospective period (as much as 9 yr in cases), and reliance on surrogate sources (62.3% and 65.1% by spouses or 26.6% and 23.6% by child in cases and decedent controls respectively).
Total carotenoids and β-carotene were significantly lower in lung cancer cases than in their matched controls. There were no differences between total cancer cases and controls. There was significantly reduced risk associated with increased total carotenoid levels; a similar trend ($p > 0.07$) for β-carotene. There was a nonsignificant trend towards lower intake of β-carotene. Serum levels of α-tocopherol were not related to cancer of any site.	This was a prospective cohort study of CHD from which data on cancer was extracted. All subjects were at risk for CHD, 63% were smokers, therefore the generalizability of these results is suspect. There was a potential impact of blood sample storage time on outcomes. Reliability of a single 24-hr dietary recall was questionable. Many of the "controls" may have been in early stages of cancer (7 died of cancer after the cutoff date for inclusion).
Consumption of preformed vitamin A and β-carotene was significantly and independently associated with epidermoid lung cancer. The effect did not change with the inclusion of potential confounders, e.g., smoking, into the model.	Estimated intake of vitamin A; no portion sizes used on food-frequency questionnaire; reference period relative to hospitalization rather than onset of disease; unknown duration or stage of disease in cases. No community-based controls. No supplementation data.
An inverse association was found between vitamin C intake and specific types of LC (squamous and small cell). A similar though not as strong effect was found for vitamin A (carotene). There was a significant inverse relationship between retinol intake and adenocarcinoma in blacks.	Time from diagnosis for either group not given. No community-based control group. Since comparisons were based on tertiles of intakes for control group, there may have been an underestimation of intake and associated risk due to low intakes by hospital controls. Portion sizes were not estimated by subjects; extrapolated from data on "typical serving." No comparable reference period for controls. No data on supplement use. No descriptive data reported for nutrient intake. No comparisons to intake standards, e.g., RDA. No biochemistry.
Significantly reduced risk associated with increased intake of vegetables. No association between risk and total vitamin A, retinol, vitamin C, or fruit. There was an irregular nonsignificant decrease in risk associated with β-carotene. In the small number of supplement users, there was a significant inverse relationship between vitamin A and risk. The form or amount of vitamin A was not available.	Large portion of cases used proxy interviews; 52% of ♀ case interviews were by spouses. Unknown time period between diagnosis and interview in cases could have resulted in long retrospective reference period. Most of the cases (92.5%) were smokers as opposed to 61% of controls.

(continued)

APPENDIX TABLE   (*continued*)

Study	Type/Location	Subject Number and Description	Methods
Koo et al., 1988	Case–control Hong Kong	88 cases of lung cancer. 137 district-matched controls. All subjects were ♀ with no known history of smoking.	All subjects were interviewed for demographic data including household number and/or a food-frequency questionnaire. Cases asked about intake 1 yr prior to diagnosis. Controls asked about current intake and were interviewed within 6 wk of matched cases.
Kune et al., 1989	Case–control Melbourne, Australia	64 cases of lung cancer, consecutively admitted, histologically confirmed. 63 hospital controls. All subjects were ♂ and not matched for age or any other variables.	All subjects given an interview that included a food-frequency questionnaire of unspecified length. Reference period was not reported. Blood samples were drawn from cases within a few days of diagnosis and before any treatment was initiated. Samples were drawn from controls after admission and before surgery. Fasting status and time between sampling and analysis were not mentioned.
LeGardeur et al., 1990	Case–control Louisiana	59 cases of LC. 59 hospital controls (HC) selected in a next-patient-encountered procedure. 31 community controls (CC). Subjects were matched for age (± 5 yr), race, county.	LC and HC subjects given a structured interview to obtain data about smoking history and dietary intake (method not described, no reference period given). 20 mL non-fasting venipuncture samples were collected from all subjects. Measures included: serum ascorbate, retinol and carotenoids, vitamin E and cholesterol. Assays were done within a month of collection. CC group was not interviewed only blood was collected.
Le Marchand et al., 1989	Case–control Hawaii	432 cases of LC (230 ♂, 102 ♀). 865 community controls matched for age and sex. Cases diagnosed over 2-yr period 1983–1985.	All subjects given a structured interview to garner data on smoking and alcohol consumption history. Interviews were done at home with the subject or surrogate (29% for cases, 7% for controls). 130-item food-frequency questionnaire was given to all subjects. The reference period was a usual wk, mo, or yr before onset of symptoms for the patients and a corresponding time period for the controls.
		II. Head and Neck Cancers	
de Vries and Snow, 1990	Cross-sectional Netherlands	71 cases of squamous cell cancer of the head and neck (HNC-I), with only a single tumor. 17 cases HNC with at least one additional tumor (HNC-II).	Serum levels of vitamin A, vitamin E, and β-carotene were measured.

Results	Comments
Significantly increased risk associated with low intakes of fresh fruit and fish. Protective effect of high consumption of leafy green vegetables, carrots, tofu, fresh fruit, and fresh fish in cases of adenocarcinoma and large cell cancer. Fresh fruits were found to offer protection against squamous cell tumors.	Data analyzed by foods, no analysis for specific nutrients, no biochemistry. Retrospective data, large difference in reference intervals: cases, 1 yr prior to diagnosis, controls, current diet. Conclusions regarding potential protective effects of vitamin C, retinol, and calcium are presumptive.
Mean serum levels of β-carotene and vitamin A were significantly lower in cases than controls. No difference for serum zinc. This effect held after adjustment for age and smoking history. There were no significant associations between dietary vitamin A or dietary β-carotene and serum levels of these nutrients.	No community-based controls, no supplement data reported. Cases had very low levels of retinol (30.6 μg/dL) as compared to controls. No diet data reported. The authors contend that these results are indicative of a nutritional or metabolic response to the disease rather than a reflection of a role for vitamin A vitamer levels as risk factors. It is difficult to determine whether this is a state or trait phenomena under the conditions reported.
Mean serum levels of carotenoids, vitamin E, and total cholesterol for LC cases were significantly lower than HC. Retinol levels were lower in cases but not significantly ($p < 0.07$). Although reported as no difference, HC subjects had significantly lower levels of vitamin C and vitamin E than CC. Cholesterol adjusted serum levels of vitamin E were still significantly lower in LC cases than HC.	No diet data, no questionnaire data for CC group were reported. The CC group was compared to HC group to test for appropriateness of HC as controls for LC group. Text reported no difference. Data in table indicated significant differences in the major dependent variables vitamin C and E. LC and HC group were not matched for smoking history. In addition the nature of the illnesses (e.g., 20% CHD, 14% metabolic endocrine, or nutritional disorders) of the HC group also made it an inappropriate control. No comparisons between CC group and LC cases. Retinol binding protein was significantly associated with all variables except vitamin C; this could reflect a general malnutrition or a metabolic defect. Insufficient data to make appropriate interpretation. Given the inappropriateness of the controls and poor matching, the use of a paired T-test must be questioned.
Total vitamin A (food and supplements) was inversely associated with risk; not significantly with ♀. A dose-dependent negative association was found between dietary β-carotene and LC. All vegetables, dark green vegetables, cruciferous vegetables, and tomatoes showed stronger association than β-carotene. An inverse association between total vitamin C (from food and supplements) in ♂ only There was an apparent interaction between sex and race for vitamin C.	Did not control for ethnic differences in intake. No biochemistry. The authors concluded that the effects associated with vitamin C (resulting from interaction between sex and race) were aberrations that could not be explained by any known biological mechanism and therefore did not explore the vitamin C question further.

II. Head and Neck Cancers

Statistically significant differences between groups for serum vitamin A and vitamin E levels (HNC-I > HNC-II). No difference between groups for β-carotene.	No diet, no documentation of disease history, no supplementation data, no control group. No description of analytical methods, no time period for sampling to analysis. No demographic, no control for smoking, alcohol, or any other confounding risk factors.

(*continued*)

APPENDIX TABLE   (*continued*)

Study	Type/Location	Subject Number and Description	Methods
Drozdz et al., 1989	Case–control Poland	22 newly diagnosed cases of *larynx cancer*. 16 patients with nonmalignant laryngeal disease. 16 patients with other nonmalignant diseases including CVD or hernia.	Overnight-fasted serum samples were collected and stored at –40°C for no more than 2 wk before analysis. Serum vitamins A and E were measured fluorometrically. Serum zinc and copper were measured by atomic absorption spectrophotometry.
Franco et al., 1989	Case–control Brazil	232 cases of oral cancer. 464 hospital non-cancer controls 2/case matched for sex, age (± 5 yr), and trimester of hospital admission. Neoplastic disease and mental-disordered patients were excluded.	All subjects given a 40 to 60 min structured interview by blinded interviewers. Information included: SES, demographics, general health, environmental and occupational exposure history, tobacco and alcohol use, 20-item food-frequency questionnaire, and oral hygiene habits. No proxy interviews. No reference period reported.
Graham et al., 1990	Case–control New York	178 (136 ♂, 42 ♀) cases of *esophageal cancer* drawn from a total pool of 743 cases identified during the period of 1975–1986 from 3 counties of western New York State. 178 community-based controls matched for age, sex, race (all white), and neighborhood of residence.	Subjects given a structured interview consisting of food-frequency questionnaire covering the previous yr for controls and for cases 1 yr prior to the onset of symptoms. Photographs were used to estimate portion size. Additional information included smoking and alcohol use, occupational and health histories, seasonality of intake, preparation, and food storage.
Li et al., 1989	Case–control Linxian, China	1244 cases of cancer of the *esophagus or gastric cardia ages 35–65 yr*. 1314 controls age- and sex-matched from same geographical area.	All subjects given structured interview. Data collected included: demographics, occupation, smoking, diet history by 72-item food-frequency questionnaire, food preparation and storage methods, beverage consumption, anthropometries, and family and personal health history. Questions were referenced to 2 time periods, the late 1950s and the late 1970s.
McLaughlin et al., 1988	Case–control Four regions: New Jersey, Atlanta, Los Angeles, Santa Clara, and San Mateo in California	871 cases of *oral and pharyngeal cancer*. 979 population-based controls matched for race (all white), age, and sex.	All subjects (or next of kin in those cases who were too ill) were given a structured interview to get data on tobacco and alcohol use, diet (61-item food-frequency questionnaire), medical history, occupation, and demographics. Reference period for food was normal intake during adulthood. Intakes were adjusted for seasonal variations in availability. Vitamin supplement usage was collected but did not effect outcomes.
Brown et al., 1988	Case–control South Carolina	207 cases of *esophageal cancer* (EC) ♂, 74 hospitalized cases and 133 deaths from EC during 1977–1981. 422 controls: 157 hospitalized non-cancer and 265 non-cancer deaths. The control group for mortality study was matched for race, age, area, and year of death.	Study I: a hospital-based case control; all patients were interviewed about alcohol, tobacco, diet (65-item food-frequency questionnaire), medical and dental history, occupation, family health history, and demographics. Study II: next-of-kin (usually a spouse or close relative) of the cancer and control subjects was interviewed at home.

Results	Comments
Mean levels of vitamin A were lower in cases than either control group. β-carotene levels were also lower in cases than controls (p > 0.05). Serum RBP levels were also significantly lower in cases than either control group. There was a significant association between RBP and vitamin A in the cases but not in the controls. Zinc levels were lower and copper levels higher in cases compared to controls. Serum zinc was positively associated with RBP and vitamin A in cases but not controls. There was no difference in levels of vitamin E in any of the group comparisons.	Inappropriate control groups. No diet data or report on supplement use. No matching of groups for age, sex, smoking, occupational exposure, residence, SES. The conclusions about vitamin A or β-carotene are presumptive in the face of a lack of diet history or intake data.
Significantly reduced risk associated with smoking and alcohol (the strongest risk factors irrespective of site) adjusted intakes of citrus fruits. Without adjustment, significantly reduced risk associated with increased consumption of carotene-rich foods (e.g., carrots, pumpkins, and papaya) and citrus fruits. No protection noted for green vegetables in general	No population-based controls, no biochemistry. Retrospective diet data based on limited 20-item questionnaire. No data regarding vitamin C specifically. Conclusions regarding vitamin A or β-carotene presumptive without biochemistry or more extensive comprehensive diet analysis.
No risk was observed for vitamin A derived from vegetables or for carotene alone. There was an observation of a nonsignificant decrease in risk associated with increased intakes of vitamin A from vegetables. In a separate analysis after adjustments for sex, age, education, smoking and alcohol at intakes 1 standard deviation above the range of exposure to several vegetables (lettuce, other greens, tomatoes) were associated with decreased risk. There was a significant increase in risk associated with increased intake of vitamin A from meat and dairy foods and from retinol per se.	The sample represented a small portion (24 percent) of the larger pool of 743 cases identified. The authors discussed the potential for bias in the subjects selected.
All subjects consumed a diet low in fruits and vegetables. No association with risk. Low water and high wheat intakes were associated with increased risk.	Not designed to address specific vitamin A relationship with cancer. Not enough variability in intake to assess risk relationship. Strong genetic and/or geographical component to risk in this population.
When derived from fruit there was a significant protective effect of vitamin C, vitamin A, and fiber. There was an insignificant ↑ in risk associated with ↑ intake of preformed vitamin A (retinol). Intake of dark yellow and cruciferous vegetables was related to ↓ risk in ♂ but not ♀. Vitamin C was associated with decreased OR (odds ratios) and risk of oral cancer in ♂ and ♀. Protective effects were seen for fruit consumption. Highest quartile had 1/2 the risk of lowest. No association with calories, methods of food preservation, or cooking. This effect was not apparent for other vegetable sources of these nutrients. No effect for other vitamins or nutrients.	No biochemistry, reliance on retrospective diet data, no data on time period between diagnosis and participation (cases obtained from a cancer registry). The study not designed to address specific nutrients. Mean or median intakes for nutrients not reported.
No association between β-carotene intake and risk. High intakes of retinol were associated with higher risk. After adjustments for smoking and alcohol consumption (the leading risk factors in both studies), significantly increased risks of EC were associated with low intake of fruits, particularly citrus fruits and juices and high intakes of liver. Low vitamin C and fiber intakes were associated with increased risk.	No population-based control group or biochemistry. No portion size estimates. Reliance on retrospective diet data and the use of proxy data in the mortality study. Possibly inappropriate controls in both phases may have led to conservative estimates of effects. Duration and type of disease in controls may have affected dietary outcomes. Dietary effects may have been secondary to alcohol and tobacco use and/or related diseases.

(continued)

APPENDIX TABLE   (*continued*)

Study	Type/Location	Subject Number and Description	Methods
Stich et al., 1988	Intervention India	130 betel quid chewers with oral leukoplakia divided into 3 groups: placebo (n = 35), β-carotene (n = 35), β-carotene + vitamin A (n = 60).	Challenges given in capsules 2x/wk. Total amounts/wk: Group I, 180 mg β-carotene; group II, 180 mg β-carotene + 100,000 IU retinol. The location, size, and appearance of leukoplakia and % of micronucleated cells were evaluated at baseline and 3 and 6 mo. All subjects continued chewing the tobacco mixture throughout the trial.
Tuyns et al., 1987a	Case–control France	743 cases (704 ♂ and 39 ♀) of *esophageal cancer*. 1975 controls (922 ♂, 1053 ♀) from the same geographical region. Most of the analyses were restricted to ♂.	All subjects interviewed about usual food intake with 40-item food-frequency questionnaire. Portion sizes were estimated. Risk analysis was done first for heavy vs light consumers of individual nutrients, then in a post hoc analysis at 4 levels of consumption, adjustments were made for age and 2 levels of alcohol and tobacco consumption, and residence (rural vs urban).

III. Digestive Cancers

Study	Type/Location	Subject Number and Description	Methods
Charpiot et al., 1989	Case–control France	208 subjects: 70 cases with *digestive cancer* (DC). 34 patients w/colonic polyps. 78 healthy controls. Cases diagnosed >2 mo prior to study were excluded.	12-hr-fasted blood samples were drawn from hospitalized cases before chemical, surgical or radiological therapy. Samples were drawn from polyp and control groups just after hospitalization. Retinol and vitamin E assayed via HPLC. Other measures included RBP and prealbumin (TTR).
Coggon et al., 1989	Case–control England	95 cases (73 ♂ and 22 ♀) of newly diagnosed *stomach cancer*. 190 age- (± 2 yr) and sex-matched controls.	All subjects mailed a questionnaire about food storage and dietary habits including food-frequency questions (consumption of salted and smoked foods, fresh and frozen fruit, and salad vegetables). Follow-up at-home interview to collect or complete forms with interviewer when necessary.
Kono et al., 1988	Case–control Japan	139 cases of newly diagnosed *gastric cancer* (GC). 2574 hospital-based controls (HC). 278 randomly selected community controls (CC). Subjects matched for age and sex.	GH and HC subjects interviewed in hospital, CC at home. Data collected included occupational, smoking, and dietary histories. Reference period for all subjects was the year preceeding the interview. GC and HC subjects were interviewed before diagnosis.

Results	Comments
At 3 mo there was no difference in leukoplakia regression between groups. At 6 mo there was a significant difference in remission and appearance of new leukoplakias between the 2 active groups and the placebo. There was a significant reduction in frequency of occurrence of micronucleated exfoliated cells in both β-carotene groups as compared to controls.	Duration of chewing habit not noted. No dietary controls, no dietary history, no health history.
Higher intakes of several vitamins (retinol, β-carotene, niacin) associated with significantly decreased risk. Higher intakes of vitamin C associated with decreased risk. Significant association between vitamin E intake and relative risk. Cases consumed fewer proteins of animal origin and more proteins of vegetable origin and had a higher intake of sugars and starches of vegetable origin. Cases had a lower P:S ratio; oils associated with decreased risk, butter associated with increased risk.	No biochemistry. No control for time between diagnosis and study. No reference period. No documentation of medications or other treatment. No data on medical or family health history. Hard to determine environmental from genetic effects.

III. Digestive Cancers

Results	Comments
Retinol, RBP, TTR, and vitamin E were significantly lower in cases than controls. There were no differences between polyp group and controls. Lower carrier proteins presumed to be indicative of protein malnutrition. There were no differences between site and levels of parameters studied.	No dietary intake data or supplement use reported. Aside from a statement about a lack of "denutrition" in the control groups, there was no documentation about clinical nutrition status. Sample storage time was not given. There was no matching for sex or SES.
Significant inverse relationship between intake of salad vegetables and fruit and risk. Lettuce and tomatoes were most frequently consumed vegetables. High salt intake associated with increased risk.	Global measure of nutrient intake; conclusions about vitamin A or β-carotene would be presumptive. No data on supplement use, alcohol consumption or smoking or health history. Reference period was before onset on symptoms for cases; variable time frame between interview and reference period in cases. No reference period noted for controls.
In comparison with both control groups, there was an inverse relationship between intake of fruits and GC. Also decreased risk associated with increased intake of green tea (>10 cups/d)	No controls for SES (except approximate geographic area). No biochemistry. No data on nature of health problems in HC group. Evidence of relationship between nutrients and GC presumptive as study did not evaluate individual nutrients.

(continued)

APPENDIX TABLE   (*continued*)

		IV. Colorectal Cancer	
Study	Type/Location	Subject Number and Description	Methods
Freudenheim et al., 1990a	Case–control New York	422 cases of *rectal cancer* (277♂, 145♀). 422 sex-, race-, age (±5 yr)-, neighborhood-matched controls.	Subjects given a 2.5-hr interview consisting of food-frequency questionnaire covering the previous yr for controls and for cases a yr prior to the onset of symptoms. Additional information included smoking and alcohol use, occupational and health histories, seasonality of intake, preparation, and food storage.
Graham et al., 1988	Case–control New York	428 cases of *colon cancer* (CC). 428 controls matched for age, sex, and neighborhood.	All subjects were given a structured 2.5-hr interview similar to that used by Freudenheim et al. No reference period was noted for the diet data. No surrogates were used.
La Vecchia et al., 1988	Case–control Italy	339 cases of *colon cancer* (CC). 236 cases of *rectal cancer* (RC). 778 hospital controls admitted for acute, non-neoplastic or digestive disorders.	All subjects given a questionnaire to obtain data on: SES, smoking, alcohol, coffee and other methylxanthine-containing drinks, personal and family health history, and use of selected drugs. 29-item food-frequency questionnaire. Reference period was an unspecified period before current hospital admission. Subjects also asked to report changes over previous 10 yr.
Kune et al., 1987	Case–control Melbourne, Australia	715 cases of *colorectal cancer*, CRC (392 colon cancer, 323 rectal cancer) all histologically-confirmed new cases. 727 age- and sex-matched community controls. 159 hospital controls.	300-item food-frequency questionnaire used to ascertain usual daily consumption Serving sizes were estimated by subjects. Calculated average weekly amounts adjusted for seasonal variations. Reference period was the previous 20 yr. Data included use of vitamin supplements.
Tuyns et al., 1987b	Case–control Belgium	453 cases of *colon cancer* (CC). 365 cases of *rectal cancer* (RC). 2851 controls. All subjects were from same 2 provinces and adjusted for sex.	All subjects interviewed about diet using food-frequency questionnaire. Reference period for cases 1 wk period prior to onset of disease, controls current intake. Portion sizes were estimated using food models (pictures). Cases interviewed in hospital, controls at home.
West et al., 1989	Case–control Utah	231 cases of newly- (within 6 mo) diagnosed *colon cancer* (CC). 391 controls matched by age (± 5 yr), sex, and county of residence.	All subjects were interviewed in their homes. Questionnaire consisted of demographic, health history, current height and weight (2 yr before interview), computed body-mass index, physical activity, and dietary data. 99-item food-frequency questionnaire. Reference period was "2–3 years prior to the interview." Portion sizes were estimated with food models.

IV. Colorectal Cancer

Results	Comments
Decreased risk with increasing intake of carotenoids, vitamin C, and dietary fiber from vegetables. No association between intake of vitamin E and risk. Increased risk with increasing intakes of calories, fat, carbohydrate, and iron.	Reliance on retrospective food-frequency interviews. No data on use of supplements or stage of disease (except that "only relatively alert, healthy subjects could tolerate the 2.5 hr interview"). Well-conceived study.
No significant risks associated with intake of protein, vitamin A from vegetables and fruits, carbohydrates, vitamin C, cruciferous vegetables, calcium, or phosphorous. There was significantly reduced risk associated with high intakes of tomatoes, peppers, carrots, onions, and celery. Risk of CC was positively associated with increasing intake of total fats (predominantly animal fat) and total calories.	No reference period for food-frequency questionnaire given. No data on supplement use.
Risk of both CC and RC was inversely related to intake of green vegetables, tomatoes, melon, and coffee. There was also an inverse relationship between risk and indices of carotenoid and vitamin C intake. Consumption of pasta and rice associated with increased risk of both cancers.	No supplement data, variable reference times between cases and controls, no population-based controls. Diet database was small (only 29 items). Individual nutrient estimation unreliable due to lack of portion size information. No biochemistry. No descriptive data or comparisons to normal standards of intake.
There was a dose-dependent inverse relationship between fiber, vitamin C, β-carotene, total vegetables, and cruciferous vegetables. β-carotene was highly correlated with vegetable intake. Dietary retinol had no independent association with risk of CRC. Dietary vitamin C was protective at intakes >230 mg/d. The intake of vitamin supplements was highly protective.	Long retrospective diet period. Supplement data not clearly presented (multivitamins or individual, quantity, or interaction with diet).
Intake of retinol and vitamin B2 was higher in cases; intakes of β-carotene and vitamin C were lower in cases. Significant positive associations were found for retinol, oligosaccharides; negative associations for fiber, linoleic acid, thiamine, and iron. After adjustment for age, sex, province, and caloric intake, retinol was positively associated with CC and RC; significant negative associations with fiber, thiamine, vitamin B6, iron, and vitamin C (for RC only).	Retrospective data collection. Differences in reference period between controls and cases. Group differences by province and sex. No biochemistry, supplementation data, descriptive data on intake, demographics, smoking, alcohol, medical histories, or comparisons to normal standards for intake. Possible bias from place of interview; hospital for cases, home for controls. There was no discussion of the food sources of retinol that might have contributed to its effect. No discussion of relationship of foods and outcomes, i.e., grains as sources of thiamine, fiber, etc.
Significant protective effects of β-carotene in ♂ and ♀; cruciferous vegetables in ♂; fiber was protective in ♀.	Unknown relationship between reference period and time of diagnosis in cases.
No association between CC risk and intake of vitamin C or A (presumably retinol) after adjustment for age, BMI, fiber, and energy intakes.	No biochemistry, comparisons to intake standards or descriptive statistics. No data for SES, alcohol, smoking, or supplement history.

(continued)

APPENDIX TABLE   *(continued)*

		V. Pancreatic Cancer	
Study	Type/Location	Subject Number and Description	Methods
Burney et al., 1989.	Nested case–control Maryland	22 cases of *pancreatic cancer* (PC). 44 controls matched for age, race, sex, and hr between the blood sampling and last meal.	Subjects were drawn from the larger pool of residents who had given blood samples during the period of Sept.–Nov. 1974. Samples were frozen at –70°C until assayed for retinol, total carotenoids, β-carotene, lycopene, and α-tocopherol by HPLC.
Falk et al., 1988	Case–control Louisiana	363 cases of *pancreatic cancer* (PC). 1234 hospital-based controls (HC) matched in hospital of admittance, race, sex, and age (± 5 yr).	All subjects were given an interview to obtain data on smoking, occupational and residential history, alcohol use, family health history, medical history, leisure time activities, and diet. A 59-item food-frequency questionnaire was used. Indices for vitamins A (total) and C, retinol, and β-carotene were created. The reference period was the time (unspecified) prior to diagnosis or onset of symptoms. >50% of cases were unable to be interviewed, surrogates (next of kin, usually a spouse) were used. 3% of controls were unavailable.
Farrow et al., 1990	Case–control Washington (state)	148 married ♂ cases of PC diagnosed between 1982–1986. 188 controls randomly selected and frequency-matched by age (± 5 yr). All were married and ♂.	Data were collected from surrogates (wives) in 2 steps. A telephone interview to collect demographic data, medical and occupational history, and use of tobacco, alcohol, coffee, and vitamin supplements. Dietary questionnaire was mailed and contained a 135-item food-frequency questionnaire. Reference period was 3 yr prior to diagnosis.
Mills et al., 1988	Cohort California	Study population was 34,198 non-hispanic Seventh-Day Adventists >25 yr of age. 40 cases of death from *pancreatic cancer* (PC) occurring during the follow-up period of 1974–1982.	All subjects completed a lifestyle questionnaire, details of which were not supplied.

V. Pancreatic Cancer

Results	Comments

No differences between groups for smoking history, education, or marital status.
There were no significant differences in any measures except lycopene and selenium which were both lower in cases.
There was a protective, although not statistically significant, effect of low levels of vitamin E.

No diet or supplement use data, no medical history, or information about time of onset of PC.
Storage of serum for 12 yr can result in invalid results.

Fruit consumption (fresh and juice) was inversely related with PC. There was a smaller nonsignificant inverse association with vegetable intake. No differences in risk associated with vitamin A, retinol, or carotene intakes. Trend analysis indicated increased risk with vitamin A in both sexes (significantly in ♂); there was a ↓ trend in risk associated with carotene in ♂. After adjustment for fruit intake, a nonsignificant inverse association was found for ♂ in highest levels of carotene index.
Risks associated with consumption of fruits and with an index of vitamin C showed significant decreasing gradients across sexes. Cigarette smoking was a strong risk factor for PC.

Control diet of unknown quality used as reference
No descriptive data reported nor comparisons of diet to reference standard, i.e. RDA.
No community-based control group.
Unknown time period between time of interview and diagnosis and/or onset of symptoms.
Controls diet response reflected recent intake patterns.
No data on supplement use.
No biochemistry.
No testing for the potential interaction between smoking and vitamin C index or fruit consumption.

No association between PC risk and intake of vitamin A or total fat, saturated fat, cholesterol, ω-3 fatty acids, or vitamin C.
No difference between groups in their use of supplemental multivitamins, vitamin A, or C.

Reliability and validity of data acquisition is questionable.
Reliance on retrospective data collected from surrogates.
Reference period was 3 yr prior to diagnosis.

Current use of meat, poultry, or fish was associated with increasing risk. There was a significant increase in risk associated with increasing consumption of eggs.
Intake of vegetarian protein products, legumes, and dried fruits was significantly inversely related to risk.
No relationship between risk and intake of other fresh fruit, canned or frozen fruit, fresh citrus fruit, fresh winter fruit, green salads, or cooked green vegetables.
These results were age- and sex-adjusted.

Problems include: no comparison group, no data on quality of diet, no details on diet data, no data on individual nutrients, no data on supplement use, no biochemistry, no demographics.

(*continued*)

APPENDIX TABLE   (*continued*)

VI. Liver Cancer			
Study	Type/Location	Subject Number and Description	Methods
Kanematsu et al., 1989	Cross-sectional Japan	26 patients consecutively admitted for hepatic resection; 21 ♂ and 5 ♀ 10 cases of human hepatocellular carcinoma (HCC). 19 patients had cirrhosis, 4 had fibrosis, 1 had chronic active hepatitis, and 1 had none of these conditions.	Fasting AM blood samples were assessed for plasma levels of vitamin A (retinol) and E (presumably α-tocopherol), retinol binding protein (RBP), and pre-albumin (PA). Tissue concentrations of vitamins A and E were measured in resection samples. In HCC samples comparisons were made between malignant hepatic tumor and adjacent "normal" parenchymal tissue.
Ostrowski et al., 1987	Case–control Poland	23 cases of cancer deaths (11 ♂ and 12 ♀): 4 died from lung cancer, 4 breast cancer, 4 gastric cancer, 4 colon cancer, 3 gall bladder cancer, 3 cervical or ovarian cancers, and 1 pancreatic cancer. 19 also had metastic disease in the liver. Controls were from 34 patients who died from heart or respiratory disease, diabetes mellitus, or diseases of the CNS.	Liver necropsy samples were obtained within 24-hr postmortem and analyzed for retinol.

VII. Breast Cancer			
Basu et al., 1989	Case–control Canada	30 cases w/advanced stage *breast cancer* (BC) w/distal metastases 29 cases with benign breast disease (BBD) 30 healthy age-matched controls	All of the BC patients were drug-free for 1 mo prior to sampling. Serum samples were obtained from NCI serum bank. Analysts were blinded as to subject category. Vitamin A (retinol), vitamin E, selenium, prealbumin, RBP, and β-carotene were measured.
Brisson et al., 1989	Case–control Quebec, Canada	290 cases of newly diagnosed *breast cancer* 645 age-matched control ♀ without BC enrolled in a longitudinal BC screening program/study	All subjects were interviewed about demographics, menstrual history, height and weight, smoking history, physical activity, drug-use history, and diet history. 114-item food-frequency questionnaire. Reference period: the previous year. Food models were used to estimate the size of portions. All subjects had mammograms; for cases the unaffected breast was evaluated, for controls random selection was used. All evaluations were done blindly.

VI. Liver Cancer

Results	Comments
Statistically significant difference in levels of retinol between tumor and adjacent "normal" cells. No difference in vitamin E or cellular RBP levels. There was no correlation between blood and tissue vitamin A levels. Low levels of retinol in tumor tissue not related to availability of cellular RBP.	Not a nutrition study; no diet, no control comparisons. No comparisons reported between HCC cases and those without cancer. Within-subject comparisons are of questionable value because of the appropriateness of the adjacent tissue in cancer patients as a control specimen.
Median retinol levels were significantly lower in cases than controls. All of the cases had levels considered very low (<35 µg/g tissue). 71% of controls had low levels.	Inappropriate controls, no diet data, no nutritional or health history. Not a study of vitamin A nutrition.

VII. Breast Cancer

Levels of all nutrients studied (vitamin A, β-carotene, vitamin E, and selenium) were lower in the BC group than in controls, although not significantly. For retinol, RBP, and prealbumin the magnitude of difference was decreased in comparison of BC to BBD group. In comparison across all groups, only RBP was statistically significant.	Although BC group was drug-free, there was no mention of supplements in any group. Age was the only matching variable. No dietary intake data or nutritional history. No clinical nutrition data. All BC patients were in advanced stage and metastasizing; therefore, effects may have been secondary to disease.
↑ carotenoid and fiber intakes were associated with a ↓ in high risk features on mammograms. Retinol had no effect on mammogram features. In controls, ↑ in energy-adjusted saturated fat intake was associated with ↑ high-risk mammographic features.	No comparisons in terms of risk of BC related to intake. Analysis limited to associations between mammogram features and diet. Supplement use not reported. Dependent variables (mammogram features) were derived from subjective evaluation of the observer. The relationship of mammographic features to dietary components and breast cancer risk factors was assessed in controls only. The dietary design of this study is cross-sectional, not case–control. Potential for self-selection bias as all controls were from a pool of volunteers involved in an ongoing BC screening program.

(continued)

APPENDIX TABLE   (*continued*)

Study	Type/Location	Subject Number and Description	Methods
Ewertz and Gill, 1990	Case–control Denmark	1474 cases of *breast cancer* diagnosed over period 1983–1984 1322 age-stratified randomly-selected controls	Cases mailed questionnaire 1 yr after diagnosis. Controls matched to cases for date of diagnosis. 21-item food-frequency questionnaire designed to "include 80% of the consumption of fat and β-carotene in the study population." Food models were used to estimate portion sizes. Subjects also asked about use of supplements, caffeinated beverages, sugar and artificial sweeteners.
Hislop et al., 1990	Case–control Vancouver, Canada	124 cases of proliferative benign breast disease categorized by 2 criteria for risk. Controls were selected from a pool of participants in a breast cancer screening program. Subjects matched on year of birth (± 1 yr).	Data collected from all subjects included self-administered 39-item food-frequency questionnaire. Items selected for fat, β-carotene, and retinol content. Reference period was the previous year. Other data included family and personal history of benign breast disease, age at menarche and first pregnancy, parity, use of oral contraceptives, and estrogen use.
Howe et al., 1990	Case–control Meta-analysis of 12 studies	4437 cases of breast cancer (BC). 4341 population controls. 1754 hospital controls.	Analysis included all studies of diet and BC completed by 1986. Authors made diet data available from each of 12 studies. Where data had not been available, estimates of intake were made using food frequency answers. Data on vitamin C was available from 9 of 12 studies. Pre- and postmenopausal ♀ were analyzed separately.
Katsouyanni et al., 1988	Case–control Athens, Greece	120 breast cancer cases. 120 hospital controls (patients in orthopedic ward in a different hospital than BC cases).	All subjects interviewed before discharge on first hospital admission. Data collected included: demographics, socioeconomic, reproductive, and medical histories. 120-item food-frequency questionnaire. To assess the impact of individual nutrients on BC, nutrient intakes were calorie adjusted.
Marubini et al., 1988	Case–control Italy	214 new cases of breast cancer, treatment-naive consecutive admissions 215 controls consecutively admitted to hospital; exclusions were malignant, hepatic, vascular, or metabolic disease.	Fasted blood drawn d after admission and frozen at –18°C. Levels of retinol, β-carotene, vitamin E, vitamin C, and riboflavin were assessed. Subjects interviewed about demographics and medical history. 69-item food-frequency questionnaire was used to assess dietary habits. Reference period was the previous yr unless diet had changed, in which case subjects were asked about the previous 12 mo. Subjects estimated portion sizes.

Results	Comments

There was no association between β-carotene intake and risk of breast cancer. There was a significant trend for increased risk with increased intake of total fat. There were no changes in these findings after adjustment for SES, age at first menarche, natural menopause, parity, and age at first birth. Nonsignificant elevation in risk with the use of all common vitamin supplements. More cases (72%) than controls (67%) used supplements.

Reference period not clearly defined. The rationale stated for delay of a yr after diagnosis was "to avoid asking questions on diet during a period where adjuvant chemotherapy was administered…" This implies that the diet data referred to intake patterns after diagnosis which would not reflect risk, rather response to the disease.

Proliferative benign breast disease was inversely associated with vitamin A supplementation and frequent green vegetable consumption.
Severe changes and borderline carcinoma were significantly associated with fat consumption.
There was no relationship between vitamin A or vegetable consumption and high risk groups.

No biochemistry.
Reference period not clear with respect to health history.
No comparisons with breast cancer patients.
Self-selection bias possible as all participants were enrolled in breast cancer prevention program.
Vitamin A supplements not characterized.

Vitamin C had the most consistent statistically significant inverse association with BC risk. There were no significant changes in risk ratios associated with any nutrient in the premenopausal group. Significant negative association with risk for total vitamin A, β-carotene, fiber, and vitamin C in postmenopausal and the combined group (pre- and postmenopausal). Retinol was not associated with risk at any level. Vitamin A effect was due to β-carotene. There was a significant positive association between saturated fat intake and risk in postmenopausal cases.

Questions about the validity of meta-analysis in terms of lack of control of independent variables that could influence outcomes, i.e., socioeconomic status (SES), supplement use, clinical stage, medications, smoking habits, and reliability of dietary data.

Total vitamin A intake was inversely associated with BC risk. Cases consumed less total vitamin A and retinol than controls. There was no difference in adjusted β-carotene intake. There were no differences in actual or calorie-adjusted intakes of vitamin C between cases and controls. Similarly, there was no association between vitamin C and risk of BC.

Inappropriate controls (about 25% had osteoarthritis which is known to affect anti-oxidant vitamin status). Potential mismatching due to different cachement area of controls. No demographics; no biochemistry. Diet data was related to the period preceding the onset of the disease which was not controlled nor was it documented. Supplement use not documented. Data collected over a 12-mo period; no control for seasonal variations in intakes. Portion sizes were estimated from averages in food tables.

Mean blood levels of retinol were significantly higher in cases than controls. β-carotene levels were also higher but not significantly.
No differences in intakes of either vitamin between groups.
No difference in risk or odd ratios trend for risk between groups.

Unclear reference period.
Number of subjects with dietary changes within yr not documented.
Blood levels taken after admission to hospital + an overnight fast might not be an accurate reflection of status.
No community-based controls.
No supplement data and no analysis by food group.

(continued)

APPENDIX TABLE   *(continued)*

Study	Type/Location	Subject Number and Description	Methods
Potischman et al., 1990	Case–control Buffalo, NY	83 cases of breast cancer. 113 controls. Subjects classified according to breast biopsy. 79 controls had benign lesions.	Self-administered questionnaire about health history and dietary practices. 30-item food-frequency questionnaire (items chosen to represent 90% of variability of vitamin A intake). Reference period was period immediately prior to admission. Portion sizes estimated from "standard portion sizes." Fasting blood drawn before biopsies and stored at –80°C until the end of the study.
Rohan et al., 1990	Case–control Australia	383 biopsy-confirmed cases of benign proliferative epithelial disorders (BPED). 192 controls without BPED (confirmed by biopsy). 383 community-based controls.	All subjects given a standardized questionnaire at home. Cases and biopsy controls interviewed just after diagnosis (intervals 2.8 and 2.9 mo, respectively). 179-item food-frequency questionnaire. Cases and biopsy controls were asked to record intake prior to diagnosis and disregard any changes made subsequent to diagnosis.
Rohan et al., 1988	Case–control Australia	451 cases of breast cancer histologically confirmed. 451 controls matched by residential area (same city) and age (± 1 yr).	All subjects given a standardized interview at home. For cases the average interval between diagnosis and interview was 4.8 mo. Family and personal health history and SES data collected. Diet data collection similar to Rohan et al., 1990. Cases were asked to disregard any dietary changes made since diagnosis.
Toniolo et al., 1989	Case–control Italy	250 cases of *breast cancer* (free of metastases, except in regional lymph nodes. Controls were 499 ♀ from general population stratified by age (± 10 yr) and geographical area.	All subjects interviewed (unblinded) given modified food-frequency questionnaire structured by meals. Cases interviewed on average of 7.8 mo after diagnosis and after treatment or surgery. Indigenous foods and recipes were added to the database. General demographic data was obtained from electoral rolls. Standard portion sizes before cooking were estimated. Interview data included SES data, health, and reproductive history.
Van't Veer et al., 1990	Case–control Netherlands	133 newly diagnosed cases of breast cancer. 238 community controls.	All subjects were given a home interview about demographics, smoking history, health, and reproductive and hormone history. Cases within 6 mo of diagnosis. No interviews during chemotherapy. 236-item food-frequency questionnaire. Reference period 12 mo prior to diagnosis in cases and 12 mo preceding interview in controls. Portions were estimated by subjects using common household utensils, e.g., spoons, plates, cups.

Results	Comments

Cases had significantly lower levels of β-carotene and lycopene than controls. No difference in vitamin A intake, or blood levels of α-carotene and retinol. Adjusted multivariate analysis showed an inverse relationship between risk and levels of β-carotene that was restricted to postmenopausal ♀ (cases were significantly older than controls). No effect of plasma retinol but a significant trend with ↑ retinol and ↓ β-carotene. No association between dietary vitamin A (total or from vegetable sources) and risk.

Potentially inappropriate controls as there were no differences in known risk factors between groups (indicated that this was a high-risk group).
No community-based controls.
Self-reported diet data did not include supplement use or reference period related to disease onset.
No portion sizes reported by subjects.

Statistically significant trend towards decreased risk with ↑ intake of retinol and β-carotene when cases compared to community controls. There was a similar trend with biopsy controls but not statistically significant.
Adjustment for energy intake eliminated the β-carotene trend but not the point estimate.

Portion sizes estimated.
No analysis by food group.
No data on supplement use.
Case group may have been self-selected as they differed from controls in self-examination practices.

No change in risk associated with retinol intake. Significantly reduced risk associated with β-carotene intake across the whole sample. No effect associated with energy, protein, or total fat consumption. In premenopausal ♀, risk ↑ with ↑ retinol intake and ↓ with ↑ β-carotene intake. In postmenopausal ♀, risk was highest in the second lowest quintile of consumption.
Intakes of retinol and β-carotene were slightly higher in cases.
No difference in vitamin E or C intake between groups.
Reduced risk was associated with decreased intakes of fat especially saturated fat and animal protein.

See Rohan et al., 1990.
Study subjects were asked to record usual dietary patterns and to disregard reporting of changes in dietary patterns that occurred after diagnosis.
Reference period included time before and after diagnosis and possible treatment.
Not blinded, no biochemistry, long period of time between diagnosis or treatment and study (on average 7.8 mo after diagnosis).
Retrospective diet data not necessarily indicative of diets prior to diagnosis.
Smoking histories not reported.

There was no difference in intake of β-carotene between cases and controls. There was a nonsignificant inverse trend for risk in the age-adjusted comparison of highest to lowest intakes of β-carotene. There was a statistically significant trend for ↓ risk associated with ↑ intake of cereal (90% of cereals from bread). Cases had a statistically significant lower energy adjusted intake of dietary fiber. There was a non-significant inverse trend in risk associated with fiber intake. Non-significant lower risk with ↑ intake of β-carotene, fruit, and vegetables.

Small sample size.
Large nonresponse rate in selection of controls (238 out of a potential pool of 548) may have resulted in bias.
Cases and controls not matched on reference period, i.e., time between diagnosis and interview in cases.
No supplement data and no analysis with other risk factors, e.g., smoking, hormones

(*continued*)

APPENDIX TABLE   *(continued)*

VIII. Cervical/Ovarian Cancer			
Study	Type/Location	Subject Number and Description	Methods
Brock et al., 1988	Case–control Australia	117 cases of cervical cancer. 196 controls matched for SES, age (±5 yr) 100 of the interviewed cases agreed to blood sampling, 143 of the controls.	All subjects interviewed either at home or at work. Cases interviewed within 6 mo of diagnosis. Questioned on demographics, reproductive, contraceptive, and gynecological factors. 160-item food-frequency questionnaire with an emphasis on vitamins A, C, and folate. Reference period was the previous year. Photographs of food were used to estimate portion sizes. Blood collected after an overnight fast and assessed for β-carotene, retinol, and carotene with HPLC methods
Cuzick et al., 1990	Case–control London, England	45 controls. 30 cases of *cervical intraepithelial neoplasia* I (CIN I). 40 cases CIN III. Subjects chosen from a pool of 110 CIN I, 284 CIN III, and 833 controls involved in a larger study. Serum samples were randomly selected from an age-stratified sample.	Sera were analyzed blindly for vitamins A and E by HPLC. Samples were stored for an unspecified period at an unspecified temperature.
de Vet et al., 1991	Intervention trial randomized placebo-controlled multiblinded Netherlands	369 ♀ ages 20–65 with untreated cervical dysplasia were the subject pool.	Subjects stratified by age, hospital of diagnosis, and degree of dysplasia (3 categories). 137 received 10 mg β-carotene for 3 mo. 141 received placebo. At 2 mo, asked about diet habits.
Palan et al., 1989	Cross–sectional New York, NY	18 ♀ with uterine leiomyoma. 5 with uterine cervix cancer. 2 each with cancer of endometrium, ovary, breast, and colon and 1 each with cancer of lung, liver, and rectum.	Normal, begign and malignant tissues from uteri (hysterectomies), and various other carcinoma sites, i.e., uterine cervix, endometrium, ovary, breast, lung, liver, colon, and rectum were collected from the same group of patients. Adjacent normal tissue was used for comparison to cancer tissue within each subject. Tissues were analyzed for β-carotene content.
Palan et al., 1988	Case–control New York, NY	32 cases of cervical cancer. 72 subjects with abnormal pap smear divided into 2 groups: 37 mild and 35 severe dysplasia. 37 controls recruited from a family-planning clinic who were using barrier method of contraception.	Blood samples were collected 2–3 hr after breakfast, frozen, and stored at –80°C for not more than 1 wk prior to analysis for retinol and β-carotene. Samples were collected prior to any treatment.
Shu et al., 1989	Case–control Shanghai, China	172 cases of epithelial ovarian cancer. 172 cases matched for age (± 5 yr) and residence.	All subjects interviewed about demographics, reproductive history, personal and family health histories, occupational history, and diet. 63 indigenous item food-frequency questionnaire about normal adult consumption. Subjects were asked to estimate portion sizes.

VIII. Cervical/Ovarian Cancer

Results	Comments
Cases were not matched on sexual habits, smoking, or use of oral contraceptives. Crude risk estimates showed a significant protective effect from ↑ intakes of carotene, vitamin C, and folate. After adjustment for known risk factors the protective trends for all except vitamin C (p < 0.07) disappeared. When considered together, vitamin C, fruit juices, and plasma β-carotene showed a significant protective effect. Fruits did not show a protective effect. Current supplement use was associated with a "marginally significant" reduction in risk while past use was not. No other comparisons of supplements to intake, blood levels, or other risk factors were made.	No vitamin C biochemistry. Blood sampling of cases may have reflected state vs trait phenomena. Intakes of food or amounts or type of supplements used was not reported. Only quartile comparisons were made for intake data.
No significant differences in vitamin A were found between groups. There were no significant trends in risk associated with vitamin A. The mean levels of serum vitamin E showed a significant decreasing trend lower in cases (CIN III and I) than controls and III were less than I. Significant trends were found in vitamin E levels for both CIN I and III, with higher levels being protective. This trend was strengthened when adjustments for smoking, sexual behavior, and use of oral contraceptives were made.	No diet data or reported use of supplements. No matching for SES. Vitamin A levels not defined (presumably retinol). No discussion of β-carotene.
The number of patients who had progression was not enough for comparisons. There was no effect of supplement on regression of cervical dysplasia.	No biochemistry. Diet data collected in the middle of the trial. No baseline diet data nor was there an appropriate reference period. Selective use of food-frequency and portion-size estimation (only done for some foods).
β-carotene was significantly lower in fibroid tissue than normal myometrium. The concentrations of β-carotene were lower in all cancer tissues when compared to adjacent "normal" tissue.	Not a nutrition study. No diet data, no supplement use data. No nutritional biochemistry. Results could reflect a consequence of the disease rather than reflection of an active role of β-carotene in the cancers studied. Small sample size may be too small to establish statistical significance.
Mean plasma β-carotene was significantly lower in all dysplasias and cancers when compared to normal group. There was significant difference between mild and severe dysplasia and between both dysplasias and cancer with cancer having the lowest levels. There were no differences in plasma retinol levels between the groups.	See comments for Palan et al., 1989.
No effect of dietary vitamin A or β-carotene. Significant increased risk associated with total and saturated fat.	No time frame between interview and diagnosis given; no reference period given for cases. No biochemistry, no supplement data, no descriptive statistics or comparisons to known standards of intake. Groups were not matched for SES, cases were more educated.

(continued)

APPENDIX TABLE   (*continued*)

Study	Type/Location	Subject Number and Description	Methods
Slattery et al., 1989	Case–control Utah	85 cases of primary ovarian cancer. 492 population-based controls matched for age.	All subjects interviewed by ♀ in person at home. Data collected included demographics, smoking history, medical history, contraceptive use, pregnancy history, and anthropometries. 183-item food-frequency questionnaire used to obtain usual adult dietary habits. No reference period given. Subjects estimated portions consumed.
Verreault et al., 1989	Case–control Washington (state)	189 cases of cervical cancer. 227 controls age-matched and identified by random-digit-dialing methods.	All subjects given a telephone interview by a ♀ interviewer to collect data on demographics, reproductive history, contraceptive methods, smoking history, anthropometries (self-reported), health history, and sexual habits. 66-item food-frequency questionnaire included vitamin supplement use. Reference period was the yr prior to a reference date (date of diagnosis for cases and Dec. 31, 1981 for controls). Portion sizes were estimated by investigators.

IX. Prostate Cancers

Study	Type/Location	Subject Number and Description	Methods
Hayes et al., 1988	Case–control Netherlands	94 cases of clinical prostate cancer. 40 cases of focal prostatic cancer. 130 cases of benign prostatic hyperplasia. 130 hospital controls (admitted for either orthopedic or pulmonary surgery). Dutch literacy was required; subjects did not have to be natives. Cases were either new admissions or were identified from chart reviews.	All subjects were interviewed about demographic history, marital and sexual behavior history, and dietary history (method not described). Blood and saliva samples were collected between 9–12 AM (fasting status not indicated). Samples were "kept cool" for between 1–2 hr and then frozen at –20°C until analysis (time frame not given) for retinol, β-carotene, and α-tocopherol. Of the 134 cases of cancer, 107 had blood drawn prior to surgery. Blood from other groups was drawn within days of hospitalization.
Hsing et al., 1990a	Case–control Maryland	103 cases *prostate cancer*. 103 controls matched for race (all white), age, and sex (all ♂). Subjects drawn from a sample pool of 25,802 residents of Washington Co., MD. Cases were identified over an 11-yr period (1974–1986).	Serum samples were collected in 1974 and stored at –70°C as part of a blood banking project for cancer research. All participants were given a questionnaire that included: demographics, smoking history, medication use, and vitamin supplement use (with special reference to the 48 hr prior to blood sampling). Serum retinol, carotenoids, and vitamin E measured by HPLC. 30 cases and 30 control samples analyzed at a different lab in a pilot study. The remaining 140 samples (70/70) were analyzed as above. Inter-laboratory variations ranged from 3% for retinol to 11% for β-carotene. None reported for α-tocopherol.

Results	Comments
After adjustment for age, number of pregnancies, and the body-mass index, there was significantly reduced risk associated with β-carotene intake. No effect of vitamin C. Small non-significant decrease in risk associated with vitamins A and C and fiber.	Used nutrient analysis rather than food groups. No supplement data. Low response rate in cases.
High intakes of carotene were associated with unadjusted ↓ risk of squamous cell cancers. After adjustment for total energy intake and known risk factors there was a nonsignificant trend for ↓ risk. After adjustment for known risk factors, increased intake of dark green or yellow vegetables, and fruit juices were associated with significantly reduced risk. There was no association between retinol intake and risk. Decreased risk associated with high intakes of vitamins C and E.	No portion sizes given on food-frequency questionnaire; portion sizes estimated from food composition tables. No biochemistry. Use of a long retrospective period; the average delay between interview and reference period was 2.8 yr for cases and 2.7 yr for controls.

IX. Prostate Cancers

Mean levels of serum retinol, β-carotene and α-tocopherol were significantly lower in cases than controls. There was an unadjusted trend of increased risk for prostatic cancer in the combined cases associated with decreasing retinol levels. There was a non-significant trend when the clinical cases were analyzed alone. In more severe cases (those who had radical surgery and/or therapy), the significant trend persisted. There was no trend for β-carotene. When adjusted for age and current cigarette smoking, the trend for retinol did not reach significance.	Potential response bias indicated by different numbers of subjects giving blood in different age groups and from admitting hospital vs. cooperating hospital referrals. Other potential confounding factors include timing of blood sampling relative to hospital admission, differences in duration of disease, and nonfasted blood samples. No diet or supplement use data were reported.
No differences in mean vitamin levels between cases and controls. There was a trend for decreased risk associated with serum retinol levels; no trend associated with either β-carotene or α-tocopherol levels.	No diet or supplement use data reported. Long and variable storage time.

(continued)

APPENDIX TABLE   (*continued*)

Study	Type/Location	Subject Number and Description	Methods
Hsing et al., 1990b	Cohort/ case–control USA	149 cases of fatal prostate cancer. 17,633 controls used for computation of food-consumption quartiles. Subjects were from a pool of 26,030 holders of Lutheran Brotherhood Insurance selected in 1966 for a mortality study.	68.5% of the original cohort completed questionnaires. Comparisons of respondents to nonrespondents showed no differences in age, residence, or policy status. Questionnaire included data on demographics, alcohol and tobacco use, and diet history. Subjects asked about current (1966) intake of 35 food items. Portion sizes were estimated from survey data (NHANES II).
Kolonel et al., 1988	Case–control Hawaii	452 cases of histologically-confirmed prostatic cancer (PC). 899 age-matched controls. Subjects > 65 yr were randomly selected from a central insurance registry, those < 65 yr selected with random-digit-dialing.	All subjects given an extensive home interview to collect data on dietary, occupational, medical, social, and demographic histories. 100+ item food-frequency questionnaire was used. Reference period was a usual mo prior to onset of the disease for cases and a corresponding period for controls. Surrogates were used for those subjects who could not be interviewed.
Le Marchand et al., 1991	Case–control Hawaii	See Kolonel et al., 1988	See Kolonel et al., 1988 Data set was analyzed separately for <70 and ≥70 yr
Mettlin et al., 1989	Case–control Buffalo, NY	371 cases of histologically confirmed prostate cancer. 371 control patients with no history of cancer, matched by age. 12.1% of controls had benign prostatic hyperplasia. There were a total of 76 different diseases in this group.	All patients admitted to the Roswell Park Memorial Institute are given a lifestyle questionnaire including a 45-item food-frequency checklist. Reference period for all patients was the period preceding the onset of current illness (admission?). Portion sizes were estimated from standard food tables.
Ohno et al., 1988 Oishi et al., 1988	Case–control Japan	100 cases newly diagnosed of prostatic cancer (PC). 100 controls with benign prostatic hyperplasia (BPH). 100 hospital controls without BPH, other malignancies, liver disease, or hormonal disorder. All subjects were matched for hospital, age (± 3 yr) and date of admission (± 3 mo).	Data collected by interview upon admission to hospital included: birthplace, occupational history, marital history, religion, body type, medical history, sex-life, and dietary practices. Food-frequency questionnaire assessed dietary habits during the period 5 yr prior to current admission. Photographs were used to estimate portion sizes.

Results	Comments
No significant trends were associated with total vitamin A, retinol, or β-carotene intake.	Self-selected population. No comparison with general population, no data on mean intakes, no supplement data. The vitamin A differences in the 2 age groups could have reflected a difference in the type of foods eaten; this was not tested. Very limited food items in food-frequency questionnaire (it lacked some major sources of vitamins, e.g., liver, broccoli, spinach, and melons). Age analysis was only reported for the vitamin A intakes, not for smoking, alcohol consumption, or other foods. In 58 of the 149 fatalities, prostate cancer was not the primary cause of death. It was not clear whether prostate cancer was the primary diagnosis.

No significant trends were associated with total vitamin A, retinol, or β-carotene intake.
When analyzed by age the group < 75 yr had an ↑ risk associated with ↑ intake of total vitamin A.
In those ≥ 75 yr the trend was reversed. This pattern held true for retinol and β-carotene. There were no changes in risk associated with intake of any of 9 food groups or any individual foods.

Comments: Self-selected population. No comparison with general population, no data on mean intakes, no supplement data. The vitamin A differences in the 2 age groups could have reflected a difference in the type of foods eaten; this was not tested. Very limited food items in food-frequency questionnaire (it lacked some major sources of vitamins, e.g., liver, broccoli, spinach, and melons). Age analysis was only reported for the vitamin A intakes, not for smoking, alcohol consumption, or other foods. In 58 of the 149 fatalities, prostate cancer was not the primary cause of death. It was not clear whether prostate cancer was the primary diagnosis.

Older cases consumed significantly more saturated fat, total vitamin A, and zinc than age-matched controls. These differences were reflected in increased risk associated with saturated fat and zinc. There was a significant increase in risk with the highest quartile of total vitamin A intake as well as a trend towards increased risk. Similar finding with respect to total carotenes and β-carotene. No difference between younger subjects and their matched controls. There were no associations between risk and total vitamin C or food sources of vitamin C.
No differences found in potential confounding variables: SES, marital status, anthropometries, family history.
No significant interactions between nutrients.

Comments: Total vitamin A and total zinc included supplements. The supplements were not characterized as either individual or multivitamins/minerals. At the time of the study β-carotene was not available in Hawaii as a supplement. The older cases consumed more of all forms of vitamin A than younger cases with the exception of food sources of retinol. This would indicate a greater use of supplements or greater intakes of carotene-rich foods. The mean weekly intake of total vitamin A was 12,557 IU in the older group vs 11,028 IU in the younger cases. These intake levels are both >2x the RDA (1980 of 5000 IU/d for adult ♂). The duration of supplement use was not reported.

Main food sources of β-carotene were carrots, papaya, pumpkin, sweet potatoes, and mangoes. In < 70 yr group there was no association between risk and intake of these foods. In older group there was a strong association with papaya only.

Comments: There were no differences reported in mean intake of β-carotene rich foods between the older and younger groups. β-carotene from papaya is an unlikely cause of prostate cancer. No analysis of food and supplement separately or in interactions although at the time of the study β-carotene was not available as a supplement. Total vitamin A intake included supplements.

No differences in age, marital status, education, weight, and height. There was a geographical difference. There was a significant reduction in risk associated with the highest level of intake of β-carotene in ♂ < 68 yr but not in subjects > 68 yr. Age- and resident-adjusted risk for highest level of β-carotene for the combined age groups shows a protective effect. Increased consumption of high-fat milk was associated with increased risk. There was a non-significant trend towards increased risk associated with fat intake.

Comments: No supplement data, no population-based controls. Diet data collected during time of duress for most subjects. Variable time between first diagnosis and hospital admission.

Low intakes of vitamin A (retinol and β-carotene) were associated with increased risk.
The risk reduction associated with vitamin A and β-carotene was seen in older (70–79 yr) but not younger (50–69 yr) ♂. Vitamin A and β-carotene from green/yellow vegetables were significantly protective.
There was no association between risk and any other nutrients.

Comments: No supplement data, confusing statistics, lack of community-based controls.
Long retrospective period, 5 yr.
No smoking data.

(continued)

APPENDIX TABLE   (*continued*)

Study	Type/Location	Subject Number and Description	Methods
Reichman et al., 1990	Cohort/ case–control USA	84 cases of prostate cancer. Subjects selected from a larger cohort of 2440 ♂ ≥ 50 yr involved in the NHANES I follow-up study (NHEFS). Cases identified by hospital and/or death certificates.	NHEFS collected health outcome and dietary data on subjects who were >25 yr at time of NHANES I. The study cohort consisted of those subjects who agreed to follow-up and had blood samples taken during NHANES I. Serum samples were collected and stored at –20°C for a period < 3 mo.
Ross et al., 1987	Case–control California	179 black (BPC) of prostate cancer (PC) diagnosed between 1977–1980. 142 black controls (BC) matched for age (± 5 yr) and residence. 142 white (WPC) of PC diagnosed between 1972–1982. 142 white controls (WC).	All interviews usually done at home (all WPC and WC) or occasionally at a mutually-convenient location. A food-frequency questionnaire containing 20 categories of foods was used to estimate intake of fat, protein, and vitamin A. Reference period was time of diagnosis Portions estimated from common portion sizes
Severson et al., 1989	Cohort/ case–control Hawaii	174 cases of newly diagnosed malignant prostate cancer divided into overt PC (OPC) and latent cancer (LPC). Cohort consisted of 7999 ♂ of Japanese ancestry.	All subjects interviewed between 1965–1968 about demographics, marital, smoking, occupation, residence, education, alcohol use, and medical history. 23-item food-frequency questionnaire and 24-hr recall. Reference period was time of initial examination to time of diagnosis.

X. Bladder Cancer

Study	Type/Location	Subject Number and Description	Methods
Helzlsouer et al., 1989	Case–control Maryland	35 cases of *bladder cancer*. 70 controls (2/case) matched for nearest age, sex, race within 2 hr interval of blood sampling and last meal. Sample pool was 20,305 residents of Washington Co., MD. Cases were identified over an 11-yr period (1975–1986).	Serum samples were collected in 1974 and stored at –70°C as part of a blood-banking project for cancer research. All participants were given a questionnaire that included: demographics, smoking history, medication use, and vitamin supplement use (with special reference to the 48 hr prior to blood sampling). Serum retinol, carotenoids, and vitamin E measured by HPLC.
La Vecchia et al., 1989	Case–control northern Italy	163 cases of histologically confirmed (within 1 yr before interview) *bladder cancer* (total pool eligible not given). 181 hospital controls (HC).	All subjects interviewed about SES factors, smoking, alcohol, coffee, and other methylxanthine consumption habits, personal and family health history, and specific medication history. Frequency of consumption of 10 food items. Reference period for cases was the period before onset of symptoms; none was given for controls.
Steineck et al., 1990	Case–control Stockholm, Sweden	418 cases of urothelial cancer and or squamous cell cancer of the lower urinary tract (renal pelvis, bladder, ureter, urethra). 511 sex- and age-stratified, randomly-selected controls.	Questionnaire was mailed to all subjects and included health history, drug use, occupation, smoking, "life events," and diet. 56-item food-frequency section. Reference period was 3 yr prior to interview. Portions were estimated with photographs. Separate questions about supplement use; specifically, vitamins A, B, and C and "other kinds of supplements and tonics." Study period was 1985–1987, supplement use data after 1981 was ignored.

Results	Comments
There was a higher percentage of blacks than whites in the lower percentiles of vitamin A levels. Education, serum cholesterol, alcohol consumption, and body-mass index were all associated with vitamin A levels. Age, marital status, height, total calories, and smoking were not associated with vitamin A in this cohort. There was a statistically significant difference in mean vitamin A levels between cases and controls. There was a significant negative trend for risk of prostate cancer associated with vitamin A levels. There was no difference in risk in those over 70 yr.	No diet interactions tested. Supplement use was noted to be related to vitamin A levels; however, supplements were not characterized. No distinction made between forms of vitamin A; presumably methods used analyzed total vitamin A content.
Significant differences between races for sexual practices and incidence of venereal disease. Venereal disease (+) and circumcision (–) were significantly associated with risk in both groups. Vitamin A consumption was inconsistently related or unrelated to PC risk in both groups. Fat intake was a risk factor for both groups.	57% response rate for black cases. Variable and long reference period. Limited items on food-frequency questionnaire. Portion sizes estimated from food tables. No supplement use data. Groups differed demographically. BC were apparently not matched to BPC group demographically. There were no statistical adjustments made for any confounding variables in the diet analysis.
Individual nutrients not evaluated. No relationship between intake of total fat and protein. Intake of certain types of foods, e.g., seaweed (+) and rice (–), were associated with risk.	Reference period unclear and variable. No supplement use data; no biochemistry. Limited nutrient data. Not designed to assess vitamin A or any other specific nutrient. No comparison to general population, limited to traditional Japanese-type diet.

X. Bladder Cancer

Results	Comments
Cases had lower mean nutrient levels of all nutrients than controls. There was a significant association between vitamin E levels and supplement use, but not for any other nutrient. There were no significant differences in prediagnostic levels of any nutrients except selenium which was lower in cases. There was no difference in risk by tertiles for any serum nutrient level except selenium. Serum α-tocopherol and lycopene levels were non-significantly lower in cases.	Controls were more likely to have used supplements. There was no analysis of the vitamin E and selenium relationship. Similarly, there was no testing for interactions between any of the nutrients studied. Aside from supplement data, no dietary data was collected. Long storage time between collection and analysis. Overall sample pool characteristics were biased towards middle-aged, white, better educated, married ♀.
The frequency of consumption of green vegetables and carrots was significantly lower in cases. Estimated intakes of carotenoids and total vitamin A, but not retinoids, were significantly less in cases than controls. There was increased risk for BC associated with estimated low intakes of both carotenoids and retinol. Protective effect was stronger in current smokers. No effect from either fruit or vitamin C.	Reference period was at least 2 yr before interview for cases. Very limited number of items (10) on food-frequency questionnaire. No supplement use data. No community-based controls. Portion size was estimated by investigators.
Supplemental intake of vitamin A (uncharacterized) was inversely associated with risk. Fat and fried foods were significantly associated with increased risk.	The nature of the collection of the dietary data set was not clearly delineated. Reference period was confusing. An apparently long retrospective period between supplement use reference period and study interview. Vitamin supplements broadly categorized, e.g., vitamin A or vitamin B.

(continued)

APPENDIX TABLE (*continued*)

		XI. Skin Cancer	
Study	Type/Location	Subject Number and Description	Methods
Greenberg et al., 1990	Intervention/ randomized double-blind trial 4 clinical centers: Dartmouth, UCLA, UC-San Francisco, Univ. Minnesota	Potential subjects were patients with non-melanoma skin cancer (basal-cell or squamous cell carcinoma) since 1980. 1805 subjects were selected.	Subjects were randomized to receive 50 mg/d β-carotene or placebo. At 4-mo intervals subjects responded to a questionnaire about health, compliance, consumption of vegetables, and use of vitamins. Subjects returned annually for examination or sent detailed record of annual examination. Blood samples were collected at enrollment and annually thereafter. Plasma shipped at −20°C and subsequently stored at −70°C until assayed for β-carotene and retinol.
Stryker et al., 1990	Case–control Boston	204 cases of *malignant melanoma*. 248 control patients who were making first visit to clinic.	All subjects completed a questionnaire on diet (food frequency for 116 foods, questions on use of vitamin and mineral supplements and on type of fats used for cooking), medical history, and constitutional and lifestyle factors. Other factors collected included demographic data, pigmentation characteristics, and past medical history. Fasting serum samples stored at −70°C for up to 6 mo. Subjects estimated portion sizes. Reference period was the previous yr.

		XII. Other Studies	
Knect et al.,	Case–control Finland	766 cases of *cancer of all sites*. 1419 controls matched for age, sex, and duration of storage. Subjects drawn from a pool of 36,263 survey participants. Cases identified over a variable time period of 5–9 yr.	Baseline questionnaire included data about occupation, drug use, medical history, and smoking habits. Body-mass index was used to describe obesity. Serum samples were stored at −20°C for between 11–15 yr before analysis of retinol, RBP, β-carotene, selenium, and α-tocopherol.
Paganini-Hill et al., 1987	Cohort California	Cohort consisted of 10,473 residents of a retirement community in CA. All subjects were free of preexisting cancers. Subjects were primarily white, moderately affluent and well-educated. Median age = 74 yr ~ 67% ♀.	Subjects were mailed a questionnaire about demographics, medical history, personal habits, medical screening use, diet, and (for ♀) menstrual and reproductive history. Diet data included vitamin supplement use and a 59-item food-frequency questionnaire. Portion sizes were estimated using standard tables. Original questionnaire sent in 1981 followed by biennial questionnaires in 1983 and 1985.

XI. Skin Cancer

Results	Comments
No difference in occurrence of new non-melanoma skin cancer between groups.	38% of eligible subjects agreed to participate. No characterization of baseline or concurrent dietary habits.
Cases were more likely to be supplement users than controls. After adjustment for age, sex, plasma lipids, hair color, and tanning ability; levels of lycopene, retinol, and α-tocopherol were similar in cases and controls. Controls tended to have a greater intake of carotene and dietary vitamin E. No differences in descriptive or risk-trend analyses between groups for plasma carotenes (α-, β-, or lycopene) or retinol. There was a weak non-significant trend towards $\downarrow$ risk associated with $\uparrow$ carotene intake. There was a trend towards $\downarrow$ risk with $\uparrow$ intake of vegetable fat. Some of the higher levels of α-tocopherol were associated with a non-significant decreased risk of melanoma. Intake of vitamin E from food alone was significantly associated with a trend of decreased risk with increased intake.	Possibly inappropriate controls as all subjects were patients in skin clinic. Controls may have been more health conscious. Analyses were adjusted for age and sex but no control for SES. Subjects in case group included patients who knew their diagnosis before the study began.

XII. Other Studies

Mean β-carotene levels were significantly inversely associated with smoking. ♂ cases had significantly lower levels of retinol, RBP, and β-carotene than ♂ controls. ♀ cases had non-significantly lower levels of all vitamin A-related compounds. Among ♂ there was a significant inverse relationship between retinol and β-carotene and risk after adjustment for smoking. There was an inverse gradient between serum retinol levels and the occurrence of cancer in ♂ that was primarily concentrated in the first 2 yr of follow-up. The differences in β-carotene were reflected in risk of lung cancer. Mean serum vitamin E levels were significantly lower in cases than controls. Subjects with low level of vitamin E had about 1.5-fold risk of cancer compared to controls. ♀ with low vitamin E and low Se had a 3x higher risk of hormone-related cancer.	No diet data, supplement use data, or matching for SES. No seasonal variations in food supply and time of blood sampling reported. Long storage time. Aside from removing those who were diagnosed within 2 yr of sampling, there was no control for time to diagnosis of cancer.
By 1986, 643 cases of cancer: 56 lung, 110 colon, 59 bladder, 93 prostate, 123 ♀ breast cancer, 202 cancers of other sites. Neither vitamin or β-carotene had a statistically significant effect on overall cancer rates. For the sites considered, there was a significant trend for $\downarrow$ risk for bladder cancer in ♀ with increased consumption of dietary β-carotene. Dietary intake of vitamin A was inversely associated with smoking. The incidence rate for all cancers in ♂ who never smoked was inversely related to β-carotene and total vitamin A intakes.	Selective cohort of mid-high SES and health conscious No case–control comparisons. Supplements used not characterized. Diet data of questionable reliability. There was only a 50% agreement between the questionnaire used in the first and second follow-up.

(continued)

APPENDIX TABLE   (*continued*)

Study	Type/Location	Subject Number and Description	Methods
Stähelin et al., 1987	Prospective cohort Basel, Switzerland	2974 ♂ comprised the original pool from which 204 total cancer deaths occurred: 68 lung cancer, 20 stomach cancer, 17 colorectal, and 99 "other malignancies."	Fasting blood samples were collected over a 2-yr period (1971–1973). Analysis was done immediately.

Results	Comments
Compared to survivors, cases had significantly lower plasma carotene levels. Carotene levels were significantly lower in lung and stomach cancer cases. Vitamin C was also lower in all cancer cases than in controls. Low carotene levels were associated with ↑ risk for lung cancer after adjustment for smoking, age, and cholesterol. For all cancers the combination of low carotene and low vitamin A was associated with ↑ risk. After adjustment for smoking, vitamin C levels were significantly lower in stomach cancer deaths.	No diet data and no supplement data to control for seasonal variations in diet that might influence blood levels. Reliance on point sample procedures.

Vitamin A and Cancer: An Update

A. Catharine Ross, Ph.D.

The results of additional research using case–control or intervention designs have been reported since the 1991 literature review. The results of these studies are generally highly consistent with those discussed above and, therefore, major changes in interpretation are not required. Of note, additional studies have supported the generalizations that dietary carotenoid intake is inversely related to smoking habit (Shibata et al., 1992b), that dietary carotenoid intake is positively associated with serum carotene concentrations (Jarvinen et al., 1993; Nierenberg et al., 1991) and that smoking (Jarvinen et al., 1993; Tanabe et al., 1992; Smith and Waller, 1991) and drinking (Tanabe et al., 1992) are associated with lower serum carotene levels, even after adjustment for dietary intake (Jarvinen et al., 1993; Tanabe et al., 1992; Nierenberg et al., 1991; Palan et al.,1991). Thus the constellation of cigarette smoking, alcohol consumption and diets low in the fruits and vegetables that contain carotenoids continues to be consistently and strongly associated with lower circulating carotenoid concentrations. The epidemiological literature concerning fruit and vegetable consumption in relationship to cancer prevention was reviewed by Block et al. (1992) who concluded that "For most cancer sites, persons with low fruit and vegetable intake (at least the lower one-fourth of the population) experience about twice the risk of cancer compared with those with high intake, even after control for potentially confounding factors."

Additional work has focused on the relationship of serum concentrations or dietary intake of carotenoids and other anti-oxidant micronutrients and the risk of cancer of the oral cavity, pharynx and lung. Zheng et al. (1993) reported a negative association between serum carotenoid concentrations, particularly ß-carotene, and the risk of oral and pharyngeal cancer in a case–control study in western Maryland. The results of a case–control study of squamous cell lung cancer in Japan supported a significant, inverse association between serum micronutrients (vitamins A, E, carotene and selenium), with the highest relative risk associated with the lowest tertile for any three or all four of these micronutrients (Tominaga et al., 1992). Likewise, Negri et al. (1992) inferred from a case–control study of esophageal cancer conducted in greater Milan that elimination of smoking, drinking and an increased consumption of fruits and vegetables would significantly reduce this disease in both men and women.

Additional studies of the case–control design (Huang et al., 1992) further support an inverse association of dietary β-carotene intake and the risk of lung cancer. However, further analysis (Shibata et al., 1992a) of the data from a California retirement community cohort reported earlier by Paganini-Hill et al. (1987) in which no evidence for significant protection was found, showed only a modest, nonsignificant, negative association between lung cancer and the intake of β-carotene from foods or supplements containing vitamins A, C and E. Serum β-carotene was low in patients already diagnosed with lung cancer and was lower in a control group consisting of family members of cases than in a control group of hospitalized patients without cancer (Smith and Waller, 1991). From a case–control study of 96 men with lung cancer, 75 men with other epithelial cancers and 97 hospital controls, Harris et al. (1991) calculated that the smoking-adjusted odds ratio was 0.67 for men in the middle tertile of carotene intake and 0.45 in the upper tertile as compared to men in the lowest tertile. These authors reported that the protective effect of

106

dietary carotene, estimated from intake during the year before the diagnosis of lung cancer, was stronger than that estimated from the total intake of vegetables and fruits rich in carotene.

The question of whether supplemental β-carotene can protect against oral cancer in individuals at high risk due to smoking or areca (betel) nut chewers has continued to be of interest. In an intervention study by van Poppel et al. (1993), supplementation with 20 mg/d of β-carotene reduced the microscopic evidence of DNA damage, namely the frequency of micronuclei in exfoliated cells of the oral cavity, in heavy smokers. Supplementation resulted in a 13-fold increase in serum β-carotene and a decrease of approximately 27 percent in the number of micronuclei in the treated group as compared to the placebo group at the end of the 14-week trial. The same investigators, however, did not observe a protective effect of β-carotene when sister chromatid exchange in lymphocytes was studied as the outcome variable to assess DNA damage (van Poppel et al., 1992). In a study of β-carotene as a treatment for oral leukoplakia, eight of 18 subjects with leukoplakia responded to treatment with 90 mg/d of β-carotene (Toma et al., 1992). Stich et al. (1991) reported a lower frequency of micronucleated mucosal cells and remission of leukoplakia in chewers of tobacco-containing betel quids who were treated with β-carotene (180 mg/wk), vitamin A (100,000 or 200,000 IU/wk), or the combination of β-carotene and 100,000 IU of vitamin A/wk over a 3- or 6-month period. However, discontinuation of treatment resulted in recurrence of micronucleated cells and leukoplakia in men who continued to chew.

Additional clinical intervention trials focusing on lung cancer or cancer of all sites are underway (Omenn et al.,1991). CARET (β-Carotene and Retinol Efficacy Trial), conducted in the Seattle area, is designed as a double-blind, randomized chemoprevention trial of the efficacy of β-carotene (30 mg/d) combined with retinyl palmitate (25,000 IU/d) to decrease the incidence of lung cancer in heavy smokers and workers exposed to asbestos who have smoked. The Harvard Physicians Study will assess the effect of β-carotene on overall cancer incidence in U.S. physicians, while the α-Tocopherol–β-Carotene Study will test the combination of β-carotene plus vitamin E in the chemoprevention of lung cancer in Finland. Results of these studies will not be available for several years. Although each study is expected to help address the question of whether β-carotene is effective in chemoprevention, the quantities of carotene used are well outside the dietary range and in two of these studies the effect of β-carotene will be confounded with that of supplemental retinol or α-tocopherol.

From the 1991 review of literature on cervical cancer, it was concluded that the results of recent studies of diet and cervical cancer provide little, if any, support for a protective role of β-carotene-rich foods. In a recent case–control study, de Vet et al. (1991) found no relationship between cervical dysplasia and the intake of retinol or vitamin C, but for β-carotene there was a significant increase in risk with increasing dietary intake. Palan et al. (1991) reported lower levels of β-carotene and α-tocopherol in women with histologically diagnosed cervical dysplasia or cancer. The concentration of these micronutrients correlated inversely with the histological grade of disease. Thus, even with new research concerning β-carotene's role in protection against this form of cancer, the literature still has not approached a consensus.

Overall, the conclusion that frequent consumption of fruits and vegetables reduces cancer risk remains highly consistent and strong. Whether this benefit results from the provision of β-carotene, other carotenoids, other anti-oxidant vitamins and/or minerals or other factors in fruits and vegetables remains unsettled. It is quite clear that serum levels of β-carotene are directly affected by the quantities of dietary or supplemental β-carotene that are consumed, although individual differences in response are significant. It is also clear that serum retinol concentration is not responsive to increased intakes of pro-vitamin A or preformed retinol within the range found in normal diets. Thus, the focus of research on carotenoids as compared to retinol is appropriate at this time. The clinical trials that are now underway may help to identify particular micronutrients that are able to provide protection from cancers of the oral cavity, lungs and other sites. The results of the large majority of studies are consistent with the prediction that the burden of cancer in the U.S. and abroad will be reduced significantly by behavioral modifications that include smoking cessation, moderation of alcohol consumption and a shift in dietary patterns to include frequent consumption of fruits and vegetables as part of a calorically balanced diet.

Bibliography

Block, G.; Patterson, B. and Subar, A. 1992. Fruit, vegetables, and cancer prevention: A review of the epidemiological evidence. *Nutr. Cancer* 18:1–29.

Harris, R.W.; Key, T.J.; Silcocks, P.B.; Bull, D. and Wald, N.J. 1991. A case–control study of dietary carotene in men with lung cancer and in men with other epithelial cancers. *Nutr. Cancer* 15:63–68.

Huang, C.; Xhang, X.; Quao, Z.; Guan, L.; Peng, S.; Liu, J. and Xie, R. 1992. A case–control study of dietary factors in patients with lung cancer. *Biomed. Environ. Sci.* 5:257–265.

Jarvinen, R.; Knekt, P.; Seppanen, R.; Heinonen, M. and Aaran, R.K. 1993. Dietary determinants of serum beta-carotene and serum retinol. *Eur. J. Clin. Nutr.* 47:31–41.

Negri, E.; La Vecchia, C.; Franceschi, S.; Decarli, A. and Bruzzi, P. 1992. Attributable risks for oesophageal cancer in northern Italy. *Eur. J. Cancer* 28A:1167–1171.

Nierenberg, D.W.; Stukel, T.A.; Baron, J.A.; Dain, B.J. and Greenberg, E.R. 1991. Determinants of increase in plasma concentration of beta-carotene after chronic oral supplementation. The skin cancer prevention study group. *Am. J. Clin. Nutr.* 53:1443–1449.

Omenn, G.S.; Goodman, G.; Grizzle, J.; Thornquist, M.; Rosenstock, L.; Barnhart, S.; Anderson, G.; Balmes, J.; Cherniack, M.; Cone, J.; et al. 1991. CARET, the beta-carotene and retinol efficacy trial to prevent lung cancer in asbestos-exposed workers and in smokers. *Anti-Cancer Drugs* 2:79–86.

Paganini-Hill, A.; Chao, A.; Ross, R.K. and Henderson, B.E. 1987. Vitamin A, β-carotene, and the risk of cancer: A prospective study. *J.N.C.I.* 79:443–448.

Palan, P.R.; Mikhail, M.S.; Basu, J. and Romney, S.L. 1991. Plasma levels of antioxidant beta-carotene and alpha-tocopherol in uterine cervix dysplasias and cancer. *Nutr. Cancer* 15:13–20.

van Poppel, G.; Kok, F.J.; Duijzings, P. and deVogel, N. 1992. No influence of beta-carotene on smoking-induced DNA damage as reflected by sister chromatid exchange. *Int. J. Cancer* 51:355–358.

van Poppel, G.; Kok, F.J. and Hermus, R.J. 1993. Beta-carotene supplementation in smokers reduces the frequency of micronuclei in sputum. *Br. J. Cancer* 66:1164–1168.

Shibata, A.; Paganini-Hill, A.; Ross, R.K. and Henderson, B.E. 1992a. Intake of vegetables, fruits, beta-carotene, vitamin C and vitamin supplements and cancer incidence among the elderly: A prospective study. *Br. J. Cancer* 66:673–679.

Shibata, A.; Paganini-Hill, A.; Ross, R.K. and Henderson, B.E. 1992b. Dietary beta-carotene, cigarette smoking, and lung cancer in men. *Cancer Causes Control* 3:207–214.

Smith, A.H. and Waller, K.D. 1991. Serum beta-carotene in persons with cancer and their immediate families. *Am. J. Epidemiol.* 133:661–671.

Stich, H.F.; Mathew, B.; Sankaranarayanan, R. and Nair, M.K. 1991. Remission of oral precancerous lesions of tobacco–areca nut chewers following administration of beta-carotene or vitamin A, and maintenance of the protective effect. *Cancer Detect. Prev.* 15:93–98.

Tanabe, N.; Toyoshima, H.; Hayashi, S.; Miyanishi, J.K.; Funazaki, T.; Obata, A.; Wakai, S.; Enoik, S.; Hashimoto, S. and Kamimura, K. 1992. Effects of smoking and drinking habits and vitamin A intake on serum concentrations of beta-carotene and retinol. *Jap. J. Hygiene* 47:679–687.

Toma, S.; Benso, S.; Albanese, E.; Palumbo, R.; Cantoni, E.; Nicolo, G. and Mangiante, P. 1992. Treatment of oral leukoplakia with beta-carotene. *Oncology* 49: 77–81.

Tominaga, K.; Saito, Y.; Mori, K.; Miyazawa, N.; Yokoi, K.; Koyama, Y.; Simamura, K.; Imura, J. and Nagai, M. 1992. An evaluation of serum microelement concentrations in lung cancer and matched non-cancer patients to determine the risk of developing lung cancer: A preliminary study. *Jap. J. Clin. Oncology* 22:96–101.

de Vet, H.C.; Knipschild, P.G.; Grol, M.E.; Schouten, H.J. and Sturmans, F. 1991. The role of beta-carotene and other dietary factors in the aetiology of cervical dysplasia: Results of a case–control study. *Int. J. Epidem.* 20:603–610.

Zheng, W.; Blot, W.J.; Diamond, E.L.; Norkus, E.P.; Spate, V.; Morris, J.S. and Comstock, G.W. 1993. Serum micronutrients and the subsequent risk of oral and pharyngeal cancer. *Cancer Res.* 53:795–798.

Chapter 3

Vitamin C and Cancer

Howerde E. Sauberlich, Ph.D.

I. Introduction

This evaluation of the relationship of vitamin C with cancer will review reports of human studies published since 1987. Occasional reference will be made to those reviews that have considered the vitamin C and cancer literature prior to 1988 (Block and Menkes, 1989; Stähelin et al., 1987, 1989; Ziegler, 1986). The rationale for the 1988 cutoff was that information prior to 1988 on vitamin C and cancer was considered in the following benchmark references: *The Surgeon General's Report on Nutrition and Health* (U.S. Department of Health and Human Services, 1988); *Diet and Health: Implications for Reducing Chronic Disease Risk* (National Research Council, 1989a); *Recommended Dietary Allowances*, 10th ed., (National Research Council, 1989b), *Nutrition and Your Health: Dietary Guidelines for Americans* (U.S. Department of Agriculture and U.S. Department of Health and Human Services, 1990), *Healthy People 2000: National Health Promotion and Disease Prevention Objectives* (U.S. Department of Health and Human Services, 1991).

A. Benchmark Conclusions

In 1988, a report of the Surgeon General (U.S. Department of Health and Human Services, 1988) concluded that human studies did show a protective association between foods containing vitamin C and cancers of the esophagus, stomach, and cervix. However, while many studies supported a role of vitamin C in reducing risk of various cancers, no wholly consistent view of the role of vitamin C in human cancers had been defined at that time. The National Research Council's Diet and Health report (1989a) concluded that epidemiological studies did suggest vitamin C-containing foods such as citrus fruits and vegetables may offer protection against stomach cancer, the evidence linking vitamin C or foods containing vitamin C with other cancers was more limited and less consistent. However, the report did note that animal investigations had shown protective effects of vitamin C against nitrosamine-induced stomach cancer. The Diet and Health report (National Research Council, 1989a) also pointed out that the association of vitamin C and various cancers was indirect, in that evidence was primarily from epidemiological studies concerning foods known to contain high or low levels of vitamin C rather than measured levels of vitamin C intake.

The Report of the Dietary Guidelines Advisory Committee on the Dietary Guidelines for Americans (U.S. Department of Health and Human Services, 1990) has provided two guidelines to ensure receiving the Recommended Dietary Allowances (RDA) for vitamin C: (a) eat a variety of foods and (b) choose a diet with plenty of vegetables, fruits, and grain products. Although comments were provided regarding diet and hypertension, heart disease, diabetes, and obesity, only a passing mention was given to cancer and diet in the context of fat intake.

Attainment of the RDA for vitamin C of 60 mg/d for adults can be readily accomplished with a diet containing fresh fruits, vegetables, and citrus juice (e.g., cooked fresh broccoli, peppers, Brussels sprouts, carrots, orange juice, strawberries, tomato, cantaloupe, etc.) (Block and Sorenson, 1987). Intakes of 100–200 mg of vitamin C are commonly observed in dietary intake surveys. However, inadequate intakes often due to poor food choices or specific food aversions are also frequently encountered. The Joint Nutrition Monitoring and Evaluation Committee expressed concern about the adequacy of vitamin C, among other nutrients, in the diets of many Americans (Block, 1991b; Patterson et al., 1990). The NHANES II survey, using 24-hour dietary recall data, estimated that 45 percent of the population had no servings of fruit or juice, and 22 percent had no servings of a vegetable on the recall day (Patterson et al., 1990).

B. Vitamin C: Metabolism

Vitamin C present in foods appears to be readily available and absorbed (Sauberlich, 1985). Intakes up to 100 mg/d of ascorbic acid are 80 to 90 percent absorbed by an active transport system. However, with intakes above 500 mg, efficiency of absorption of the vitamin rapidly declines. Vitamin C is metabolized to oxalate, 2,3-diketogulonic acid, and several other known metabolites which are excreted in the urine. Excess intakes of the vitamin are excreted unchanged.

Intakes of ascorbic acid of up to 1 g/d are well tolerated (Rivers, 1989). Occasionally, intakes above this may be associated with nausea and diarrhea. However, intakes of 4 g/d of ascorbic acid were used in a long-term intervention trial on rectal polyps without adverse effects. Ingestion of high doses of vitamin C should probably be avoided by patients on anticoagulant therapy, with renal impairment, recurrent renal stone formation, or disposed to chronic hemochromatosis.

The average adult has a body pool of vitamin C of 1.2–2.0 g that may be maintained with 75 mg/d of ascorbic acid. Approximately 140 mg/d of ascorbic acid will saturate the total body pool of vitamin C (Sauberlich, 1990). The vitamin is widely distributed throughout the body with concentrations ranging considerably among tissues. The highest concentrations are in the pituitary gland, leukocytes, liver, and brain. The major portion of the body vitamin C pool is located in the skeletal muscle, liver, and brain (Sauberlich, 1990).

C. Vitamin C: Functions

Although the essentiality of vitamin C for humans to prevent scurvy has long been recognized, the biochemical functions of the vitamin have been not been fully elucidated. It is now recognized that the vitamin has diverse roles in the body besides its role in collagen synthesis. Various dioxygenases and monooxygenases are stimulated by ascorbic acid. Thus, for example, collagen synthesis is dependent upon the action of prolyl-4-hydroxylase, prolyl-3-hydroxylase, and lysyl hydroxylase.

A prime function of vitamin C is that of an antioxidant (Padh, 1991). As an antioxidant, vitamin C can also serve as an effective free-radical scavenger to protect cells from damage by oxidants. It is in this capacity that vitamin C may provide protection against the influence of potential carcinogens. Vitamin C can inhibit nitrosation, particularly in the stomach, and thereby can serve as a blocking agent for the formation of potentially carcinogenic N-nitroso compounds (Schorah et al., 1991; Sobala et al., 1991; Tannenbaum, 1991). Hence, vitamin C could have a protective role against stomach cancer. The vitamin appears to be excreted into the gastric lumen which may enhance its protective capability. Overall, it has been suggested that vitamin C plays a role in maintaining the integrity of the intracellular matrix and enhancement of the immune system.

II. Issues in Study Selection and Interpretation

A. Inclusion Criteria

The cancer studies included in this report were restricted primarily to case–control and prospective studies published since 1987. As seen in the Appendix Table, the studies reviewed were presented by cancer site which included breast, head and neck, lung, stomach, pancreas, colon and rectum, prostate, cervix, and bladder. Studies not designed specifically to investigate the association between vitamin C and cancer but which contained sufficient information relevant to this issue were included in the review. Human cancer studies that did not contain vitamin C-related data were omitted from this report.

The studies selected contained a component on diet or on dietary intake of specific nutrients (occasionally including non-nutrients) and an association with a form of cancer. The studies considered had a substantial number of subjects that could provide meaningful information for application to a larger population. Single case-type reports were not considered. Foreign studies and reports on ethnic or racial populations were included to indicate the possible effects of different cultural practices, environments, and dietary habits on the occurrence of cancer.

The cancer cases had to be properly diagnosed and matched with appropriate controls. Unfortunately, only a few studies reported on biochemical parameters associated with vitamin C that could be utilized to establish nutritional status and nutrient intakes of the vitamin. Studies with detailed dietary intake data derived from extensive food-frequency questionnaires containing specific food-intake habits, food frequency, and accurate portion size estimations were emphasized; however, it was necessary to consider studies that provided only general data on dietary habits based on the frequency of consumption of selected food groups (e.g., citrus fruits, fruit juices, vegetables, etc.). In some instances, only frequency of consumption of selected food groups was reported. Studies in which the data collected could not supply an accurate estimate of the intake of individual nutrients, such as vitamin C or carotene, were of limited use and provided only putative unsubstantiated evidence of an association.

B. Types of Studies Reviewed

Investigations of the possible relationship between diet and the etiology of cancer have used (a) correlational studies, (b) case–control studies, (c) prospective cohort studies, and (d) intervention trials (Vogel and McPherson, 1989). Each of these approaches has weaknesses or limitations.

Descriptive and correlational studies are useful for generation of hypotheses that may be examined with intervention trials; however, they provide little direct evidence as to the existence of an etiologic relationship between a particular dietary component, such as vitamin C, and the occurrence of cancer. Case–control studies are limited in their ability to obtain accurate dietary intake data by the reliance on retrospective food-frequency questionnaires and interviews. In many cases, the reference period for the dietary data collection extends over a long period of time. Yet, despite investigators' attempts to define reference periods that are relevant to the events associated with the initiation of the cancer, those events may be associated with the diet consumed over 10 years before the onset of the disease.

The validity of prospective cohort studies and intervention trials depends on a subject pool with a wide range of nutrient intakes (e.g., vitamin C). An association between an individual nutrient and cancer risk may not be discernible when there is relative homogeneity of the diets of the population studied. Thus, if the vitamin C intake and status

114   Howerde E. Sauberlich

were excellent, any protective effect of this vitamin on cancer would not be seen. Similarly, if the vitamin C status was universally poor, no protective effect would be identified. This latter population could be appropriate for an intervention trial. Intervention trials are further hampered by problems of noncompliance and with changes in dietary habits and practices that might occur during the study. Additional concerns about prospective studies and intervention trials are expense and time required.

C. Methodological Considerations

Each study included in this report was evaluated as to adequacy of experimental design. Particular consideration was given to the length of study, adequacy of sample size, use of suitable controls, and appropriateness of methodology. Since the majority of the studies considered were case–control investigations, of particular concern were the adequacy and reliability of the dietary intake information (Hartman, 1990; Mertz, 1991; National Research Council, 1981). Unfortunately, a number of the studies reviewed had inadequate dietary intake information so that only qualified evaluations were possible.

Many of the studies reviewed were not designed to investigate vitamin C per se, but were an attempt to obtain information on general food intakes or frequency of intakes of selected representative food items or food groups. For some studies, vitamin C intakes were estimated from recorded portions of individual foods and adjusted for portion sizes. The adequacy of dietary intake data is dependent on the extensiveness and appropriateness of the items on the food-frequency questionnaire. Unfortunately, even when data are obtained with the use of extended diet records, food intakes may be over- or underestimated (Hartman et al., 1990; Mertz et al., 1991; National Research Council, 1981).

Additional concerns in the assessment of nutrient intakes, especially in studies that rely on retrospective data, are changing food consumption patterns and modifications in the availability of specific food items. For example, for the U.S. adult population, the consumption of 15 food items accounted for over 80 percent of the vitamin C consumed in the diet (Block and Sorenson, 1987). In fact, six food items contributed 60 percent of the vitamin C in the diet. Orange juice alone provided approximately 25 percent of the vitamin C in the diet. However, among the lower income populations, vitamin C intake patterns were considerably lower. Consequently, demographics, cultural practices, and seasonal variations in food availability were considered as important variables to be considered in the evaluation of these studies.

Dietary intake data provide no direct measurement of nutritional status or status for a given nutrient. However, poor food intakes may provide presumptive evidence of poor nutritional status. The reverse may be true if the nutrient intakes meet certain dietary criteria. However, factors seldom considered in the collection of dietary intake data include such confounding factors as nutrient interactions, bioavailability of nutrients, individual differences in nutrient requirements, or changing food usage and patterns with time. Hence, considerable caution needs to be used in the interpretation of dietary intake data.

Frequently, other nutrients, such as carotenoids and folate, are obtained from the same foods that provide vitamin C. With only dietary data, one cannot be entirely certain that an observed protective effect was due to vitamin C alone or to a combination of factors. Vitamin C and vitamin E have been postulated to counteract, simultaneously, tumor initiation and promotion through their synergistic properties against lipid peroxidation (Sies, 1989; Stähelin, 1987). In this context, vitamin E protects the lipid-soluble phase, and vitamin C interacts at the interface and in the water-soluble compartments.

An important consideration in drawing conclusions about the vitamin C and cancer relationship was the weight of evidence supplied by the number of studies conducted which focused on a specific type of cancer. Factors considered included consistency of findings among numerous studies of the same organ, the direction and strength of the effect, the generalizability of the effects across ethnic and racial groups, cultures, locations, and how the effects were reported (e.g., relative risks, odds ratios or correlations) and their significance.

Some reports were weakened by the limited amount of dietary information provided or by the methodology employed. Greater emphasis and reliance were placed on those epidemiology studies that made a concerted effort to obtain adequate and reliable dietary intake information, particularly with respect to vitamin C and associated nutrients (e.g., β-carotene, retinol, vitamin E). Whether or not statistical adjustments were made for such potentially confounding variables as occupation, smoking, alcohol use, age, sex, and demographic histories also influenced the interpretation and validity of the studies reviewed.

The general nutritional status of the population pool from which cases and controls were drawn was considered in weighting the evidence from a given study. In those populations that are well-supplied with vitamin C, any protective effect against cancer would already have occurred and thus any impact of the vitamin on a cancer would be masked (Block and Sorenson, 1987); however, the reverse could be true in a population with a marginal vitamin C status. Thus, if a high-risk population was studied where the subject pool may have a very low intake of vitamin C, negative results may be observed that cannot be interpreted with respect to a protective effect of ascorbic acid. Conversely, if all of the cases and controls were highly nourished with respect to vitamin C, the effect of "low" levels of vitamin C may not reveal an increased risk. The low levels under these conditions may have already provided optimum protection. Unfortunately, biochemical information, such as plasma ascorbate concentrations, was seldom available to provide a more direct confirmation of the vitamin C nutritional status. A greater emphasis was placed on those reports where biochemical data were available.

Intervention trials with vitamin C could have provided definitive information as to the protective effects of the vitamin on cancer risk. Unfortunately, only two small intervention trials, with design deficiencies, were reported during the review time period.

III. Vitamin C and Human Cancer

A. Breast Cancer

While both epidemiological and animal studies have suggested an association of high fat intake with increased risk of breast cancer (Willett, 1989), there was no evidence noted from these studies of a link between vitamin C and breast cancer. Toniolo et al. (1989), for instance, compared 250 cases of women with breast cancer with 499 community-based control women in Vercelli, Italy. Nutrient intakes were calculated from information obtained from a dietary questionnaire modified to include foods indigenous to that section of Italy. The study revealed no evidence of an association of vitamin C intake with breast cancer. However, a reduced risk of breast cancer was associated with a reduced consumption of fat, particularly of animal fat and saturated fat.

In a case–control study from Athens, Greece, Katsouyanni et al. (1988) compared 118 patients with histologically confirmed breast cancer to 115 hospital-based control patients with orthopedic disorders selected from a different hospital. Over a period of 12 months, all subjects completed a 120-item food-frequency questionnaire referenced to the period prior to the onset of their diseases. The calculated mean intakes of vitamin C were similar for both cases and controls (133 mg and 138 mg/d, respectively). No evidence was found of an association between vitamin C intake and the incidence of breast cancer. When adjusted for calorie intake, an increased intake of vitamin A was associated with a decreased risk of breast cancer. The study had weaknesses in the nutrient intake procedures and in the appropriateness of the controls used.

Recently, Howe and collaborators (1990) performed a meta-analysis of 12 case–control studies of diet and breast cancer. Original individual data records for all studies were used. Nine of the studies provided data on vitamin C. Overall, these studies were conducted in populations with very different breast cancer risks and dietary habits. The only U.S. population included in the analysis was a comparison of Japanese Hawaiians (183 cases, 183 population controls, 183 hospital controls) with a group of white Hawaiians (161 cases, 161 population controls, 161 hospital controls).

The meta-analysis, which included a total of 4437 cases of breast cancer, 4341 population controls, and 1754 hospital controls, demonstrated a consistent protective effect for a number of markers of fruit and vegetable intake. Of importance was the observation that vitamin C intake had the most consistent and statistically significant inverse association with breast cancer risk (RR = 0.69, for highest versus lowest quintile of vitamin C intake; $p < 0.0001$). The highest quintile represented an intake of 300 mg/d of vitamin C. Although the effects were less than that observed for vitamin C, dietary fiber and β-carotene also showed an inverse relationship with risk. In contrast, an increase in intake of saturated fat was associated with a significant increase in the risk for breast cancer (RR = 1.00 to 1.46; $p = 0.0002$ for trend). The findings of Howe et al. (1990) emphasize the need for further investigation of the role of diet in the control of breast cancer.

B. Esophageal and Oral Cancers

Rates of esophageal cancer vary more than 500-fold among countries, with particularly high rates in males in parts of Africa, Asia, Iran, and the Soviet Union (Ghadirian et al., 1988). Esophageal cancer has been found to be strongly associated with the consumption of alcohol and the use of tobacco and is more likely to occur in males than females. Several reviews have examined earlier (pre-1987) studies on the relationship of diet with oral cancer (Block, 1991a; Block and Menkes, 1989).

Brown et al. (1988) investigated the problem in South Carolina where the incidence of esophageal cancer among the black male population is markedly above the national rates. In this case–control study 207 cases of esophageal cancer (159 black, 48 white) and 422 control subjects (324 black, 98 white) were interviewed. All subjects were from eight coastal counties of South Carolina. The study consisted of two components. One part was a hospital-based incidence study that enrolled patients during the period of 1982–1984. The second part was a next-of-kin mortality study that covered deaths from esophageal cancer during 1977–1981. For the incident study, two control patients per case were identified through admission records at the same hospital in the same time period. The controls were similar to the patients with respect to age and race. For the mortality study, two control subjects for each case were selected that were matched for race, age, county of residence, and year of death. Healthy population-based controls were not used in either phase. The 65-item dietary questionnaire used placed an emphasis on citrus fruits and juices (oranges, grapefruit, orange juice, grapefruit juice, and lemonade).

Tobacco and alcohol were found to be major determinants of esophageal cancer risk. However, the dietary questionnaire information indicated that increased risk also existed with a low intake of fresh fruits. After adjustment for smoking and drinking, the odds ratio (OR) for vitamin C for subjects with the highest intake was approximately one-half the OR for subjects with the lowest intake ($p < 0.01$ for trend). A similar effect was observed in subjects with the highest intakes of fiber. Approximately a twofold increase in risk was seen for subjects with the highest intakes of retinol compared with the lowest intake of the vitamin (primarily related to intakes of liver). The frequency of intake of vegetables and of β-carotene-rich fruits was not significantly associated with esophageal cancer risk.

Esophageal cancer is considered the second leading cause of death from cancer in China. Li et al. (1989) conducted a case–control study in Linxian, a rural county in north central China with an exceedingly high mortality rate from esophageal cancer. The study involved interviews with 758 male and 486 female cases of esophageal cancer and 1314 population-based controls (789 males, 525 females). Dietary information was obtained with the use of questionnaires administered by trained interviewers. Seventy-two food items common to the Linxian diet were included in the questionnaire.

The results indicated little or no association with fresh fruit consumption. However, the overall consumption of fresh fruits was low. Seventy-seven percent of the esophageal cancer patients and controls either never consumed fresh fruits or consumed them fewer than 35 times per year. Even the highest quartile of intake of fresh fruits appeared unsatisfactory to meet accepted criteria of an adequate diet. Of note, a high percentage of the Linxian population had deficiencies of many vitamins, including vitamin C. Despite the large patient population studied, the cause of the high incidence of esophageal cancer in Linxian remains undetermined. It may relate to unknown environmental factors or a genetic component.

Subsequently, Guo et al. (1990) reported on a broader study of diet and esophageal cancer mortality that was based on a 65-county nutrition survey conducted in the fall of 1983 in China. The counties were selected on the basis of their observed cancer mortality rates. Within this population, annual cumulative mortality rates from esophageal cancer ranged from 0.4 to 153 per 1000 population among the males and 0 to 99.8 per 1000 among the females. From each county, 100 persons were selected with a balance in age and sex. Each person was administered a food-frequency questionnaire that provided information on intakes of fruits, green vegetables, moldy pickled vegetables, other foods, alcohol, and smoking. Blood specimens were obtained for the measurement of plasma vitamin C, retinol, β-carotene, α-tocopherol, and other nutrients.

Data analysis revealed that the esophageal cancer mortality rates between counties had a strong inverse association with plasma vitamin C and fruit consumption in both sexes. The standardized regression coefficients between county esophageal cancer mortality rates and vitamin C were –0.36 for males and –0.31 for females. Correlations between esophageal cancer mortality and fruit intake were –0.37 for males and –0.37 for females. Esophageal cancer mortality rates were 3.3 times (males) and 2.6 times (females) higher in counties with the lowest plasma vitamin C levels when compared with the highest quartile levels. Mean plasma concentrations of ascorbic acid by quartile were 0.53, 0.84, 1.17, and 1.63 mg/dL among males and 0.68, 1.07, 1.38, and 1.95 mg/dL among females. These plasma levels of ascorbic acid appear unusually high in view of the low frequency of fruit intake. Cross-classification of the cancer rates by vitamin C level and fruit intake revealed separate effects.

Although the study suggests that low levels of intake of vitamin C and fruit may be involved in an increased risk of esophageal cancer, other factors may be involved as well. Included are the intakes of moldy pickled vegetables, wheat consumption, low intakes of selenium, riboflavin, and fluids. Information was not available on the dietary practices or other environmental factors possibly affecting individual esophageal cancer patients. No case–control comparisons were reported.

Tuyns et al. (1987a) reported on a case–control study conducted in the Calvados region of France where a high mortality rate for esophageal cancer occurs among the male population. The study considered 704 male and 39 female cases of esophageal cancer compared with a control group of 922 males and 1053 females from the same region.

The results presented related primarily to the males studied. From a 40-item diet questionnaire, the frequency of consumption per week of each item and an estimate of the portion size were obtained. The daily intakes of nutrients were computed from these data with the use of food composition tables. For each nutrient, relative risks were derived for heavy and moderate consumers versus light consumers. Adjustments were made for alcohol and tobacco use, age, and residential area.

High intakes of several vitamins, as calculated, were associated with a reduction of risk of esophageal cancer. The relative risks were significantly lower with high intakes of vitamins C, E, and niacin. However, high intakes of retinol were associated with an increased risk, while carotene decreased the risk. In view of the possible errors in the estimation of retinol intakes, the investigators suggested that the risk associated with retinol should be disregarded. Use of vegetable oils decreased the risk while butter increased the risk.

High intakes of citrus fruits and vegetables were associated with a reduced risk. While citrus fruits serve as a rich source of vitamin C, they provide little carotene or vitamin E. The protective effect of vegetable oils may have been associated with their significant vitamin E content. Although certain foods appeared to provide protective effects against esophageal cancer, high alcohol consumption is largely responsible for the high frequency of this cancer in the Calvados area of France.

Incidence rates for oral cancer are high in certain areas of the world, such as in parts of India and France and metropolitan areas of Brazil. Franco et al. (1989) conducted a case–control study of potential risk factors for oral cancer in Brazil. Dietary information, as well as health and demographic characteristics were obtained from interviews with 232 cases of oral cancer and 464 hospital-based controls. The dietary habits were based on past consumption frequency for only 20 food items.

Of the factors studied, tobacco use and alcohol consumption were the strongest risk factors. However, a decrease in risk was observed with the more frequent use of citrus fruits (adjusted RR = 0.5; p = 0.03). Although it was not possible to calculate vitamin C intakes in this study, the protective effect may have been a reflection of intake of this vitamin. Reductions in risk were also associated with more frequent consumption of carotene-rich foods, such as carrots, papaya, and pumpkins. The association was of less strength than that observed for citrus fruits (smoking and alcohol adjusted associations: p = 0.06 for carotene vs p = 0.03 for citrus fruits).

In the study by McLaughlin et al. (1988), 871 pathologically confirmed cases of oral and pharyngeal cancer were ascertained from the population-based cancer registries of New Jersey; Atlanta, Georgia; and the Santa Clara, San Mateo, and Los Angeles counties of California. The 979 population-based controls were selected in an age- and sex-stratified manner. All subjects were white. A 61-item food- frequency questionnaire was used to determine dietary habits with specific reference to foods that were sources of vitamins C and A and carotene. Fruit and vegetable intakes were adjusted for seasonal variations. Information was obtained on vitamin supplement use, but their use did not affect the results.

These investigators observed a strong protective effect for citrus fruits and vitamin C from fruits on the incidence of oral cancer (OR = 0.5; p = 0.001 for trend). The decreased risk occurred in both men and women. A comparable protective effect was also obtained from the carotene and fiber derived from the fruits consumed. Vitamin C, carotene, and fiber derived from the vegetables consumed provided little protective effect on oral cancer. This suggested to the investigators that additional components present in fruits may contribute to the reduced risk of oral cancer. Phenols, aromatic isothiocyanates, flavones, and other non-nutritive compounds were suggested as possible contributing factors present in fruits. However, since McLauglin et al. (1988) did not report on the mean or median intakes for any of the vitamins, no comparison can be made between the level of intake of vitamin C and carotene provided by the fruits and the amounts provided by the vegetables. In general, vegetables are not the major contributors of vitamin C to the diet. Furthermore, the absence of biochemical confirmation of vitamin status renders any conclusions about vitamin C presumptive.

C. Lung Cancer

Earlier epidemiologic studies of the relationship between vitamins and lung cancer reviewed by Ziegler (1986) and Fontham (1990) found no association between vitamin C or fruit intake and the risk of lung cancer.

Byers et al. (1987) compared 450 Caucasian lung cancer cases (296 males and 154 females) diagnosed between August 1980 and July 1984, with 902 race-, sex-, and residentially-matched controls (587 males and 315 females) from three western New York counties. All subjects were given a standardized interview of approximately 2.5 hours duration designed to obtain information on occupation; tobacco, drug, and alcohol use; oral health; and medical and dietary history. The interviews for both the cases and controls were conducted between August 1980 and August 1984.

The dietary history used a 129-item food-frequency questionnaire to determine average frequency of consumption and portion size. Nutrient supplements were included. The reference period for the cases was the year before the onset of symptoms of the lung cancer, while the controls reported on their dietary habits up to the time of the interview. The dietary focus was on total vitamin A, vitamin A from fruit and vegetable sources, vitamin C, vitamin E, calories, fat, cholesterol, protein, and dietary fiber. Vitamin A and carotene intakes were calculated from food composition tables. Case–control comparisons were made on quartiles for the nutrient intakes with relative risks computed for each quartile. No biochemical assessments were performed.

No protective effect was observed between dietary vitamin C (estimated intakes) and lung cancer. Similarly, no association was observed between lung cancer and retinol intakes (vitamin A from animal sources). However, an inverse association was found between lung cancer and carotene intakes (calculated from fruit and vegetable intakes). The strongest protective association of carotene was with the squamous cell carcinoma cases, with a weaker association with adenocarcinoma cases. The greatest effect of carotene on lung cancers was for those over 60 years of age. For this group, the relative risk with the lowest quartile of carotene intake was 3.1 for men and 2.0 for women. The greatest reduction in risk was apparent in those individuals who never smoked or were ex-smokers (quit for > 3 yrs). No data were presented as to a quantitative estimate of the intakes of vitamin C, carotene, or other nutrients. Thus, the level of intake of nutrients that may provide a protective effect cannot be computed. It was noted that risk estimates were not substantially affected by the addition of supplements to the nutrient indices.

In 1988, Fontham et al. conducted a hospital-based incidence case–control study of lung cancer over a period of 28 months in a high-risk region of southern Louisiana. The controls were subjects admitted to the same hospitals and matched by race, sex, and age within 5 years. Dietary intakes of vitamin C, carotene, and retinol were estimated from food-frequency questionnaires administered to 1253 cases and 1274 controls. The questionnaire provided information on the frequency of consumption of each of the 59 food items on a monthly basis before the onset of illness or symptoms. Additional information was obtained on the use of tobacco, occupation, residence, and medical history. Indices for vitamin C, carotene, and retinol intake were created by summing the frequency of consumption of each of the food items multiplied by the median nutrient content of a typical serving. The nutrient indices were stratified into tertiles. The upper tertile consumed 150 mg of vitamin C per day, while the lower tertile consumed less than 90 mg per day.

Although an inverse association was found between the level of carotene intake and lung cancer (squamous and small cell carcinomas), a stronger protective effect for these tumors was associated with dietary vitamin C intake. An odds ratio of 0.65 (confidence interval 0.50–0.87, for highest vitamin C intake) was reported. Fruit consumption adjusted for vegetable intake remained a protective factor for all lung cancers combined. No protective effects of carotene or vitamin C were observed for adenocarcinoma. However, an inverse relationship between dietary retinol and adenocarcinoma was observed, particularly for the black males. The investigators suggest that the protective effect associated with vitamin C may be expressed only in populations with a relatively low intake of the vitamin as apparently occurs in the Louisiana population studied. Fontham (1990) recently reviewed epidemiological studies on the effects of dietary components on lung cancer risk. The majority of these studies focused on the protective effects of retinol and β-carotene.

It should be noted that only 51 of the cases never smoked compared to 388 of the controls. The majority of the cases were current smokers. Although not considered, the intakes of vitamin C by the hospital controls may not reflect the intakes of the general population. Blood levels of vitamin C would have given more information about adequacy of the intakes of the vitamin and the impact of smoking on vitamin C levels and the relationship between these levels and cancer risk.

Koo (1988) conducted a retrospective study in which 88 lung cancer patients and 137 matched controls were interviewed concerning the effect of diet on lung cancer risk among Chinese women from Hong Kong who never smoked. The diet information was obtained by food-frequency inquiry. The cases provided information on their usual food habits one year before the diagnosis of cancer, while the controls provided information on their current eating habits. The assessment focused on the consumption patterns of broad groups or types of foods in order to accommodate Chinese cooking habits.

A higher consumption of leafy green vegetables, carrots, fresh fruits, tofu, and fresh fish was inversely associated with development of adenocarcinoma and large cell tumors. Of the dietary components investigated, only the consumption of fresh fruit showed a negative relationship against squamous or small cell tumors. The protective effect was reflected in a relative risk of 0.42 (trend p = 0.014). Sources of vitamin C also conferred some protection against adenocarcinomas. No quantitative information was provided regarding the intakes of vitamin C. Any protective effects on vitamin C must be considered presumptive.

Le Marchand et al. (1989) investigated the effect of vegetable consumption on lung cancer risk in a Hawaiian population. Interviews were conducted on 230 men and 102 women with lung cancer and 597 men and 268 women as controls. The cases were identified by the Hawaii Tumor Registry and had been diagnosed during the period of March 1983 and September 30, 1985. Difficulties occurred in obtaining suitable controls that resulted in an imbalance in the ethnic composition of the study groups. Age, sex, smoking, alcohol consumption, and occupation were factors considered in the conduct of the study. A quantitative dietary history using a 130-item food-frequency questionnaire was completed to assess the usual intake of foods rich in vitamins C and A and carotenoids. The interviews were conducted at home with the subject or a surrogate.

Total vitamin C (from food sources and supplements) was inversely associated with lung cancer risk among males only. A reverse effect was observed for Caucasian women. The investigators considered the results an aberration and did not explore them further. No biochemical data were available on plasma levels of vitamin C that could have been used to explore the relationship of the vitamin and smoking to lung cancer risk. A significant negative association between dietary β-carotene and lung cancer was observed in males only. However, all vegetables, dark green vegetables, cruciferous vegetables, and tomatoes were found to have a stronger inverse association with risk than β-carotene.

LeGardeur et al. (1990) measured serum vitamins C, A (retinol), E, and carotenoids in 59 cases of newly diagnosed lung cancer, 59 matched hospital controls, and 31 community-based controls. Information on smoking habits and dietary intakes was obtained from the lung cancer cases and the hospitalized controls but not the non-institutionalized subjects.

Serum levels of vitamin C were significantly lower in the lung cancer patients when compared to the hospital controls (0.41 + 0.04 mg/dL vs 0.59 + 0.06 mg/dL; p = 0.014). Correcting for smoking may have eliminated these differences. However, the investigators did not comment on these findings. Their emphasis was placed on the observed lower serum levels of vitamin E and carotenoids found in the lung cancer patients. This study had serious problems in design and analysis that are noted in Appendix Table 3.

D. Gastric Cancer

Because ascorbic acid can function as a free radical scavenger and can block the formation of nitrosamines in the stomach, various studies have investigated the possible role of vitamin C or dietary sources of the vitamin in stomach cancer (Leaf et al., 1987; Stähelin et al., 1987). Many of these studies have been reviewed by Block (1991a) and Block and Menkes (1989). Recently, additional studies have examined the relationship between ascorbic acid's interference in the formation of *N*-nitroso compounds and their by-products and the occurrence of stomach cancer (Schorah et al., 1991; Sobala, 1991). This is the only case of a plausible explanation of the protective effect of vitamin C for a specific cancer type.

You et al. (1988) interviewed 564 diagnosed stomach cancer patients and 1131 population-based controls in Linqu, a rural county in Shandong Province in northeast China. This area has an exceptionally high rate of stomach cancer. A structured questionnaire was used that provided information on dietary habits and on the frequency of consumption and portion size of 85 food items that had been eaten several years before the start of the investigation.

The findings indicate that dietary factors contribute, but only partially, to the high rates of stomach cancer in this population. Increased intakes of fresh fruits and total fresh vegetables reduced the risk of stomach cancer (OR = 0.5–0.6). Increased intakes of vitamin C (estimated) also conferred a protective effect (OR = 0.5; 95 percent confidence interval = 0.3–0.6). Increased intakes of carotene were also associated with a protective effect on stomach cancer. The effect of vitamin C was independent of the carotene effect. However, the study suggests a complex of dietary variables which may relate to the high rates of stomach cancer in this area of China.

Japan continues to have a high incidence of stomach cancer. Kono et al. (1988) conducted a case–control study of stomach cancer and diet in northern Kyushu, Japan, during the period of 1979 to 1982. The study involved 139 cases of newly diagnosed stomach cancer at a single institute, 2574 hospital controls, and 278 controls from the area. A questionnaire was employed that provided information on dietary habits and on the frequency of consumption of food items. Analysis of the data revealed a protective effect against stomach cancer with increased frequency of consumption of fruits, mandarin oranges, and green tea (an important source of vitamin C in the Japanese diet). The relative risk of stomach cancer with the upper tertile frequency of consumption of these food items ranged from 0.4 to 0.6 (p < 0.05). Because of the design of the study, vitamin C intakes were not estimated. Although a role for vitamin C is suggested, it must be considered presumptive as the study focused on food groups and could not estimate intakes of individual nutrients.

Buiatti et al. (1989) conducted a case–control study in areas of Italy with either a high or low risk for stomach cancer. The study involved 1016 histologically confirmed stomach cancer cases and 1159 population controls. Dietary patterns were obtained with the use of a structured 146-item food-frequency questionnaire. Consistent throughout the several areas of Italy studied was the decreased risk of stomach cancer with increasing consumption of citrus fruits, other fresh fruits, and raw vegetables. Relative risks for the highest tertile of consumption for these food groups ranged from 0.4 to 0.6 (p = 0.001 for trend). The protective effect of fresh fruits appeared to be at least partially independent of the effect of raw vegetables. High consumption of both food groups resulted in a relative risk of 0.3. Hence, a participation of vitamin C in the protective effect was suggested.

Data from this study were also used to examine a possible relationship between diet and stomach cancer (Buiatti et al., 1990). Estimates of intake of individual nutrients were calculated from the food-frequency data. The results suggested that the lowered risk associated with increasing intake of fresh fruits, fresh vegetables, and olive oil may result from the vitamin C and vitamin E present in these items. Notably, the most significant effect was the geographical gradient in vitamin C intake; the highest consumption was found in the areas with lowest risk. Estimates of the intake of nitrates and nitrites were calculated for the several geographic areas studied. The results indicated an increasing relative risk of stomach cancer with an increasing consumption of nitrites and protein. The risk decreased with increased intakes of ascorbic acid and α-tocopherol both for male and female subjects.

In a similar study, Boeing and Frentzel-Beyme (1991) investigated risk factors for stomach cancer in high- and low-risk areas of Germany. In this case–control study conducted during 1985–1987, 143 cases and 579 hospital- and community-based controls from three high-risk regions and one low-risk region were interviewed about sociodemographic characteristics, occupation, medical and smoking histories, water supply, food conservation methods, and intake of food for the 5 years prior to the onset of their disease.

Risk of stomach cancer was associated with several factors including: vitamin C intake, type of water supply, type of wood used for smoking meats, and years of refrigerator use. When compared with a central water supply, the use of well water was associated with an increased risk of stomach cancer (relative risk = 2.17). Although not assessed, this risk may have been the consequence of nitrate in the well water. Use of spruce wood rather than other types for smoking meats was also associated with increased risk (relative risk = 3.32). Long-term availability of a home refrigerator was associated with a lower relative risk (1.0 vs 1.33). Low intakes of vitamin C were associated with an increased risk of stomach cancer with the lowest quintile of intake associated with significant elevation in risk (relative risk = 2.32). However, no information was provided as to how the vitamin C intakes of the cases and controls were estimated. Similarly, there were no biochemical measures of vitamin C status. There was little detail supplied about methods of diet assessment or subject selection.

Chyou et al. (1990) initiated a case–cohort study during the period of 1965 to 1968 on 8006 Hawaiian men of Japanese ancestry. Each subject was interviewed during this period with the use of a 24-hour dietary-recall questionnaire. Over the next 18 years, 111 stomach cancer incident cases were identified. Dietary data from these cases and from 361 cancer-free men revealed that the consumption of all types of vegetables was protective against stomach cancer. Subjects with the highest vegetable consumption had a relative risk for stomach cancer of 0.6 (95 percent confidence interval = 0.3–0.9) in comparison with non-consumers. A protective effect against stomach cancer was also observed with increased intake of fruits (p = 0.05), although this trend was weakened when cigarette smoking was taken into account. From the limited data presented, an association of stomach cancer with foods containing vitamin C, vitamin A, and β-carotene was suggestive, although the intake of individual nutrients such as vitamin C and vitamin A was not assessed.

Coggon et al. (1989) examined the influence of food storage habits, i.e., fresh versus frozen or preserved, on the development of stomach cancer by comparing 95 patients with cancer identified during 1985–1987 and 190 controls from two areas of the United Kingdom. As part of the investigation, a questionnaire was completed by each subject that provided information regarding the frequency of consumption of selected food items, including fresh and frozen fruit and salad vegetables. Evaluation of the data indicated a protective effect against stomach cancer by an increased frequency of consumption of fresh or frozen fruit (RR = 0.4; 95 percent confidence interval = 0.2–0.8) and by salad vegetables (RR = 0.2; 95 percent confidence interval = 0.1–0.5). Because of the design of the study, the effect of individual nutrients was not addressed. A more detailed cohort study is in progress by these investigators.

Burr et al. (1987) conducted a cross-sectional study in two British towns (Bath and Caerphilly) with regard to vitamin C status and stomach cancer and atrophic gastritis. Bath (southwest England) has a low mortality rate for stomach cancer, while Caerphilly (south Wales) has a high mortality incidence. For the study, 4078 men in Bath and 2789 men in Caerphilly, aged 65–74 years, were identified. From these groups, 267 persons from Bath and 246 persons from Caerphilly were selected for study. A questionnaire was completed that provided information on height and smoking, as well as limited dietary information. Blood samples were obtained at least two hours after the last meal for ascorbate and pepsinogen measurements. Serum pepsinogen levels served to diagnose atrophic gastritis. The participants were classified into social classes as well as manual workers and non-manual workers.

The Bath subjects, who were of somewhat higher social class, had significantly higher plasma ascorbate concentrations than those from Caerphilly (0.37 mg/dL vs 0.24 mg/dL). The consumption of fruit was considerably higher for the Bath men and the plasma ascorbate concentrations were directly associated with the frequency of fruit consumption (r = 0.274, p < 0.01). This relationship has been reported also by other investigators, particularly with respect to intakes of citrus fruits and juices.

The incidence of smoking was about 25 percent higher among the Caerphilly participants. Smoking commonly lowers plasma ascorbate concentrations. The influence of smoking on the plasma ascorbate levels in the populations studied was not considered. Since no estimates of vitamin C intakes were made, no consideration can be made as to the level of intake of the vitamin necessary to provide an apparent protection.

Severe atrophic gastritis, as assessed by pepsinogen concentrations, was nearly twice as common among the subjects from Caerphilly as from Bath. This difference did not appear to be related to plasma ascorbate levels. Mortality incidence (standard mortality ratio of 138) of stomach cancer was high in Caerphilly, while Bath had a low mortality rate for stomach cancer (standard mortality ratio of 77). The inverse relationship of ascorbate status to the occurrence of stomach cancer supports the concept of a role for vitamin C in the prevention of this cancer. Since the intake and status for other nutrients such as vitamin E and carotenoids were not investigated, their participation in the prevention of stomach cancer remains uncertain.

E. Pancreatic Cancer

The etiology of pancreatic cancer is unknown. Pancreatic cancer is common in developed countries, such as Japan, where a sharp increase in the disease has occurred in recent years (Boyle et al., 1989; Hirayama, 1989). In a large-scale cohort study conducted in Japan by Hirayama (1989), the occurrence of pancreatic cancer was observed to have a close association with cigarette smoking and the daily consumption of meat. Information was not reported whereby any association with vitamin C could be evaluated.

La Vecchia et al. (1990) conducted a hospital-based case–control study in northern Italy on 247 patients with pancreatic cancer and on 1089 age- and sex-matched hospital-based controls with acute, non-digestive, non-neoplastic diseases. Information was obtained by interview about sociodemographic characteristics, medical history, smoking habits, alcohol and coffee intakes, and on 14 selected indicator foods that included the major sources of vitamin A, fats, and fibers. A more frequent consumption of fish, oil (presumably vegetable, although not described), and fresh fruit was inversely associated with risk. Relative risk estimate decreased to 0.65–0.68 with an increased intake of fresh fruit (trend 4.53, $p < 0.05$). The data collection did not have a particular focus on vitamin C intake. Consequently, without additional information, any association of a vitamin C effect would be presumptive.

Mills et al. (1988) examined dietary habits and risk of pancreatic cancer in a prospective study of fatal pancreatic cancer among 34,000 non-Hispanic Seventh-Day Adventists during the period of 1974–1982. Forty deaths from pancreatic cancer occurred during this period. An increased consumption of vegetable protein products, beans, lentils or peas, and dried fruits was inversely associated with risk of fatal pancreatic cancer. The consumption of fresh fruits (fresh citrus and fresh winter fruit) was associated with a non-significant protective effect suggestive of a prophylactic role for vitamin C in pancreatic cancer; however, because of the limited data, confounding variables, and inadequate dietary information, such a role for vitamin C is conjecture.

Farrow and Davis (1990) investigated the relationship between diet and risk of pancreatic cancer in a population-based case–control study in western Washington. One hundred forty-eight married men diagnosed with pancreatic cancer and 188 controls were studied. Wives of the cases and controls were mailed a self-administered 135-item food-frequency questionnaire to provide information on the dietary intakes of their husbands for the previous 3 years. Dietary information was provided for 68 percent of the cases. No association was found between pancreatic cancer risk and the intake of total fat, saturated fat, cholesterol, vegetables, all fruits, citrus fruits, and vitamin C (calculated). The investigators recognized several limitations in their data. Information collected from surrogate respondents may be susceptible to recall bias related to the long retrospective period, and a larger portion of the cases were deceased than in the control group.

Falk et al. (1988) described a hospital-based, incident case–control study of pancreatic cancer, conducted between 1979 and 1983 in a high risk area of southern Louisiana. The study involved 363 cases and 1234 race-, sex-, and age-matched controls admitted to the same hospital. Because of the rapid fatal course of the disease, data from 50 percent of the cases were provided by the spouse or relatives. A 59-item food-frequency questionnaire was used to obtain dietary patterns prior to illness or onset of symptoms.

Of the dietary food items included, fruit consumption (oranges, bananas, orange juice, etc.) exhibited a protective effect against pancreatic cancer in both men and women. An odds ratio of 0.63 (95 percent confidence interval = 0.49–0.82) was reported. The highest risk was associated with an estimated intake of 65 mg/d of vitamin C and the lowest risk with an estimated intake above 150 mg/d. Smoking in both sexes was related to a significant trend for increased risk.

F. Colorectal Cancer

Epidemiological studies of colon cancer have implicated diet as a causative factor. Evidence is strong that the occurrence of colon cancer may be reduced in diets containing less animal fat and more fruit and vegetables (Willett, 1989). Several reviewers have considered the causative factors associated with colorectal cancers (Bingham, 1988; Block, 1991a; Block and Menkes, 1989; Hargreaves et al., 1989; Vogel and McPherson, 1989; Walker and Segal, 1989; Willett, 1989). As was the case with gastric cancer, the possible protective effect of vitamin C in colorectal carcinogenesis could be associated with its prevention of the formation of fecal N-nitrosamines or by action against other fecal mutagens (Block, 1991a; Block and Menkes, 1989; Schiffman, 1987).

Freudenheim et al. (1990) conducted a case–control study on primary rectal cancer in 277 case–control pairs of males and 145 case–control pairs of females in western New York. Extensive testing of the dietary intake assessment tools and interviewers was performed to ensure the reliability of the data. The focus of the interview was on the usual intake of 129 foods. The reference period was the usual intake in the year prior to interview for the controls and for the cases, a year prior to the onset of symptoms. During the 2.5 hour interview, information was also obtained on tobacco and alcohol use, occupation, health history, seasonal effects on diet, food preparation, and storage.

Although the study was well conceived, the duration of the interviews and the reliance on retrospective food frequency information may have limits. The dietary information provided evidence of a reduction in risk of rectal cancer with an increasing intake of vitamin C for both sexes. However, the protective effect was statistically significant for females only (OR = 0.45; 95 percent confidence interval = 0.24–0.85). Increased dietary intakes of carotenoids and fiber from vegetables were also associated with a decreased risk of rectal cancer. In an earlier separate report by Graham et al. (1988) using an approach similar to that used by Freudenheim et al. (1990), vitamin C and carotenoids were not found to be associated with a lowered risk of colon cancer.

The relationship between dietary factors and the risk of colorectal cancer in northern Italy was investigated in a case–control study conducted on 339 cases of colon cancer, 236 cases of rectal cancer, and 778 controls selected from hospital patients admitted for acute non-neoplastic or digestive disorders (La Vecchia et al., 1988). No population-based controls were used. Information was obtained on the current frequency of consumption per week of only 29 selected food items. Additional information was obtained about tobacco and alcohol use, consumption of coffee and methylxanthine-containing drinks, and health histories.

These investigators found that frequent consumption of green vegetables conveyed significant protective effect against both colon cancer (RR = 0.50) and rectal cancer (RR = 0.51). However, no significant protective effect was observed for either type of cancer with increased levels of intake of total fresh fruit, citrus fruit, or dietary vitamin C. With age and sex adjustments, an inverse relationship existed between risk and indices of carotenoid and vitamin C.

The limitations in the study included:

1) a limited number of food items in the food-frequency questionnaire;

2) no quantitative estimate of portion size;

3) a focus on current dietary practices rather than a reference period that may have been more relevant to initiation of colorectal cancers; and

4) reliance on hospital-based controls with no community-based control group.

Adenomatous polyps have been presumed to be precursor lesions for colorectal cancer. Several researchers have investigated the effect of vitamin C and other vitamin supplements in patients with colorectal polyps (DeCosse et al., 1989; McKeown-Eyssen et al., 1988; McLaughlin et al., 1988; Meyskens, 1990; Mills et al., 1988; Neugut et al., 1988). During the period of 1983–1985, Neugut et al. (1988) interviewed 244 women from New York who had undergone a colonoscopy. The cases consisted of 105 patients with adenomatous polyps, 56 patients with colon cancer, and 83 women without colorectal neoplasia on colonoscopy. Information was obtained from the women about their use of supplemental vitamins A, C, and E. Approximately 20 percent of the subjects in each group used vitamin C supplements. Information was not obtained as to the quantitative contribution of the supplements to the intake of vitamin C or of other vitamins. The study failed to demonstrate significant benefits from any of the vitamin supplements in preventing colon polyps or cancer.

Tuyns et al. (1987b) conducted a case–control study on colorectal cancer in the Belgian provinces of Oost-Vlaanderen and Liege. For the study, 453 colon cancer patients and 365 rectal cancer patients were selected along with 2851 controls from the adult populations of the two provinces. Approximately equal numbers of males and females were studied. Food consumption data were obtained from all subjects with the use of a previously tested dietary history procedure referenced to the week prior to onset of the disease symptoms for the cases and current intakes for the controls. Portion weights were estimated with the use of photographs of standard portions. Seasonal foods, such as fruits and vegetables, were considered in frequency of consumption data. Average daily intakes of individual nutrients were calculated with the use of Dutch food composition tables.

The average intakes for vitamin C and β-carotene were slightly lower in the cancer patients. This difference was not significant in view of the considerable age and sex differences associated with the food intake data. The average intake of vitamin C for the populations studied ranged from 91 to 109 mg per day. The relative risks (odds ratios) for vitamin C intake did not indicate a protective effect of the vitamin against rectal or colon cancer. While fiber in the diet had a protective effect, the investigators did not observe an association of fats with rectal or colon cancers. The effect of food groups, sources of vitamin C, vitamin supplements, smoking, and alcohol consumption were not considered as to their possible association with rectal or colon cancers.

West et al. (1989) conducted a case–control study in Utah between July 1979 and June 1983 in which 231 cases of colon cancer and 391 matched controls were interviewed. A comprehensive food frequency questionnaire was used to obtain information on foods eaten in the 2 to 3 years prior to the interview. Results indicated a protective effect against colon cancer was provided by fiber, β-carotene, and cruciferous vegetables. However, intake of vitamin C did not provide any protection against colon cancer after adjustment for body-mass index, age, crude fiber, and energy intake.

McKeown-Eyssen et al. (1988) conducted a double-blind randomized trial in Toronto, Canada, to examine the effect of vitamin C and vitamin E on the rate of recurrence of colorectal polyps. The study included 185 cases presumed to be free of polyps after the removal of at least 1 colorectal polyp. The subjects received either a supplement of 400 mg each of ascorbic acid and α-tocopherol (n = 96) or a placebo (n = 89) for up to 2 years. Random urine samples were collected to test for compliance. The findings of the investigation suggest that the vitamin C and vitamin E supplements produced very little, if any, effect in the reduced rate of polyp recurrence. Of the 137 (75 percent) subjects that completed the study, polyps were observed in the second colonoscopy in 41.4 percent of 70 subjects on vitamin supplements and in 50.7 percent of 67 subjects on placebo.

Whether this small reduction in the rate of polyp recurrence is of significance would require a larger study.

DeCosse et al. (1989) studied the effects of ascorbic acid plus α-tocopherol with and without grain-fiber supplements on rectal polyps. Over a period of 4 years, 58 patients from the New York City area with familial adenomatous polyposis were followed in a random, double-blind, placebo-controlled trial. There were 3 treatment groups: 22 patients received 8 capsules daily of a lactose placebo along with 2.2 grams of a low-fiber supplement; 16 patients received 8 capsules that provided 4 g of ascorbic acid, 400 mg of α-tocopherol and 2.2 g of the low-fiber supplement per day; and 20 patients received both vitamins at the same dosage as for the second group, plus 22.5 g of a high-fiber supplement. In addition, all groups received 30 mg of ascorbic acid, 2000 IU of vitamin A, and equivalent amounts of several other vitamins and minerals approximating 30 percent of the Recommended Dietary Allowances. Over the 4 years of the trial, each patient underwent proctosigmoidoscopy every 3 months and provided extensive food consumption information that included a 3-day diet diary recorded during the week preceding each examination and a food frequency questionnaire completed at the time of the examination.

The results did not indicate any protective effect of the vitamin C and vitamin E supplements on the occurrence of rectal polyps. A beneficial effect was obtained from the high-fiber supplements, particularly during the middle 2 years of the trial. Compliance for all groups decreased over the course of the trial. No biochemical measurements were performed, either at baseline or during the trial, that could indicate the level of compliance or the response to the supplements. Since all subjects received some vitamin supplements, their independent effects cannot be ascertained.

G. Prostate Cancer

Prostate cancer is the leading cancer in incidence in black men and the second leading cancer in white men. The 1985 estimated cancer incidence by site for men was lung cancer, 22 percent; prostate cancer, 19 percent; and colon cancer and rectal cancer combined, 15 percent (Horn et al., 1984). The possible role of diet in the etiology of prostate cancer has been investigated in several studies.

Kolonel et al. (1988) conducted a well-designed case–controlled study on diet and prostate cancer in Hawaii that covered the period of 1977–1983. Four hundred fifty-two cases of prostate cancer, identified through the population-based Hawaii Tumor Registry, were compared to 899 age-matched controls. A detailed quantitative dietary history method was used that included information on vitamins C and A. The results showed no effect on risk from either total (food plus supplements) or food sources of vitamin C in younger or older men irrespective of ethnic group. The mean total vitamin C intake ranged from 357 to 428 mg/d, representing a high intake.

Vitamin C intake of 100 prostate cancer patients and 2 different control groups (100 benign prostatic hyperplasia patients and 100 general hospital patients) was compared in a case–control study in Kyoto, Japan, from January 1981 to December 1984 (Ohno et al., 1988). No community-based control subjects were used. Quantitative food frequency information obtained from each subject showed that the mean daily intake of vitamin C was comparable for the 3 groups (92–103 mg/d). Contributions of vitamin supplements were not provided. No significant association of vitamin C intake and prostate cancer risk was observed. Following a more detailed analysis of information on dietary habits of participants in this study (Oishi et al., 1988), the conclusion concerning vitamin C remained unchanged.

H. Cervical/Ovarian Cancer

Cervical cancer rates in the U.S. are generally elevated in regions of low socioeconomic status. An association of diet with the risk of cervical cancer and cervical dysplasia, a premalignant lesion of the uterine cervix, has been proposed. Studies on the role of vitamin C and other vitamins in the development of cervical cancer have been reviewed recently (Block, 1991a; Block and Menkes, 1989; Schneider and Shah, 1989; Ziegler, 1986). These reviews suggested a consistent correlation between an increased prevalence of cervical neoplasia and low tissue concentrations, low serum levels, and low intakes of vitamin C, β-carotene, or folate.

During the years 1980–1983, Brock et al. (1988) conducted a study on 117 confirmed in situ cervical cancer patients and on 196 matched community controls in Sydney, Australia. Blood samples were obtained in 100 of the cases and 143 of the controls. Dietary patterns over the previous year were established with the use of a 160-item quantitative food-frequency questionnaire specifically designed to cover the significant dietary sources of retinol, carotene, vitamin C, and folate in the Australian diet. Reliability was evaluated by a repeated interview. Information was also obtained on smoking, sexual habits, and contraceptive use, and on the use of vitamin supplements. Fasting plasma levels were measured for retinol, total carotenes, and β-carotene, but not for vitamin C.

Dietary intakes of vitamin C, derived by calculation, suggested that an increased intake of the vitamin provided a protective effect. Plasma β-carotene levels and dietary intakes of vitamin C and fruit juices showed protective effects. The higher plasma β-carotene levels were associated with a reduced risk of 80 percent, while a higher intake of vitamin C reduced risk by 60 percent and fruit juices by 50 percent. With a calculated intake of vitamin C of 170 mg and above per day, the relative risk was 0.5 when adjusted for smoking, contraceptive use, and sexual habits. However, the trend was not significant. It is unfortunate that plasma ascorbate levels were not measured; these may have more accurately reflected the vitamin C status and dietary intakes.

Similar results were obtained by Verreault et al. (1989) who conducted a case–controlled study that involved 189 women diagnosed with cervical carcinoma between 1979 and 1983 in Seattle, Washington, and 227 randomly selected age-matched controls. A food frequency questionnaire was used to obtain intake information on 66 food items. Data were obtained on demographic characteristics, reproductive history, contraceptive use, smoking history, sexual habits, and anthropometries. All subjects were asked to refer to the time prior to a reference date (date of diagnosis for cases and December 1981 for controls). The average delay between the reference date and the interview was 2.8 years for the cases and 2.7 years for the controls.

This study found a significant inverse relationship between calculated vitamin C intake and the risk of cervical cancer. The adjusted relative risk (RR) was 0.5 (95 percent confidence interval = 0.2–1.0, p = 0.04 for trend) for the highest quartile of intake of vitamin C. The estimated intake of vitamin C for this quartile was 77 mg and above per day. The effect of fruit juices was even stronger with an RR of 0.3 (p < 0.01). After adjustment for known risk factors, frequent consumption of dark green or yellow vegetables and of fruit juices was related to a reduced risk of cervical cancer. High intakes of vitamin E and of carotene were also associated with a lower risk of cervical cancer. However, plasma levels of vitamin C, vitamin E, or carotene were not determined.

These studies offer considerable evidence of a protective effect for vitamin C in cervical cancer. Nevertheless, carefully conducted longitudinal and prospective cohort studies are needed to establish the significance of vitamin C as a protective factor against cervical cancer. Such studies should include multiple measurements of ascorbic acid levels in plasma and blood components as indicators of vitamin C status and its relationship to protective effects.

Contrasting results were obtained by Ziegler et al. (1990) in a case–control study of invasive cervical cancer among white women in five U.S. metropolitan areas (Birmingham, Chicago, Denver, Miami, and Philadelphia) during the period 1982–1983. The study involved an examination of dietary habits and information on the frequency of consumption of 75 food items and vitamin supplements by 271 cases and 502 matched controls. Information was also obtained on demographic characteristics, sexual behavior, use of contraceptives and female hormones, reproductive and menstrual history, personal and familial medical history, and smoking.

In this study, the risk of invasive cervical cancer was not affected by increased consumption of fruits, vegetables, dark green vegetables, dark yellow-orange vegetables, or legumes. No increased risk of cervical cancer could be associated with a decreased intake of vitamin A, vitamin C, carotenoids, or folate. However, among heavy smokers, vitamin C intake appeared to be protective. The contrast of these findings to those obtained in previous epidemiologic studies is not readily explained.

Cigarette smoking has been hypothesized to be a causative factor in the development of cervical cancer. Of interest is the study of Basu et al. (1990) on the influence of cigarette smoking on ascorbic acid levels in plasma, leukocyte, and cervicovaginal cells from 16 women who smoked and 30 women who did not. The levels of ascorbic acid in the cervicovaginal cells and in the plasma were significantly lower in the smokers when compared to the nonsmokers ($p < 0.001$, $p < 0.01$, respectively).

Ovarian cancer is considered responsible for more cancer deaths in women than any other cancer in the female genital tract. A few studies have reported an association between ovarian cancer and specific nutrients (Shu et al., 1989; Slattery et al., 1989). Recently, Slattery et al. (1989) conducted a population-based, case–control study in Utah to examine the association between nutrient intake and ovarian cancer. During 1984 and 1987, information on contraceptive use, smoking history, demographics, anthropometrics, medical history, and pregnancy history, plus detailed dietary information was obtained on 85 first primary ovarian cancer cases and 492 population-based, age-matched controls. The questionnaire contained 183 food items. Vitamin C intake appeared to decrease slightly the risk of ovarian cancer, but the magnitude of the effect was small, with an adjusted odds ratio of 0.7. Similar slight non-significant increases in risk were observed with a decreased intake of vitamin A or of fiber. A protective effect was observed between dietary β-carotene and ovarian cancer.

In Shanghai, Shu et al. (1989) investigated dietary factors and epithelial ovarian cancer in a population-based, case–control study of 172 cases and 172 controls matched for age and residence. Dietary information was obtained on the frequency of consumption of 63 food items. A slight protective effect was observed with high intakes of total vegetables. However, no protective effect was associated with an increased intake of vitamin C. High fat intake was significantly related to an increased risk of ovarian cancer (trends in risk for total fat: $p = 0.03$; for animal fat: $p = 0.07$). Again, the lack of biochemical analyses, accurate portion size estimations, and the limited number of food items assessed attenuates the interpretation of these results

I. Other Cancers

La Vecchia et al. (1989) studied the relationship between bladder cancer risk and vitamin A and other dietary factors in a case–control study of histologically confirmed invasive bladder cancer in 136 male and 27 female cases below the age of 75 years, recruited from hospitals in Milan, Italy. The age-matched controls (129 males, 52 females) admitted for traumatic conditions (fractures and sprains), surgical conditions, non-traumatic orthopedic disorders, or other illnesses were recruited from the same hospitals.

A structured questionnaire was used to obtain information on sociodemographic factors, smoking, consumption of alcohol, coffee, and methylxanthine-containing beverages, family medical history, and drug use. Dietary information was limited to the frequency, but not quantity, of consumption of only 10 selected foods items (milk and dairy products, meat, fish, liver, ham, eggs, carrots, green vegetables, and fruits) prior to the onset of the disease or condition which led to their admission. The results presented focused on vitamin A and provitamin A with no mention of vitamin C. Mean monthly intakes of carotenoids and retinoids were lower for the cases, but the differences were statistically significant only for the carotenoids. Intakes of green vegetables and carrots were significantly lower for the cases, but the consumption of fresh fruits was essentially the same for the cases and controls. The risk of bladder cancer decreased with increasing intakes of carotenoids and retinoids. Consumption of fresh fruits did not appear to be associated with a reduction of risk for bladder cancer in this study.

Stähelin et al. (1987, 1989) reported on 2975 male participants evaluated between 1971–1973 who had taken part in a large prospective cohort study of cardiovascular disease, the Basel Study, begun in 1960. Blood concentrations and dietary intakes of vitamin C, vitamin E, vitamin A, and β-carotene were evaluated in this prospective study of cancer deaths. By 1980, a total of 102 cancer cases occurred which consisted of 37 lung cancers, 17 stomach cancers, 9 colorectal cancers, and 39 cancers of other sites.

Compared to survivors, the plasma concentrations of vitamin C were significantly lower (p < 0.05) in all death cases (n = 286, 9 percent of the cohort), all cancer cases, and stomach cancer. After adjustment for smoking, the impact of all studied vitamins on mortality was markedly diminished and for vitamin C, a significantly lower plasma concentration was observed only for stomach cancer. For stomach cancer, vitamin C and β-carotene, as well as vitamin C and vitamin E, appeared to act independently yet synergistically (Stähelin et al., 1987, 1989). Subjects with low plasma vitamin C and vitamin E values had a high risk ratio (2.39), while subjects with high levels of these two vitamins had a lower risk ratio (0.68). In this study, neither food consumption data nor estimates of the intake of these vitamins were provided. Thus, it is not possible to relate the amount of vitamin C, β-carotene, or vitamin E that might provide a protective effect against stomach cancer.

IV. Conclusions and Recommendations

A. General Conclusions and Recommendations

The majority of the investigations on the association of vitamin C with various types of cancer are epidemiologic studies that have depended on retrospective questionnaires, usually food-frequency techniques, in order to examine this relationship. The retrospective nature of these studies is necessitated by the long period that may elapse between induction and the appearance of a specific cancer. Although studies reported protective effects against specific types of cancer with an increased frequency of use of vegetables, fresh green leafy vegetables, fresh fruit, and citrus fruit/juices, collection of data on the actual intakes of specific nutrients was not possible. Plasma levels of ascorbic acid were rarely measured. Calculated estimates occasionally provided an indication of the association of vitamins C, A, and E, and β-carotene. For some studies, it was not possible to discern whether the suggested protective activity was due to the presence of vitamin C or β-carotene, or a combined effect of both or of additional factors, such as fiber. In some of the investigations, however, a specific effect from vitamin C alone was evident.

It is well recognized that the multistage process of carcinogenesis permits various opportunities for the intervention of nutrients such as vitamin C to prevent or impede the transformation of a normal cell into a cancer cell. But how specific nutrients may participate in this process remains to be clarified. To date, an over-reliance has probably been placed on the outcomes of epidemiology studies. Such data are necessary in order to conceive intervention and preventive strategies against cancer. Knowledge gained from the studies reviewed should provide guidance in the design and conduct of needed cancer intervention trials with vitamin C.

However, the design and implementation of controlled intervention trials are difficult and exceedingly expensive. The ability to attain replicate data about the influence of any single nutrient factor on cancer development is difficult for several reasons:

1) more than one nutrient factor may be involved;

2) there may be differences in the racial/ethnic makeup of the population sample; and

3) results may be further confounded by geographic and demographic patterns of dietary intake.

Similarly, while few studies have paid attention to the relationship of diet to the occurrence of cancer in various racial and ethnic groups in the U.S. (Hargreaves et al., 1989), the overall incidence of cancer is much lower in American Indians than in whites, blacks, and other racial and ethnic groups in the U.S. Yet, the potential role of diet in the higher prevalence of certain cancers in groups such as Native American Indians remains unresolved. The results of the several human intervention trials in progress may provide definitive and quantitative assessments as to the role of vitamin C in cancer prevention (Boone et al., 1990; Costa et al., 1990). In the meantime, in view of the consistency of dietary findings, it seems appropriate and prudent to direct efforts towards increasing the consumption of fruits and vegetables.

In addition, evidence suggests that vitamin C may interact with other dietary components in the prevention of cancer. Thus, for example, both vitamin C and β-carotene have been reported to reduce the risk of cervical dysplasia (Basu et al., 1990; Brock et al., 1988). Other studies indicate a protective role for folate. Interactions of vitamin C with nutrients, such as vitamin E, vitamin A, carotenoids, and fiber require a better understanding in order to appreciate the role of vitamin C in cancer prevention. Furthermore, mechanisms other than the nitrosamine inhibition, whereby vitamin C may produce an anti-cancer effect, require investigation. A better understanding of the functions of vitamin C would clarify the magnitude of influence of the vitamin on tumorigenesis.

Finally, among the plethora of studies reviewed, few have attempted to quantify the actual intakes of vitamin C and associate the level of intakes with cancer prevention. An optimum intake of vitamin C for cancer prevention is therefore uncertain. Intakes of vitamin C that maintain blood vitamin C concentrations (plasma, leukocytes, etc.) at the concentrations associated with reduced cancer risk may serve as an initial guide as to desired intakes. For example, in the Basel Study, men with stomach cancer had a mean plasma vitamin C concentration of 35.8 μmol/L (Stähelin et al., 1987, 1989). Subjects free of cancer had a vitamin C concentration of 47.0 μmol/L. A plasma vitamin C concentration of approximately 40 μmol/L may be attained in men with a daily intake of 75 mg of ascorbic acid. This level of intake has been reported to maintain the high levels of ascorbic acid present in leukocytes and to provide for optimum immunocompetence.

Individuals who smoke require an increased intake of vitamin C to attain these blood concentrations.

B. Specific Conclusions

1. Effects of vitamin C in reducing the occurrence of *breast cancer* remain uncertain at present. Two studies (Katsouyani et al., 1988; Toniolo et al., 1989) indicated no protective effect. While a meta-analysis of 12 case–controlled studies by Howe et al. (1990) found that nine studies indicated a consistent protective effect of diets with calculated high vitamin C intakes, Howe et al. (1990) concluded that the inverse association between breast cancer and markers of fruit and vegetable consumption lent support to the hypothesis that increased consumption of these foods may reduce breast cancer risk.

2. Citrus fruits provided a significant negative association with risk of *oral cancer* (Franco et al., 1989; McLaughlin et al., 1988). The design of the studies, i.e., the lack of direct measures of vitamin C intake and/or status, provides only presumptive evidence that vitamin C was the active agent.

   Risk of *esophageal cancer* was reduced with higher intakes of vitamin C-rich fruits and juices (Brown et al., 1988; Li et al., 1989; Tuyns et al., 1987a). In one study (Li et al., 1989), the high incidence of esophageal cancer found in China appeared to be unrelated to vitamin C; however, in another (Guo et al., 1990) there was a significant association between both intake and serum levels of vitamin C and esophageal cancer. The vitamin C status of the first population studied (Li et al., 1989) appeared poor, so that a protective effect of the vitamin may not have been discernible. Further, that study was not designed to address specifically the relationship of vitamin C and cancer.

3. Although not consistent, some studies have demonstrated an inverse association between *lung cancer* risk and vitamin C (Fontham et al., 1988; Koo et al., 1988; LeGardeur et al., 1990; Le Marchand et al., 1989); however, the studies reviewed had design problems, e.g., lack of community-based control groups, focus on food groups rather than accurate estimates of intakes of individual nutrients, and lack of biochemical confirmation of vitamin C status, that precluded a definitive link with vitamin C.

4. One of the most consistent epidemiological findings has been an association with high intakes of vitamin C or vitamin C-rich foods and a reduced risk of *stomach cancer*. This relationship may have been mediated through the action of vitamin C in blocking the formation of nitrosamines and other carcinogens in the stomach. Considerable biochemical and physiological evidence exists to support this action of vitamin C.

5. For *pancreatic cancer,* the effect of vitamin C was equivocal, although a presumptive protective effect was observed in two studies (Falk et al., 1988; La Vecchia et al., 1990). Difficulties of design similar to those previously discussed were found in the investigations of dietary associations with this form of cancer.

6. Vitamin C appeared to provide no protection against *colon cancer* (Graham et al., 1988; Tuyns et al., 1987b; West et al., 1989). Weak protection was observed in one study against rectal cancer (Freudenheim et al., 1990). No benefit was observed from the use of vitamin C and other vitamin supplements on colorectal cancer or on the incidence of recurrence of polyps (McKeown-Eyssens et al., 1988; DeCosse et al., 1989).

7. Low intakes of vitamin C were associated with an increased risk of *cervical cancer* in two of three studies reported (Brock et al., 1988; Verreault et al., 1989). This relationship

deserves further study, because results of these studies suggest that several nutrients either individually or in synergy may impart a protective effect.

8. Vitamin C was not associated with reproducible significant changes in risk for *ovarian, prostate, bladder, or other cancers.*

V. Bibliography*

Basu, J.; Mikhail, M.S.; Payraudeau, P.H.; Palan, P.R.; Romney, S.L. 1990. Smoking and the antioxidant ascorbic acid: plasma, leukocyte, and cervicovaginal cell concentrations in normal healthy women. *Am. J. Obstet. Gynecol.* 163:1948–1952.

Bingham, S.A. 1988. Meat, starch, and nonstarch polysaccharides and large bowel cancer. *Am. J. Clin. Nutr.* 48:762–767.

Block, G. 1991a. Dietary guidelines and the results of food consumption surveys. *Am. J. Clin. Nutr.* 53:356S–357S.

Block, G. 1991b. Vitamin C and cancer prevention: the epidemiologic evidence. *Am. J. Clin. Nutr.* 53:270S–282S.

Block, G.; Menkes, M. 1989. Ascorbic acid in cancer prevention. In: Moon, T.E.; Micozzi, M.S., eds. *Diet and cancer prevention: investigating the role of micronutrients.* New York: Marcel Dekker. p. 341–388.

Block, G.; Sorenson, A. 1987. Vitamin C intake and dietary sources by demographic characteristics. *Nutr. Cancer* 10:53–65.

Boeing, H.; Frentzel-Beyme, R. 1991. Regional risk factors for stomach cancer in the FRG. *Environ. Health Perspect.* 94:83–89.

Boone, C.W.; Kellof, G.J.; Malone, W.E. 1990. Identification of candidate cancer chemopreventive agents and their evaluation in animal models and human clinical trials: a review. *Cancer Res.* 50:2–9.

Boyle, P.; Hsieh, C.-C.; Maisonneuve, P.; La Vecchia, C.; Macfarlane, G.J.; Walker, A.M.; Trichopoulos, D. 1989. Epidemiology of pancreas cancer (1988). *Int. J. Pancreatol.* 5:327–346.

Brock, K.E.; Berry, G.; Mock, P.A.; MacLennan, R.; Truswell, A.S.; Brinton, L.A. 1988. Nutrients in diet and plasma and risk of in situ cervical cancer. *J. Natl. Cancer Inst.* 80:580–585.

Brown, L.M.; Blot, W.J.; Schuman, S.H.; Smith, V.M.; Ershow, A.G.; Marks, R.D.; Fraumeni, J.F. 1988. Environmental factors and high risk of esophageal cancer among men in coastal South Carolina. *J. Natl. Cancer Inst.* 80:1620–1625.

Buiatti, E.; Palli, D.; Decarli, A.; Amadori, D.; Avellini, C.; Bianchi, S.; Biserni, R.; Cipriani, F.; Cocco, P.; Giacosa, A.; Marubini, E.; Puntoni, R.; Vindigni, C.; Fraumeni, J.; Blot, W. 1989. A case–control study of gastric cancer and diet in Italy. *Int. J. Cancer* 44:611–616.

Buiatti, E.; Palli, D.; Decarli, A.; Amadori, D.; Avellini, C.; Bianchi, S.; Bonaguri, C.; Cipriani, F.; Cocco, P.; Giacosa, A.; Marubini, E.; Minacci, C.; Puntoni, R.; Russo, A.; Vindigni, C.; Fraumeni, J.F.; Blot, W.J. 1990. A case–control study of gastric cancer and diet in Italy. II. Association with nutrients. *Int. J. Cancer* 45:896–901.

Burr, M.L.; Samloff, I.M.; Bates, C.J.; Holliday, R. 1987. Atrophic gastritis and vitamin C status in two towns with different stomach cancer death-rates. *Br. J. Cancer* 56:163–167.

Byers, T.E.; Graham, S.; Haughey, B.P.; Marshall, J.R.; Swanson, M.K. 1987. Diet and lung cancer risk: findings from the western New York diet study. *Am. J. Epidemiol.* 125:351–363.

Chyou, P.-H.; Nomura, A.M.Y.; Hankin, J.H.; Stemmermann, G.N. 1990. A case–cohort study of diet and stomach cancer. *Cancer Res.* 50:7501–7504.

*This bibliography contains all refence citations that are either in the text or the appendix table or both.

Coggan, C.; Barker, D.J.P.; Cole, R.B.; Nelson, M. 1989. Stomach cancer and food storage. *J. Natl. Cancer Inst.* 81:1178–1182.

Costa, A.; Santoro, G.; Assimakopoulos, G. 1990. Cancer chemoprevention. *Rev. Oncol.* 29:657–663.

DeCosse, J.J.; Miller, H.H.; Lesser, M.L. 1989. Effect of wheat fiber and vitamins C and E on rectal polyps in patients with familial adenomatous polyposis. *J. Natl. Cancer Inst.* 81:1290–1297.

Falk, R.T.; Pickle, L.W.; Fontham, E.T.; Correa, P.; Fraumeni, J.F. 1988. Life-style risk factors for pancreatic cancer in Louisiana: a case–control study. *Am. J. Epidemiol.* 128:324–336.

Farrow, D.C.; Davis, S. 1990. Diet and the risk of pancreatic cancer in men. *Am. J. Epidemiol.* 132:423–431.

Fontham, E.T. 1990. Protective dietary factors and lung cancer. *Int. J. Epidemiol.* 19(Suppl. 1):S32–S42.

Fontham, E.T.; Pickle, L.W.; Haenszel, W.; Correa, P.; Lin, Y.; Falk, R.T. 1988. Dietary vitamins A and C and lung cancer risk in Louisiana. *Cancer* 62:2267–2273.

Franco, E.L.; Kowalski, L.P.; Oliveira, B.V.; Curado, M.P.; Pereira, R.N.; Silva, M.E.; Fava, A.S.; Torloni, H. 1989. Risk factors for oral cancer in Brazil: a case–control study. *Int. J. Cancer* 43:992–1000.

Freudenheim, J.L.; Graham, S.; Marshall, J.R.; Haughey, B.P.; Wilkinson, G. 1990. A case–control study of diet and rectal cancer in western New York. *Am. J. Epidemiol.* 131:612–624.

Ghadirian, P.; Vobecky, J.; Vobecky, J.S. 1988. Factors associated with cancer of the oesophagus: an overview. *Cancer Detect. Prevent.* 11:225–234.

Graham, S.; Marshall, J.; Haughey, B.; Mittelman, A.; Swanson, M.; Zielezny, M.; Byers, T.; Wilkinson, G.; West, D. 1988. Dietary epidemiology of cancer of the colon in western New York. *Am. J. Epidemiol.* 128:490–503.

Guo, W.; Li, B.; Blot, W.J. 1989. A case–control study of cancer of the esophagus and gastric cardia in Linxian. *Int. J. Cancer Res.* 43:755–761.

Hargreaves, M.K.; Banquet, C.; Gamshadzahi, A. 1989. Diet, nutritional status, and cancer risk in Americn blacks. *Nutr. Cancer* 12:1–28.

Hirayama, T. 1989. Epidemiology of pancreatic cancer in Japan. *Jpn. J. Clin. Oncol.* 19:208–215.

Horn, J.W.; Asire, A.J.; Young, J.L. 1984. *National Cancer Institute Surveillance, Epidemiology and End Results (SEER) Program: cancer incidence and mortality in the United States, 1973–1981.* NIH Publication No. 85-1837. Available from: U.S. Government Printing Office, Washington, DC.

Howe, G.R.; Hirohata, T.; Hislop, T.G.; Iscovich, J.M.; Yuan, J.-M.; Katsouyanni, K.; Lubin, F.; Marubini, E.; Modan, B.; Rohan, T.; Toniolo, P.; Shunzhang, Y. 1990. Dietary factors and risk of breast cancer: combined analysis of 12 case–control studies. *J. Natl. Cancer Inst.* 82:561–569.

Katsouyanni, K.; Willett, W.; Trichopoulos, D.; Boyle, P.; Trichopoulou, A.; Vasilaros, S.; Papadiamantis, J.; MacMahon, B. 1988. Risk of breast cancer among Greek women in relation to nutrient intake. *Cancer* 61:181–185.

Kolonel, L.N.; Yoshizawa, C.N.; Hankin, J.H. 1988. Diet and prostatic cancer: a case–control study in Hawaii. *Am. J. Epidemiol.* 127:999–1012.

Kono, S.; Ikeda, M.; Tokudome, S.; Kuratsune, M. 1988. A case–control study of gastric cancer and diet in northern Kyushu, Japan. *Jpn. J. Cancer Res.* 79:1067–1074.

Koo, L.C. 1988. Dietary habits and lung cancer risk among Chinese females in Hong Kong who never smoked. *Nutr. Cancer* 11:155–172.

La Vecchia, C.; Negri, E.; D'Avanzo, B.; Ferraroni, M.; Gramenzi, A.; Savoldelli, R.; Boyle, P.; Franceschi, S. 1990. Medical history, diet, and pancreatic cancer. *Oncology* 47:463–466.

La Vecchia, C.; Negri, E.; Decarli, A.; D'Avanzo, B.; Franceschi, S. 1989. Dietary factors in the risk of bladder cancer. *Nutr. Cancer* 12:93–101.

La Vecchia, C.; Negri, E.; Decarli, A.; D'Avanzo, B.; Gallotti, L.; Gentile, A.; Franceschi, S. 1988. A case–control study of diet and colo-rectal cancer in northern Italy. *Int. J. Cancer* 41:492–498.

Leaf, C.D.; Vecchio, A.J.; Roe, D.A.; Hotchkiss, J.H. 1987. Influence of ascorbic acid dose on *N*-nitrosoproline formation in humans. *Carcinogenesis* 8:791–795.

LeGardeur, B.Y.; Lopez, S.A.; Johnson, W.D. 1990. A case–control study of serum vitamins A, E, and C in lung cancer patients. *Nutr. Cancer* 14:133–140.

Le Marchand, L.; Yoshizawa, C.N.; Kolonel, L.N.; Hankin, J.H.; Goodman, M.T. 1989. Vegetable consumption and lung cancer risk: a population-based case–control study in Hawaii. *J. Natl. Cancer Inst.* 81:1158–1164.

Li, J.-Y.; Ershow, A.G.; Chen, Z.-J.; Wacholder, S.; Li, G.-Y.; Guo, W.; Li, B.; Blot, W.J. 1989. A case–control study of cancer of the esophagus and gastric cardia in Linxian.

Malone, W.F. 1991. Studies evaluating antioxidants and β-carotene as chemopreventives. *Am. J. Clin. Nutr.* 53:305S–313S.

McKeown-Eyssen, G.; Holloway, C.; Jazmaji, V.; Bright-See, E.; Dion, P.; Bruce, W.R. 1988. A randomized trial of vitamins C and E in the prevention of recurrence of colorectal polyps. *Cancer Res.* 48:4701–4705.

McLaughlin, J.K.; Gridley, G.; Block, G.; Winn, D.M.; Preston-Martin, S.; Schoenberg, J.B.; Greenberg, R.S.; Stemhagen, A.; Austin, D.F.; Ershow, A.G.; Blot, W.J.; Fraumeni, J.F. 1988. Dietary factors in oral and pharyngeal cancer. *J. Natl. Cancer Inst.* 80:1237–1243.

Meyskens, F.L., Jr. 1990. Coming of age—the chemoprevention of cancer. *N. Engl. J. Med.* 323:825–827.

Mills, P.K.; Beeson, W.L.; Abbey, D.E.; Fraser, G.E.; Phillips, R.L. 1988. Dietary habits and past medical history as related to fatal pancreas cancer among Adventists. *Cancer* 61:2578–2585.

National Research Council, Committee on Diet, Nutrition and Cancer. 1989. *Cancer*. Diet and health: implications for reducing chronic risk. Washington, DC: National Academy Press. p. 593–605.

National Research Council, Food and Nutrition Board. 1989. *Recommended dietary allowances*. 10th ed. Washington, DC: National Academy Press.

Neugut, A.I.; Johnsen, C.M.; Forde, K.A.; Treat, M.R.; Nims, C. 1988. Vitamin supplements among women with adenomatous polyps and cancer of the colon: preliminary findings. *Dis. Colon Rectum* 31:430–432.

Ohno, Y.; Yoshida, O.; Ioshi, K.; Yamabe, H.; Schroeder, F.H. 1988. Dietary β-carotene and cancer of the prostate: a case–control study in Kyoto, Japan. *Cancer Res.* 48:1331–1336.

Oishi, Y.; Okada, K.; Yoshida, O.; Yamabe, H.; Ohno, Y.; Hayes, R.B.; Schroeder, F.H. 1988. A case–control study of prostatic cancer with reference to dietary habits. *Prostate* 12:179–190.

Padh, H. 1991. Vitamin C: newer insights into its biochemical functions. *Nutr. Rev.* 49:65–70.

Patterson, B.H.; Block, G.; Rosenberger, W.F.; Pee, D.; Kahle, L.L. 1990. Fruit and vegetables in the American diet: data from the NHANES II Survey. *Am. J. Publ. Health* 80:1443–1449.

Rivers, J.M. 1989. Safety of high-level vitamin C ingestion. *Int. J. Vitam. Nutr. Res.* 30:95–102.

Sauberlich, H.E. 1985. Bioavailability of vitamins. *Prog. Food Nutr. Sci.* 9:1–33.

Sauberlich, H.E. 1990. Ascorbic acid. In: Brown, M.L., ed. *Present knowledge in nutrition*. Washington, DC: Nutrition Foundation. p. 132–141.

Schiffman, M.H. 1987. Diet and faecal genotoxicity. *Cancer Surv.* 6:653–672.

Schneider, A.; Shah, K. 1989. The role of vitamins in the etiology of cervical neoplasia: an epidemiological review. *Arch. Gynecol. Obstet.* 246:1–13.

Schorah, C.J.; Sobala, G.M.; Sanderson, M.; Collis, N.; Primrose, J.N. 1991. Gastric juice ascorbic acid: effects of disease and implications for gastric carcinogenesis. *Am. J. Clin. Nutr.* 53:287S–293S.

Shu, O.X.; Gao, Y.T.; Yuan, J.M.; Ziegler, R.G.; Brinton, L.A. 1989. Dietary factors and epithelial ovarian cancer. *Br. J. Cancer* 59:92–96.

Sies, H. 1989. Relationship between free radicals and vitamins: an overview. *Int. J. Vitam. Nutr. Res. Suppl.* 30:215–223.

Slattery, M.L.; Schuman, K.L.; West, D.W.; French, T.K.; Robison, L.M. 1989. Nutrient intake and ovarian cancer. *Am. J. Epidemiol.* 130:497–502.

Sobala, G.M.; Pignatelli, B.; Schorah, C.J.; Bartsch, H.; Sanderson, M.; Dixon, M.F.; Shires, S.; King, R.F.G.; Axon, A.T.R. 1991. Levels of nitrite, nitrate, *N*-nitroso compounds, ascorbic acid and total bile acids in gastric juice of patients with and without precancerous conditions of the stomach. *Carcinogenesis* 12:193–198.

Stähelin, H.B.; Gey, K.F.; Brubacker, G. 1987. Plasma vitamin C and cancer death: the prospective Basel study. *Ann. N.Y. Acad. Sci.* 498:124–131.

Stähelin, H.B.; Gey, F.; Brubacker, G. 1989. Preventive potential of antioxidative vitamins and carotenoids on cancer. *Int. J. Vitam. Nutr. Res.* 30:232–241.

Tannenbaum, S.R.; Wishnok, J.S.; Leaf, C.D. 1991. Inhibition of nitrosamine formation by ascorbic acid. *Am. J. Clin. Nutr.* 53:247S–250S.

Toniolo, P.; Riboli, E.; Protta, F.; Charrel, M.; Cappa, A.P. 1989. Calorie-providing nutrients and risk of breast cancer. *J. Natl. Cancer Inst.* 81:278–286.

Tuyns, A.J.; Haelterman, M.; Kaaks, R. 1987. Colorectal cancer and the intake of nutrients: oligosaccharides are a risk factor, fats are not. A case–control study in Belgium. *Nutr. Cancer* 10:181–196.

Tuyns, A.J.; Riboli, E.; Doornbos, G.; Péquignot, G. 1987. Diet and esophageal cancer in Calvados (France). *Nutr. Cancer* 9:81–92.

U.S. Department of Agriculture and U.S. Department of Health and Human Services. 1990. *Nutrition and your health: dietary guidelines for Americans.* 3rd ed. Home and Garden Bulletin No. 232. Available from: U.S. Government Printing Office, Washington, DC.

U.S. Department of Health and Human Services. 1991. *Healthy people 2000: national health promotion and disease prevention objectives.* Available from: U.S. Government Printing Office, Washington, DC.

U.S. Department of Health and Human Services. 1988. *The Surgeon General's report on nutrition and health.* Available from: U.S. Government Printing Office, Washington, DC.

Vogel, V.G.; McPherson, R.S. 1989. Dietary epidemiology of colon cancer. *Hematol. Oncol. Clin. North Am.* 3:35–63.

Walker, A.R.P.; Segal, I. 1989. Puzzles in the epidemiology of colon cancer. *J. Clin. Gastroenterol.* 11:10–11.

West, D.W.; Slattery, M.L.; Robison, L.M.; Schuman, K.L.; Ford, M.H.; Mahoney, A.W.; Lyon, J.L.; Sorensen, A.W. 1989. Dietary intake and colon cancer: sex- and anatomic site-specific associations. *Am. J. Epidemiol.* 130:883–894.

Willett, W. 1989. The search for the causes of breast and colon cancer. *Nature* 338:389–393.

You, W.C.; Blot, W.J.; Chang, Y.-S.; Ershow, A.G.; Yang, Z.-T.; An, Q.; Henderson, B.; Xu, G.-W.; Fraumeni, J.F.; Wang. T.-G. 1988. Diet and high risk of stomach cancer in Shandong, China. *Cancer Res.* 48:3518–3523.

Ziegler, R.G. 1986. Epidemiologic studies of vitamins and cancer of the lung, esophagus, and cervix. In: Poirier, L.A.; Newberne, P.M.; Pariza, M.W.; eds. *Essential nutrients in carcinogenesis.* New York: Plenum Press.

Ziegler, R.G.; Brinton, L.A.; Hamman, R.F.; Lehman, H.F.; Levine, R.S.; Mallin, K.; Norman, S.A.; Rosenthal, J.F.; Trumble, A.C.; Hoover, R.N. 1990. Diet and the risk of invasive cervical cancer among white women in the United States. *Am. J. Epidemiol.* 132:432–445.

Appendix

Criteria for Inclusion of Articles in Appendix Tables

Articles in peer-reviewed journals related to the topic of this review were selected primarily on the basis of date and content. In general, papers appearing in 1987 or thereafter were included, provided that they presented original data from studies in humans. Certain items tabulated for the sake of completeness may not have been cited in the body of the text if their weight or relevance did not add significantly to development of the author's argument. Reviews have not been listed except as they included new data or useful meta-analyses.

APPENDIX TABLE 1   Vitamin C and Breast Cancer

Study	Type/Location	Subject Number and Description	Methods
Howe et al., 1990	Case–control Meta-analysis of 12 studies	4437 cases of *breast cancer* (BC). 4341 population controls. 1754 hospital controls.	Analysis included all studies of diet and BC completed by 1986. Authors made diet data available from each of 12 studies. Where data had not been available, estimates of intake were made using food frequency answers. Data on vitamin C were available from 9 of 12 studies. Pre- and postmenopausal women were analyzed separately.
Katsouyanni et al., 1988	Case–control Athens, Greece	120 BC cases. 120 hospital controls (patients in orthopedic ward in a different hospital than BC cases).	All subjects interviewed before discharge on first hospital admission. Data collected included demographics, socioeconomic, and reproductive and medical histories. Dietary histories were collected with a 120-item food-frequency questionnaire. To assess the impact of individual nutrients on BC, nutrient intakes were adjusted for calories.
Toniolo et al., 1989	Case–control Italy	250 cases of *breast cancer* (free of metastases, except in regional lymph nodes. Controls were 499 ♀ from general population stratified by age (± 10 yr) and geographical area.	All subjects interviewed (unblinded) given modified food frequency questionnaire structured by meals. Indigenous foods and recipes were added to the database. General demographic data were obtained from electoral rolls. Interview data included SES data, and health and reproductive histories.

Results	Comments
Vitamin C had the most consistent statistically significant inverse association with BC risk. There was a significant positive association between saturated fat intake and risk in postmenopausal cases. Other markers of fruits and vegetable consumption, e.g., β-carotene, fiber, and carotenoids also showed an inverse relationship with risk.	Questions about the validity of meta-analysis in terms of lack of control of independent variables that could influence outcomes, i.e., socioeconomic status (SES), supplement use, clinical stage, medications, and smoking habits. Reliability of dietary data.
There were no differences in actual or calorie-adjusted intakes of vitamin C between cases and controls. Similarly there was no association between vitamin C and risk of BC. Total vitamin A intake was inversely associated with BC risk.	Inappropriate controls (about 25% had osteoarthritis which is known to affect vitamin C metabolism). No biochemistry. Diet data was related to the period preceding the onset of the disease which was not controlled nor was it documented. Supplement use not documented. Data collected over a 12-mo period with no control for seasonal variations in intakes.
No difference in vitamin E intake between groups. Reduced risk was associated with decreased intakes of fat, especially saturated fat and animal protein.	Not blinded, no biochemistry, long period of time between diagnosis or treatment and study (on average 7.8 mo after diagnosis). Retrospective diet data not necessarily indicative of diets prior to diagnosis. Smoking histories not reported.

APPENDIX TABLE 2   Vitamin C and Head and Neck Cancer

Study	Type/Location	Subject Number and Description	Methods
Brown et al., 1988	Case–control South Carolina	207 cases of *esophageal cancer* (EC) all♂: 74 hospitalized cases and 133 deaths from EC during the period of 1977–1981. 422 controls: 157 hospitalized without cancer and 265 non-cancer related deaths. All subjects were from the same 8 coastal counties in SC. The control group for the mortality study was matched for race, age, residence, and year of death.	There were two studies: a hospital-based case–control in which all patients were interviewed about alcohol, tobacco, and diet (65-item food-frequency questionnaire) medical and dental history, occupation, family health history (with specific reference to cancer), and other demographics. In the second phase, next-of-kin (usually a spouse or close relative) of the cancer and control subjects were interviewed at home.
Franco et al., 1989	Case–control Brazil	232 cases of oral cancer (tongue, gum, floor of the mouth, and other parts of the oral cavity). 464 hospital non-cancer controls, 2/case matched for sex, age (± 5 yr), and trimester of hospital admission. Patients with neoplastic disease and mental disorders were excluded.	All subjects given a 40 to 60 min structured interview by interviewers blinded to case–control status. Information included SES and demographics, general health, environmental and occupational exposure history, tobacco and alcohol use, 20-item food-frequency questionnaire and oral hygiene habits.
Li et al., 1989	Case–control Linxian, China	1244 cases of cancer of the *esophagus or gastric cardia,* ages 35–65 yr. 1314 controls age- and sex-matched from same geographical area.	All subjects given structured interview. Data collected included demographics, occupation, smoking, diet history (72-item food frequency questionnaire), food preparation and storage methods, beverage consumption, anthropometries, and family and personal health history. Questions were referenced to 2 time periods, the late 1950s and the late 1970s.
McLaughlin et al., 1988	Case–control 4 regions: New Jersey; Atlanta, GA; Los Angeles, Santa Clara, and San Mateo in CA.	871 cases of *oral (and pharyngeal) cancer.* 979 population-based controls matched for race (all white) age and sex.	All subjects (or next-of-kin in those cases who were too ill) were given a structured interview to get data on tobacco and alcohol use, diet (61-item food-frequency questionnaire), medical history, occupation, and demographics. Reference period for food was normal intake during adulthood. Intakes were adjusted for seasonal variations in availability. Vitamin supplement usage was collected but did not affect outcomes.
Tuyns et al., 1987a	Case–control France	743 cases (704 males and 39 females) of *esophageal cancer.* 1975 controls from the same geographical region.	All subjects interviewed about usual food intake with a 40-item food-frequency questionnaire. Risk analysis was done for heavy vs light consumers adjusted for age and 2 levels of alcohol and tobacco consumption, and residence (rural vs urban).
Guo et al., 1990	Cross-sectional survey China	Survey of 65 counties in China selected for their high incidence of certain types of cancer. 100 subjects were randomly selected from each county, with equal distributions of ♂ and ♀ grouped into three age brackets: 35–44, 45–54, 55–64.	A fasting 10 mL blood sample was drawn from each subject. Aliquots were formed by pooling plasma samples from individuals in the same age-sex group within each county and stored at −30°C. Red blood cells were similarly aliquoted. Diet data regarding frequency of intake of selected foods was collected at time of blood sample. Nutrients assessed included: plasma vitamin C, β-carotene, α-tocopherol, zinc, selenium, and erythrocyte glutathione reductase (an indicator of riboflavin status).

Results	Comments
After adjustments for smoking and alcohol consumption (the leading risk factors in both studies), significantly increased risks of EC were associated with low intake of fruits, particularly citrus fruits and juices and high intakes of liver. Low vitamin C and fiber intakes were associated with increased risk. High intakes of retinol were associated with higher risk.	No population-based control group or biochemistry. Reliance on retrospective diet data and the use of proxy data in the mortality study. Possibly inappropriate controls in both phases may have lead to conservative estimates of effects. Duration and type of disease in controls may have affected dietary outcomes. Dietary effects may have been secondary to alcohol and tobacco use and/or related diseases.
Significantly reduced risk associated with intake of citrus fruits adjusted for smoking and alcohol (the strongest risk factors irrespective of site). Without adjustment, significantly reduced risk associated with increased consumption of carotene-rich foods (e.g., carrots, pumpkins, and papaya) and citrus fruits. No protection noted for green vegetables in general.	No population-based controls, no biochemistry. Retrospective diet data based on limited (20-item) questionnaire. No data regarding vitamin C specifically.
All subjects consumed a diet low in fruits and vegetables. No association with risk. Low water and high wheat intakes were associated with increased risk.	Not designed to address specific vitamin C relationship with cancer. Not enough variability in intake to assess risk relationship. Strong genetic and or geographical component to risk in this population.
Vitamin C was associated with decreased OR (odds ratios) and risk of oral cancer in men and women. Protective effects were seen for fruit consumption. Highest quartile had 1/2 the risk of lowest. No association with calories, methods of food preservation, or cooking. When derived from fruit, there was a significant protective effect of vitamin C, vitamin A and fiber. This effect was not apparent for vegetable sources of these nutrients. No effect for other vitamins or nutrients.	No biochemistry, reliance of retrospective diet data, no data on time period between diagnosis and participation (cases obtained from a cancer registry). The study not designed to address vitamin C specifically. Mean or median intakes for nutrients not reported.
Higher intakes of vitamin C associated with decreased risk. Significant association between vitamin E intake and relative risk. Higher intakes of several other vitamins (retinol, β-carotene, niacin) also associated with significantly decreased risk. Cases consumed fewer proteins of animal origin and more proteins of vegetable origin and had a higher intake of sugars and starches of vegetable origin. Cases had a lower P:S ratio, oils associated with decreased risk, butter associated with increased risk.	No biochemistry. No control for time between diagnosis and study. No documentation of medications or other treatment. No data on medical or family health history. Hard to determine environmental from genetic effects.
Correlations between county esophageal cancer mortality rates and nutritional data indicated that the strongest association was with plasma vitamin C and dietary fruit consumption. These associations were significant across sexes. Riboflavin status was also inversely related to risk of esophageal cancer but only in ♂. Consumption of moldy pickled vegetables was significantly associated with risk.	No information about the composition of the subject pool. There was no data regarding health status of subjects. Small diet database.

APPENDIX TABLE 3   Vitamin C and Lung Cancer

Study	Type/Location	Subject Number and Description	Methods
Byers et al., 1987	Case–control western New York	450 cases of *lung cancer* (LC) 296♂, 154 ♀ diagnosed between 1980 and 1984. 902 controls matched for sex, age (± 5 yr), and neighborhood of residence. Subjects were white and from the same 3-county area of western N.Y.	A structured interview (c. 2.5 hr) containing information about demographics, occupation, health history, oral health, drug, alcohol, and tobacco use, and occupational exposures was given to all subjects. Interviews occurred typically within 3 mo of diagnosis for cases. Diet history was collected with a modified 129-item food-frequency questionnaire. Subjects were asked to give average frequency of consumption and typical serving size. Reference time for cases was a year before the appearance of symptoms; for controls the period just prior to the interview.
Fontham et al., 1988	Case–control Los Angeles	1253 cases of *lung cancer*. 1274 controls matched for race, sex, and age (± 5 yr) were all admitted to the same hospitals as cases. There were significantly more non-smokers in the control group (31.6% vs. 4.3%).	All subjects were given a questionnaire containing diet and tobacco history, occupational, residential, medical and family health histories. A 59-item food-frequency questionnaire was given with the reference period being before appearance of symptoms. Surrogates were interviewed in both cases (26.7%) and controls (11.5%) when subjects were unable to respond.
Koo et al., 1988	Case–control Hong Kong	88 cases of *lung cancer*. 137 district-matched controls. All subjects were ♀ with no known history of smoking.	All subjects were interviewed for demographic data, including household number, and a food frequency questionnaire. Cases asked about intake 1 yr prior to diagnosis. Controls asked about current intake and were interviewed within 6 wk of matched cases.
LeGardeur et al., 1990	Case–control Los Angeles	59 cases of *lung cancer*. 59 hospital controls (HC) selected in a next-patient-encountered procedure. 31 community controls (CC) subjects were matched for age (± 5 yr), race, county.	LC and HC subjects given a structured interview to obtain data about smoking history and dietary intake (method not described). 20 mL non-fasting venipuncture samples were collected from all subjects. Measures included serum ascorbate, retinol and carotenoids, vitamin E and cholesterol. Assays were done within a month of collection. CC group was not interviewed, only blood was collected.
Le Marchand et al., 1989	Case–control Hawaii	432 cases of *lung cancer* (230♂, 102♀). 865 community controls matched for age and sex. Cases diagnosed over 2-yr period 1983–1985.	All subjects given a structured interview to garner data on smoking and alcohol consumption history. Interviews were done at home with the subject or surrogate (29% for cases, 7% for controls). 130-item food-frequency questionnaire was given to all subjects. The reference period was a usual wk, mo, or yr before onset of symptoms for the patients and a corresponding time period for the controls.

Results	Comments
The age and smoking history (pack-years) adjusted risk analysis showed no difference in vitamin C intake between groups. There was a significantly reduced risk associated with vitamin A (carotene) intake and lower quartiles of fat consumption. The vitamin A association was statistically significant for ♂, for those with squamous cell carcinoma, for light or ex-smokers, and for those >60 yr.	Retrospective food frequency was only source of diet data, no data on supplement use. Much longer period between interview for cases than controls. Mean nutrient data not given. No descriptive statistics (t-tests) given. Health history of controls not reported. No biochemistry.
An inverse association was found between vitamin C intake and specific types of LC (squamous and small cell). A similar, though not as strong, effect was found for vitamin A (carotene). There was a significant inverse relationship between retinol intake and adenocarcinoma in blacks.	Time from diagnosis for either group not given. No community-based control group. Since comparisons were based on tertiles of intakes for control group, there may have been an underestimation of intake and associated risk due to low intakes of hospital controls. No data on supplement use. No descriptive data reported for nutrient intake. No comparisons to intake standards, e.g., RDA. No biochemistry.
Protective effect of high consumption of leafy green vegetables, carrots, tofu, fresh fruit, and fresh fish in cases of adenocarcinoma and large cell cancer. Fresh fruits found to offer protection against squamous cell tumors.	Data analyzed by foods, no analysis for specific nutrients, no biochemistry. Retrospective data, large difference in reference intervals: cases, 1 yr prior to diagnosis, controls, current diet. Conclusions regarding potential protective effects of vitamin C, retinol and calcium are presumptive.
Mean serum levels of carotenoids, vitamin E, and total cholesterol for LC cases were significantly lower than HC. Although reported as not different, HC subjects had significantly lower levels of vitamin C and vitamin E than CC. Cholesterol-adjusted serum levels of vitamin E were still significantly lower in LC cases than HC.	No diet data reported. No questionnaire data for CC group. The CC group was compared to HC group to test for appropriateness of HC as controls for LC group. Text reported no difference. Data in table indicated significant differences in the major dependent variables, vitamins C and E. LC and HC group were not matched for smoking history. In addition the nature of the illnesses (e.g., 20% CHD, 14% metabolic, endocrine, or nutritional disorders) of the HC group also made it an inappropriate control. No comparisons between CC group and LC cases, although the LC cases did have lower levels of vitamins E and C and retinol and carotenoids. Retinol binding protein was significantly associated with all variables except vitamin C; this could reflect a general malnutrition or a metabolic defect. Insufficient data to make appropriate interpretation. Given the inappropriateness of the controls and poor matching, the use of a paired t-test must be questioned. Poorly designed study.
An inverse association between total vitamin C (from food and supplements) in males only. Total vitamin A (food and supplements) was also inversely associated with risk, but not significantly, in ♀. There was an apparent interaction between sex and race for vitamin C. A dose-dependent negative association was found between dietary β-carotene and LC. All vegetables, dark green vegetables, cruciferous vegetables, and tomatoes showed stronger association than β-carotene.	Did not control for ethnic differences in intake. No biochemistry. The authors concluded that the effects associated with vitamin C (resulting from interaction between sex and race) were aberrations that could not be explained by any known biological mechanism and therefore did not explore the vitamin C question further.

144   *Howerde E. Sauberlich*

APPENDIX TABLE 4   Vitamin C and Gastric Cancer

Study	Type/Location	Subject Number and Description	Methods
Boeing and Frentzel-Beyme, 1991	Case–control Germany	142 cases of stomach cancer. 579 controls, either patients or visitors to local hospital. No other details supplied.	Subjects selected from either 3 counties with high incidence or 1 with low incidence. All subjects given an interview about demographics, residential, occupational, medical and smoking histories, water supply, food conservation methods. Reference period for dietary questions was 5 yr prior to onset of a severe disease. No other details about dietary information given.
Buiatti et al., 1989, 1990	Case–control Italy	1016 cases of gastric cancer (GC) histologically confirmed between 6/85 and 12/87. 1159 controls matched for age (5-yr strata) and sex. All subjects chosen from area surrounding the clinical centers involved.	All subjects given a structured interview to garner data about demographics, socioeconomic status, occupational histories, smoking and medical histories, and diet. 146-item food-frequency questionnaire used. Reference period for cases and controls was the 12-mo period 2 yr prior to the interview. 94% of cases were interviewed in hospital, 63% of controls interviewed at home, 30% of controls interviewed at local health department.
Chyou et al., 1990	Case–cohort Hawaii	111 cases of GC. 361 controls. All subjects came from a larger cohort of 8006 American ♂ of Japanese ancestry interviewed from 1965–1968. Cases were identified from 1966–1983.	All subjects from original cohort were interviewed and examined and gave a 24-hr dietary recall which is the source of the data for this report. Recalls were originally used as a food frequency questionnaire; for this report recalls were recoded recording actual items consumed rather than food groups. Relative risk (RR) estimates were adjusted for age at interview and smoking status.
Kono et al., 1988	Case–control Japan	139 cases of newly diagnosed GC. 2574 hospital-based controls (HC). 278 randomly selected community controls (CC). Subjects matched for age and sex.	GC and HC subjects interviewed in hospital, CC at home. Data collected included occupational, smoking, and dietary histories. Reference period for all subjects was the year preceding the interview. GC and HC subjects were interviewed before diagnosis.
You et al., 1988	Case–control China	564 cases of GC. 1131 population-based controls matched for age and sex. Cases identified over a 2.5-yr period.	All subjects given a structured interview to collect data about demographics, medical history, occupation, smoking history, and diet. 85-item food-frequency questionnaire. Reference period "several years prior to the interview (about 1980) and just prior to the Cultural Revolution (1965)." The majority of subjects were interviewed at home (96% cases, 75% controls). Data presented represented 1980 interviews.
Burr et al., 1987	Cross-sectional England and Wales, UK	♂ ages 65–74 yr from 2 towns with differing death rates from stomach cancer (1 high-risk, 1 low-risk compared to relative rates for England and Wales) were compared. Random selection from pools of 4078 in the low-risk town and 2789 eligible ♂ in the high-risk town resulted in samples of 267 and 246 subjects used for comparisons.	Data included items from a standardized questionnaire and anthropometric measures. Blood samples were taken for assessment of ascorbate and pepsinogen. Samples were collected "at least 2 hours after last meal."

Results	Comments
Vitamin C, the type of water supply (well vs public), years of refrigerator use, and type of wood used for smoking meat were associated with risk. Other factors such as smoking, food groups, and alcohol consumption were not considered because "of their uncertain mode of action or the possibility of spurious associations." Use of spruce wood, well water, limited refrigerator use, and low intake of vitamin C were all associated with increased risk for stomach cancer.	Limited data on methods used for collection of dietary data and no description of how the vitamin C intake levels were derived. No biochemical assessment of vitamin C status. Limited description of subjects with no description of duration or stage of disease in cases. The control group contained both hospital patients and visitors (presumably healthy). There was no reference period given for the healthy controls.
In the 1989 report on foods only, there was significantly reduced risk associated with increased intakes of raw vegetables, fresh fruit and citrus fruits. Increased risk with consumption of traditional soups, meat, salted dried fish and a combination of cold cuts and seasoned cheeses. The 1990 report focused on individual nutrients and found risk decreased in proportion to intake of vitamin C, β-carotene, α-tocopherol, and vegetable fat. Vitamin C had the largest geographical gradient with highest consumption in lowest risk areas.	Long time period between reference period and interview. Reliance on retrospective data. No biochemistry. Stage of disease of cases not reported. No descriptive statistics. There was an apparent difference (no statistics) in SES with cases being lower than controls. No means given to compare with known standards of intake, e.g., RDA. Control group diet is of unknown quality.
There were no significant differences in age-adjusted mean nutrient intakes between groups. Cases consumed significantly less vegetables than controls. There was a non-significant difference in fruits (cases < controls, p < 0.07).There was a statistically significant inverse relationship between risk of GC and intake of all vegetables. There was also an inverse relationship between fruit consumption and GC but that failed to reach significance after adjustment for cigarette smoking.	No matching for SES or any other demographic factors. Variable period between interview and diagnosis in cases. No biochemistry. Association with vitamin C is presumptive as study did not assess specific nutrients.
In comparison with both control groups, there was an inverse relationship between intake of fruits and GC. Also, there was decreased risk associated with increased intake of green tea (>10 cups/day).	No controls for SES (except approximate geographic area). No biochemistry. No data on nature of health problems in HC group. Evidence of relationship between vitamin C and GC presumptive as study did not evaluate individual nutrients.
There was a decline in risk of GC with increased consumption of carotene, vitamin C, and calcium which was associated with high intakes of fresh vegetables and fruits.	Very long time between reference period and interview for all subjects. No biochemistry. No descriptive statistics given to indicate mean intakes of nutrients. The control group's intake was of unknown quality.
Plasma ascorbate levels and fruit intake were significantly higher in the low-risk sample. There was no direct relationship between ascorbate levels and the presence of severe atrophic gastritis.	No diet data given. Nature of the food frequency-questionnaire not described. Significant difference between towns in terms of SES. No matching of subjects in terms of smoking, demographics, or health history. Significant difference in gastric surgery incidence and severe atrophic gastritis between towns. Case–control comparison within and between towns might have garnered more useful data.

APPENDIX TABLE 5   Vitamin C and Pancreatic Cancer

Study	Type/Location	Subject Number and Description	Methods
Falk et al., 1988	Case–control Louisiana	363 cases of pancreatic cancer (PC). 1234 hospital-based controls (HC) matched on hospital of admittance, race, sex, and age (± 5 yr).	All subjects were given an interview to obtain data on smoking, occupational and residential history, alcohol use, family health history, medical history, leisure time activities, and diet. A 59-item food-frequency questionnaire was used. The reference period was the time (unspecified) prior to diagnosis or onset of symptoms. >50% of cases were unable to be interviewed personally, necessitating the use of surrogates (next-of-kin, usually a spouse), 13% of controls were unavailable.
Farrow and Davis, 1990	Case–control western Washington	148 married ♂ cases of PC diagnosed between 1982–1986. 188 married ♂ controls randomly selected and frequency matched by age (± 5 yr).	Data from all subjects was collected from surrogates (wives). Two-stage data collection: 1) a telephone interview was used to collect demographic data, medical and occupational history, and use of tobacco, alcohol, coffee, and vitamin supplements, and 2) a dietary questionnaire containing a 135-item food-frequency questionnaire was mailed. Reference period was 3 yr prior to diagnosis.
La Vecchia et al., 1990	Case–control Italy	247 cases of PC. 1089 age- and sex-matched hospital-based controls with acute non-digestive, non-neoplastic disease.	All subjects were given a structured interview to obtain data on SES, smoking, alcohol and coffee intake, medical history, and dietary intake of 14 "indicator foods." Reference period 1 yr prior to treatment.
Mills et al., 1988	Cohort California	Study population was 34,198 non-Hispanic, Seventh-Day Adventists >25 yr of age. 40 cases of death from PC occurring during the follow-up period of 1974–1982.	All subjects completed a lifestyle questionnaire, details of which were not supplied.

Results	Comments
Fruit consumption (fresh and juice) showed a significant inverse relationship with PC. There was a smaller inverse association with vegetable intake.	Control diet of unknown quality used as reference. No descriptive data reported nor comparisons of diet to reference standard, i.e., RDA.
Risks associated with consumption of fruits and with an index of vitamin C showed significant decreasing gradients across sexes. Cigarette smoking was a strong risk factor for PC.	No community-based control group. Unknown time period between time of interview and diagnosis and/or onset of symptoms. Controls' diet response reflective of recent intake patterns. No data on supplement use. No biochemistry. No testing for the potential interaction between smoking and vitamin C index or fruit consumption.
No association between PC risk and intake of vitamin C or total fat, saturated fat, cholesterol, ω-3 fatty acids, or vitamin A.	Reliability and validity of data acquisition is questionable. Reliance on retrospective data collected from surrogates. Reference period was 3 yr prior to interview.
Statistically significant decreased risk with increased intake of fresh fruits. Similar inverse relationship between risk and intake of fish and oil (uncharacterized).	No biochemistry, long period between reference period and interview, no adjustment in analysis or matching for SES or other confounding variables, i.e., smoking. No descriptive data. No community-based control or comparisons to reference standards of normal intake. Vitamin C effect would be presumptive. No assessment of individual nutrients.
Current use of meat, poultry, or fish was associated with increasing risk. There was a significant increase in risk associated with increasing consumption of eggs. Intake of vegetarian protein products, legumes, and dried fruits were significantly inversely related to risk. No relationship between risk and intake of other fresh fruit, canned or frozen fruit, fresh citrus fruit, fresh winter fruit, green salads, or cooked green vegetables. These results were age- and sex-adjusted.	Problems include no comparison group, no data on quality of diet, no details on diet data, no data on individual nutrients, no data on supplement use, no biochemistry, and no demographics.

APPENDIX TABLE 6 Vitamin C and Colorectal Cancer

Study	Type/Location	Subject Number and Description	Methods
DeCosse et al., 1989.	Intervention-randomized double-blind, placebo-controlled. New York, NY	58 patients with *familial adenomatous polyposis* drawn from an initial pool of 72 who had total colectomy and ileorectal anastomosis 1 yr prior to the study.	Control group got 8 caps placebo (lactose)/d + 2.2 g of low fiber. Vitamin group got 4 g vitamin C/d + 400 mg vitamin E/d + 2.2 g of low fiber. Fiber group got both vitamins + 22.5 g of high fiber/d. All subjects had a 3-mo placebo period, 4-yr trial. All groups received 30 mg vitamin C, 2,000 IU vitamin A and equivalent amounts of several other vitamins and minerals (about 30% RDA). Patients had 18 examinations over test period. Each completed a 3-d diet diary prior to each visit. Subjects also completed a food-frequency questionnaire at each visit.
Freudenheim et al., 1990	Case–control New York	422 cases of *rectal cancer* (277♂, 145♀) 422 sex-, race-, age- (± 5 yr), neighborhood-matched controls.	Subjects given a 2.5 hr interview consisting of food-frequency questionnaire covering the previous yr for controls and for cases a yr prior to the onset of symptoms. Additional information included smoking and alcohol use, occupational and health histories, seasonality of intake, preparation, and food storage.
Graham et al., 1988	Case–control New York	428 cases of colon cancer (CC). 428 controls matched for age, sex, and neighborhood.	All subjects given a structured 2.5 hr interview similar to that used by Freudenheim et al. (1990). No reference period was noted for the diet data. No surrogates were used.
La Vecchia et al., 1988	Case–control Italy	339 cases of colon cancer (CC). 236 cases of rectal cancer (RC). 778 hospital controls admitted for acute, non-neoplastic, or digestive disorders.	All subjects given a questionnaire to obtain data on SES, smoking, alcohol, coffee and other methylxanthine-containing drinks, personal and family health history, and use of selected drugs. 29-item food-frequency questionnaire. Reference period was an unspecified period before current hospital admission. Subjects also asked to report changes over previous 10 yr.
McKeown-Eyssen et al., 1988	Intervention (randomized double-blind trial) Toronto, Canada	185 cases with at least 1 polyp in the colon or rectum. 96 received vitamins. 89 received placebo. All subjects were presumed to be polyp-free at start of the trial.	Subjects completed questionnaire containing a limited (9-item) food-frequency questionnaire, demographic data, smoking status, bowel habits, previous polyp history, and vitamin supplement use. Subjects randomized to receive 400 mg vitamin E and C or lactose placebo over 2-yr period and re-examined (blinded). Random urine samples were collected to test for compliance. The two groups were matched for all parameters except that the vitamin group had more members who used vitamin C supplements prior to trial.
Neugut et al., 1988	Cross–sectional New York	244 ♀ who had undergone colonoscopy. 105 cases of polyps. 56 cases of colon cancer. 83 ♀ without colonic neoplasia.	All subjects were given a structured telephone interview. Information garnered included demographics, SES factors, lifestyle, personal and family health history, and reproductive history. Subjects were asked about use of multivitamins and individual vitamin supplements (A, C, E).

Results	Comments
Subject groups were comparable in demographics, median time since colectomy, median intake of fiber at baseline, and prior supplementation with vitamins C and E. There were no discernible effects for the vitamins. The high-fiber group had the stronger benefit especially during the middle years of the trial. Compliance for all groups decreased over the course of the trial.	No blood levels of the vitamins were reported for baseline or during the trial. No data of dietary vitamin intakes at baseline or during trial were reported. Because of combined use of vitamins, an analysis of independent effects or interactions of individual vitamins was not possible.
Decreased risk with increasing intake of carotenoids, vitamin C and dietary fiber from vegetables. No association between intake of vitamin E and risk. Increased risk with increasing intakes of calories, fat, carbohydrate, and iron.	Reliance on retrospective food-frequency interviews. No data on use of supplements or stage of disease (except that "only relatively alert, healthy subjects could tolerate the 2.5 hr. interview"). Well-conceived study.
No significant risks associated with intake of protein, vitamin A from vegetables and fruits, carbohydrates, vitamin C, cruciferous vegetables, calcium, or phosphorous. There was significantly reduced risk associated with high intakes of tomatoes, peppers, carrots, onions, and celery. Risk of CC was positively associated with increasing intake of total fats (predominantly animal fat) and total calories.	No reference period for food-frequency questionnaire given. No data on supplement use.
Risk of both CC and RC was inversely related to intake of green vegetables, tomatoes, melon, and coffee. There was also an inverse relationship between risk and indices of carotenoid and vitamin C intake. Consumption of pasta and rice associated with increased risk of both cancers.	No supplement data, variable reference times for cases and controls, no population-based control. Diet database was small (only 29 items). Individual nutrient estimation unreliable due to lack of portion size information. No biochemistry. No descriptive data or comparisons with normal standards of intake.
There were no differences in food frequency items. 137 subjects (75%) completed the trial. Polyps found in 41.4% of vitamin group and 50.7% of placebo.	No biochemical data either at baseline or after trial. Insufficient power due to small sample size. Because of the design, the study could not distinguish differences in effect of individual vitamins.
Significant differences in SES factors, e.g., education, between CC group and either of the others. Use of any vitamins in the 3 groups were 49% of CC compared to 61 and 59% of the other 2. This was not statistically significant.	No data on amount of supplement, current or past diet, or duration of supplement use. Reference period was after surgical procedure. No appropriate control group.

(*continued*)

APPENDIX TABLE 6   (*continued*)

Study	Type/Location	Subject Number and Description	Methods
Tuyns et al., 1987b	Case–control Belgium	453 cases of colon cancer (CC). 365 cases of rectal cancer (RC). 2851 controls. All subjects were from same 2 provinces and adjusted for age and sex.	All subjects interviewed about diet using food frequency questionnaire. Reference period for cases 1 wk period prior to onset of disease, controls current intake. Portion sizes were estimated using food models (pictures). Cases interviewed in hospital, controls at home.
West et al., 1989	Case–control Utah	231 cases of newly (within 6 mo) diagnosed colon cancer (CC). 391 controls matched by age (± 5 yr), sex, and county of residence.	All subjects were interviewed in their homes. Questionnaire consisted of demographic, health history, current height and weight (2 yr before interview), computed body-mass index, physical activity, and dietary data. 99-item food-frequency questionnaire. Reference period was "2–3 years prior to the interview." Portion sizes were estimated with food models.

Results	Comments
No association between risk for either CC or RC and vitamin C intake. Positive associations were found for retinol, oligosaccharides. Negative associations for fiber, linoleic acid, thiamine, and iron.	Retrospective data collection. Differences in reference period between controls and cases. Group differences by province and sex. No biochemistry, supplementation data, descriptive data on intake, demographics, smoking, alcohol, medical histories, or comparisons to normal standards for intake.
No association between CC risk and intake of vitamin C. Protective effects of β-carotene and cruciferous vegetables in ♂; fiber was protective in ♀.	Unknown relationship between reference period and time of diagnosis in cases. No biochemistry, comparisons to intake standards or descriptive statistics. No data for SES, or alcohol, smoking, or supplement history.

APPENDIX TABLE 7   Vitamin C and Prostate Cancer

Study	Type/Location	Subject Number and Description	Methods
Kolonel et al., 1988	Case–control Hawaii	452 cases of histologically confirmed prostatic cancer (PC). 899 age-matched controls. Subjects > 65 yr were randomly selected from a central insurance registry, those < 65 yr selected with random-digit-dialing.	All subjects were given an extensive home interview to collect data on dietary, occupational, medical, social, and demographic histories. Food-frequency questionnaire (100+ items) was used. Reference period was a usual mo prior to onset of the disease for cases and a corresponding period for controls. Surrogates were used for those subjects who could not be interviewed.
Ohno et al., 1988 Oishi et al., 1988	Case–control Japan	100 cases newly diagnosed of prostatic cancer (PC). 100 controls with benign prostatic hyperplasia (BPH). 100 hospital controls without BPH, other malignancies, liver disease, or hormonal disorders. All subjects were matched for hospital, age (± 3 yr) and date of admission (± 3 mo).	Data collected by interview upon admission to hospital included birthplace, occupational history, marital history, religion, body type, medical history, sex-life, and dietary practices. Food-frequency questionnaire assessed dietary habits during the period 5 yr prior to current admission.

Results	Comments
There were no associations between risk and either total or food sources of vitamin C. No differences found in potential confounding variables: SES, marital status, anthropometries, or family history. Older cases consumed significantly more saturated fat, total vitamin A, and zinc than age-matched controls. These differences were reflected in increased risk associated with saturated fat and zinc. No differences in younger subjects.	Total vitamin C (food + supplements) intakes ranged from 2500–3000 mg/wk across all groups. This is a well-designed and executed study.
Intake of vitamin C from foods was not significantly associated with PC risk. Low intakes of vitamin A (retinol and β-carotene) were associated with increased risk. The risk reduction associated with vitamin A and β-carotene was seen in older but not younger ♂.	No supplement data, confusing statistics, lack of community-based control. Long retrospective period, 5 yr. No smoking data.

APPENDIX TABLE 8   Vitamin C and Cervical/Ovarian Cancer

Study	Type/Location	Subject Number and Description	Methods
Brock et al., 1988	Case–control Australia	117 cases of cervical cancer. 196 controls matched for SES, age (± 5 yr). 100 of the interviewed cases and 143 of the controls agreed to blood sampling.	All subjects interviewed either at home or at work. Cases interviewed within 6 mo of diagnosis. Questioned on demographics, reproductive, contraceptive, and gynecological factors. 160-item food-frequency questionnaire with an emphasis on vitamins A, C, and folate. Blood collected after an overnight fast and assessed for β-carotene, retinol, and other carotenes with HPLC methods.
Shu et al., 1989	Case–control Shanghai, China	172 cases of epithelial ovarian cancer. 172 controls matched for age (± 5 yr), residence.	All subjects interviewed about demographics, reproductive history, personal and family health histories, occupational history, and diet. 63-item food-frequency questionnaire.
Slattery et al., 1989	Case–control Utah	85 cases of primary ovarian cancer. 492 population-based controls matched for age.	All subjects interviewed in person at home by ♀. Data collected included demographics, smoking history, medical history, contraceptive use, pregnancy history, and anthropometries. 183-item food-frequency questionnaire used to obtain usual adult dietary habits. No reference period given.
Verreault et al., 1989	Case–control Washington (state)	189 cases of cervical cancer. 227 controls, age-matched and identified by random-digit-dialing methods.	All subjects were given a telephone interview by a female interviewer to collect data on demographics, reproductive history, contraceptive methods, smoking history, anthropometries (self-reported), health history, and sexual habits. 66-item food-frequency questionnaire included vitamin supplement use. Reference period was the year prior to a reference date (date of diagnosis for cases and Dec. 31, 1981 for controls).
Ziegler et al., 1990	Case–control Cross-sectional multicenter study: Chicago, IL, Birmingham, AL, Denver, CO, Miami, FL, Philadelphia, PA	271 cases of cervical cancer. 502 controls matched by age, race, and telephone exchange. All subjects were white, non-Hispanic.	All subjects interviewed at home. Data collected included demographics, sexual behavior, reproductive and menstrual history, use of contraceptives and female hormones, personal and family health history, smoking habits, and diet. 75-item food-frequency questionnaire about usual adult intake of foods and vitamin supplements. Subjects asked about number of servings per d, wk, mo, or yr.

Results	Comments
Cases were not matched on sexual habits, smoking, or use of oral contraceptives. Crude risk estimates showed a significant protective effect from carotene, vitamin C, and folate. After adjustment for known risk factors the protective trends for all except vitamin C (p < 0.07) disappeared. When considered together, vitamin C, fruit juices, and plasma β-carotene showed a significant protective effect. Fruits did not show a protective effect.	No data on amount or type of supplements used nor were any comparisons made with regard to dietary intake or blood levels. No vitamin C biochemistry. Blood sampling of cases may have reflected state vs trait phenomena.
No effect of dietary vitamin C. Significantly increased risk associated with total and saturated fat.	No time frame between interview and diagnosis given; no reference period given for cases. No biochemistry, no supplement data, no descriptive statistics or comparisons to known standards of intake. Groups were not matched for SES, cases were more educated.
No effect of vitamin C. Small non-significant decrease in risk associated with vitamins A, C, and fiber. Adjusted risk reduced for high intakes of β-carotene.	Used nutrient analysis rather than food groups. No supplement data. Low response rate in cases.
Decreased risk associated with high intakes of vitamin C. After adjustment for known risk factors, increased intakes of dark green or yellow vegetables and fruit juices were associated with significantly reduced risk.	No portion sizes given on food-frequency questionnaire; portion sizes estimated from food composition tables. No biochemistry. Use of a long retrospective period; the average delay between interview and reference period was 2.8 yr for cases and 2.7 yr for controls.
No effect of either vitamin C or vitamin C-rich foods or any other foods or nutrients.	No reference period relative to onset of symptoms or diagnosis in cases. Cases were histologically confirmed during period 4/82–12/83.

APPENDIX TABLE 9   Vitamin C and Other Cancers

Study	Type/Location	Subject Number and Description	Methods
La Vecchia et al., 1989	Case–control northern Italy	163 cases of *bladder cancer* histologically confirmed within 1 yr before interview (total pool eligible not given). 181 hospital controls (HC).	All subjects given interview to obtain information about SES factors, smoking, alcohol, coffee and other methylxanthine consumption habits, personal and family health history, and specific medication history. Subjects were asked about frequency of consumption of 10 food items. Reference period for cases was the period before onset of symptoms; none was given for controls.
Stähelin et al., 1989	Prospective cohort study Basel, Switzerland	2975 ♂ comprised the original pool from which 102 total cancer deaths occurred (37 lung cancer, 17 stomach cancer, 9 colorectal cancer, and 39 cancers at "other sites").	Samples were collected over a 2-yr period (1971–1973). Analysis was done immediately.

Results	Comments
No effect from either fruit or vitamin C. The frequency of consumption of green vegetables and carrots was lower in cases; increased risk for BC associated with low intake. Protective effect was stronger in current smokers.	Reference period was at least 2 yr before interview for cases. Very limited number of items (10) on food-frequency questionnaire. No supplement use data.
After adjustment for smoking, blood vitamin C was significantly lower in stomach cancer deaths.	No diet data, no supplement data, and no control for seasonal variations in diet that might influence blood vitamin levels. Reliance on point-sample procedure.

Vitamin C and Cancer: An Update

Howerde E. Sauberlich, Ph.D.

Subsequent to the preparation of the above manuscript, additional cancer studies became available. These reports are briefly summarized by cancer site and supplement the information previously presented.

A. Breast Cancer

Several additional reports have been made on breast cancer and diet in populations outside of the U.S. Zaridze et al. (1991) conducted a case–control study on the effect of diet on risk of breast cancer in women from Moscow. The study involved 139 case–control pairs matched by age and neighborhood. Dietary information was obtained with the use of a food frequency questionnaire that incorporated 145 food items. Blood samples were not obtained for analysis of nutrients.

An increase in risk of breast cancer was associated with high intakes of fat and animal products and a lower risk with high intakes of vegetables and fruits. The effects of diet appeared to be more important for the risk of breast cancer in postmenopausal than for premenopausal women. Although the dietary information was limited, data evaluations indicated a decreased risk of postmenopausal breast cancer with high intakes of β-carotene (odds ratio [OR] = 0.09) and vitamin C (OR = 0.20).

Richardson and associates (1991) investigated the role of diet on breast cancer in women from Montpelier, France. The case–control study involved 409 cases and 515 controls and was designed to study specifically the role of dietary fat, animal protein and vitamin intake. Dietary information was obtained by interviews and use of a food frequency questionnaire that covered 55 food items. Although information was provided on retinol, β-carotene and vitamin E intakes, data on vitamin C intakes were not presented. No evidence was obtained of a risk reduction with increased consumption of vegetables, vitamin E or β-carotene. Evidence was presented, however, of a positive association between dietary fat and breast cancer. This association was particularly evident with an increased intake of saturated fat in postmenopausal women.

Morales and Llopis (1992) conducted an epidemiological study during the period of 1977–1985 on the role of diet and breast cancer in Spain. Breast cancer has increased from 15 to 21 cases per 100,000 inhabitants within the last several years. Data relating to food consumption and nutrients were obtained from family surveys for the years 1980 and 1981. Limited dietary information was provided, and of the vitamins, only vitamin C was considered. Although information was included on the mortality and morbidity rates for the 50 Spanish provinces, correlations of diet with these rates were not provided. Nevertheless, without supporting data, the investigators stated that the correlations were low. They also indicated that the most significant correlations were with increased mortality with an increased total lipid intake. Higher intakes of vitamin C were associated with lower mortality rates.

Although some investigators consider fibroadenoma of the breasts as a benign breast disease, others have found the risk of breast cancer was increased two- to sevenfold among women with fibroadenoma. Yu et al. (1992) examined risk factors for fibroadenoma in a case–control study conducted in Adelaide, Australia, between the period of January 1983 and

October 1985. For the study, 117 confirmed fibroadenoma cases participated. Two control groups were selected for the study. One group was a matched population control. The other group was an unmatched biopsy control group of 189 women. Their first biopsy for benign breast disease was performed in the same laboratory during the same time period as those of the cases, but did not show evidence of epithelia proliferation. Food intake information was obtained from a self-administered food frequency questionnaire that listed 179 food items.

From the results of the study, it was concluded that an increased consumption of vitamin C was associated with a decreased risk of fibroadenoma (OR = 0.5; 95 percent confidence interval [CI] = 0.2–1.1). However, plasma levels of vitamin C that could have helped substantiate these findings were not determined. Intakes of other nutrients examined did not appear to be associated with an altered risk of fibroadenoma (e.g., vitamin A, β-carotene, fat, alcohol).

B. Esophageal and Oral Cancers

The incidence and mortality rates for oral and pharyngeal cancer among black men in the U.S. have risen over the past decade. Gridley et al. (1990) investigated the influence of diet in oral and pharyngeal cancer among blacks. The case–control study consisted of 190 cases (142 male and 48 female) and 201 controls (139 male and 62 female). The cases were diagnosed during the period of January 1, 1984–March 31, 1985. The cases were obtained from population-based cancer registries of New Jersey, Atlanta, Los Angeles and Santa Clara and San Mateo counties of California. Controls were selected by using random-digit-dialing and were matched based on sex and age. Dietary information was obtained with the use of a food frequency questionnaire that contained 61 food items.

In men, an increased consumption of fruit, vegetables and fish was associated with a decreased risk of oral cancer. The consumption of fruits had an OR of 0.2 (p = 0.006). For calculated nutrient intakes, an increased intake of carotene, vitamin C and dietary fiber was associated with significantly reduced risks among men. The OR for vitamin C was 0.3 (p = 0.004), for carotene 0.2 (p = 0.001), and for fiber 0.3 (p = 0.001). For women, an increased intake of vitamin C and fiber was associated with a nonsignificant reduced risk. No blood specimens were obtained for the measurement of plasma vitamin C and other nutrients. Although diet may influence the risk of oral and pharyngeal cancer, tobacco and alcohol were the strongest risk factors for both men and women. The OR for combined tobacco and alcohol use were by quartile 1.0, 2.2, 4.2 and 19.6.

Freudenheim et al. (1992) conducted a case–control study among white men in western New York during the period of 1975–1985 to examine diet and other risk factors for laryngeal cancer. Although 938 eligible white cases were identified, only 250 men were successfully studied. The high percentage of refusals to participate may have introduced a bias to the study. An equal number of controls were matched to cases based on race, sex, age and neighborhood. An in-depth food frequency questionnaire was used to obtain diet information. Data were also obtained on tobacco usage and alcohol consumption.

Smoking was found to be the overwhelming risk factor for laryngeal cancer. The increase in risk among the heaviest smokers was 12-fold. No relationship was observed between laryngeal cancer and vitamin C, vitamin E or dietary fiber. A reduced risk was associated with the highest intake levels of carotenoids. Plasma levels of these nutrients were not measured.

Zheng and associates (1993) conducted a nested case–control study to investigate the relationship between serum micronutrients and the subsequent risk of oral and pharyngeal cancer. A cohort of 25802 adults from Washington County, Maryland, volunteered blood samples in 1974. Of these volunteers, 28 developed oral and pharyngeal cancer during the period 1975–1990. Serum levels of β-carotene were lower among the individuals who developed oral and pharyngeal cancer than levels in 112 matched controls. High levels of α-tocopherol were associated with a lower risk of oral cancer. Unfortunately plasma analyses for vitamin C were not included in the study.

C. Lung Cancer

Jain et al. (1990) investigated associations between dietary factors and risk of lung cancer in an equal number of men and women of metropolitan Toronto between 1981 and 1985. For the case–control study, 839 cases with diagnosed lung cancer and 772 population-based controls were interviewed to obtain demographic and dietary information. From the diet history, estimates of average daily intake of nutrients were calculated. An increased consumption of vegetables was associated with a decreased relative risk (RR) of 0.60 (95% confidence limits = 0.40 to 0.88) for those in the highest compared with the lowest quartile. However, no consistent protective effect was observed with vitamin C, vitamin A or β-carotene.

Chow and colleagues (1992) reported on a cohort study of diet, tobacco use and occupation on lung cancer mortality. In 1966, 17633 U.S. white males aged 35 years and over completed a mail questionnaire that covered tobacco use, occupation and frequency of consumption of 35 food items. Nutrient intakes were calculated with the use of U.S. Department of Agriculture food consumption data.

By 1986, 219 lung cancer deaths had occurred in the subjects under study. Cigarette smoking was strongly associated with lung cancer deaths. A mild reduction in risk of lung cancer was associated with higher intakes of fruits and lesser reductions in risk for cruciferous vegetables. Intake of vitamin C was associated with a reduced risk of lung cancer death. Dietary intake of vitamin A and carotenoids had a variable association with reduced risk of lung cancer. However, overall the trends for reduced risk with these associations were not consistent and did not reach statistical significance. Limitations existed in the dietary intake information as the questionnaire used failed to include various food items rich in vitamin C and vitamin A.

D. Gastric Cancer

A number of additional studies on gastric cancer are presented in this addendum. Bulatti et al. (1991) conducted an extensive case–control study of gastric cancer in high risk areas of Italy. For this study, 923 gastric cancer cases were classified by histologic examination as intestinal type and diffuse type. Interviews were conducted with 1016 gastric cancer patients first diagnosed between June 1985 and December 1987 along with 1159 comparable controls. Dietary information was obtained with the use of a food frequency questionnaire designed to reflect the Italian food consumption pattern. The average intake of nutrients was computed with the use of Italian and English food tables.

Similar risk patterns were observed for intestinal and diffuse types of gastric cancer. For both types there were increased risks associated with a high intake of meat, salted dried fish, seasoned cheeses and traditional soups. Heavy consumption of fresh vegetables and fruits was associated with a reduced risk of both types of cancer. Based on calculated intakes, an increased consumption of vitamin C (OR = 0.5) and vitamin E (OR = 0.5) was associated with a decrease in both types of gastric cancer. Plasma levels of these two vitamins were not measured. The level of intake of β-carotene appeared to have little or no effect.

The gastric cancer patients studied by Bulatti et al. (1991) were evaluated further by Palli and co-workers (1992). The same 923 case–control gastric cancer patients were classified according to anatomic site. Sixty-eight (7.4 percent) of the cancers occurred in the gastric cardia. As with other gastric cancers, cardia tumors showed a decreased risk of occurrence with increased consumption of raw vegetables, citrus and other fresh fruit and vitamin C. When comparing the highest intake of ascorbic acid to the lowest intake of ascorbic acid, the OR for cardia cancer was 0.3 (95 percent CI = 0.2–0.8). Alpha-tocopherol intake had a lower protective effect (OR = 0.8) than ascorbic acid, while increased intakes of β-carotene failed to provide any protective effect.

Boeing et al. (1991) conducted additional studies on the stomach cancer population investigated by Boeing and Frentzel-Beyme (1991). These reports were based on a multicenter hospital-based case–control study performed during 1985–1987 in a high-risk and a low-risk area for stomach cancer in Germany. The findings were based on retrospective interviews on life-style aspects of 143 patients with incident stomach cancer and 579 controls. Cases and controls were almost equally divided between men and women. Dietary information was obtained with the use of a lengthy questionnaire. Individual nutrient intakes were derived from the German food composition table. The information presented in this report was based on the same study reported by Boeing and Frentzel-Beyme (1991). Consequently the conclusions were essentially the same.

After adjustment for other food constituents, only an increased intake of vitamin C provided a reduced risk of stomach cancer. The RR for the highest intake of vitamin C was 0.37. Carotene intake did appear to influence the risk of stomach cancer. Consumption of processed meat appeared to be associated with an increased risk of stomach cancer (RR = 2.21 at highest level of consumption). No information was provided on the intake of vitamin E, an anti-oxidant that may protect against stomach cancer.

Stomach cancer is the leading cause of cancer mortality in China, with areas of high mortality rates in west-central, northeastern and coastal areas while low rates exist in the south. The occurrence of stomach cancer in males is twice that of females. Kneller et al. (1992) reported on an ecological survey based on cancer mortality rates in 65 counties in China during the period of 1973–1975. From each of these selected counties, two townships were randomly selected. For each township an age- and sex-stratified sample of 100 residents (35–64 years of age) was chosen. Dietary and demographic information was obtained with the use of a questionnaire. Blood samples were collected on each subject and pooled on a sex- and township-specific basis. Hence, analyses on an individual basis was not possible. Analyses performed on the pooled plasma samples included selenium, vitamin C, β-carotene, and α-tocopherol.

Consumption of green vegetables was associated with a reduced mortality from stomach cancer. Counties in the lowest consumption quartile for green vegetables had cumulative mortality rates 2.3 and 1.9 times higher among men and women, respectively, compared to counties in the highest consumption quartile. In contrast, salt-preserved vegetables correlated with significantly increased mortality. Increased plasma levels of selenium were associated with a significant protective effect. For men, vitamin C showed a protect effect, while β-carotene had a borderline protective association. Information was not provided as to the actual intakes of the nutrients, but rather the data were presented as Pearson correlation coefficients or regression coefficients. Hence, the actual intake of vitamin C and other nutrients or the plasma concentrations of the nutrients could not evaluated as to the levels of intake required to impart the associated reduced risks of stomach cancer. Moreover, fruit consumption was low in most of the counties studied which may indicate an overall low intake of vitamin C. Green vegetables were probably the major source for vitamin C as well as for carotenes and α-tocopherol. Furthermore, it must be recognized that this was an ecological study that utilized data from pooled plasma samples rather than individual data. Of interest, *Helicobacter pylori* infection was associated with an elevated risk of stomach cancer, but not at a significant degree (p = 0.26).

E. Pancreatic Cancer

Recently increased attention has been given to the role of diet in the development of pancreatic cancer. Thus, Bueno de Mesquita et al. (1991) conducted during 1984–1988 a population-based case–control study in The Netherlands to investigate the role of diet in exocrine pancreatic carcinoma. A dietary questionnaire provided information on the usual diet 1 year prior to the diagnosis of the 164 pancreatic cancer cases. Interviews were also conducted on 480 general population controls who lived in the area of the cases studied.

Compared to the controls, the cases reported significantly lower mean daily consumption of vegetables, fiber and cruciferous vegetables. Thirty to forty percent of the cases and controls reported no consumption of tomatoes, fruit juices or cooked fruits. Based on the estimated intakes, vitamin C had no apparent effect on the risk of pancreatic cancer in men (OR = 1.06; 95 percent CI 0.58–1.94), but in women, a significant inverse association was observed (OR = 0.47; 95 percent CI 0.22–0.98). This effect was supported by the inverse association also noted for the consumption of fresh fruits and noncitrus fruits. Despite the inadequate dietary intake data and the lack of biochemical measurements, the study suggests an association of diet with the risk of pancreatic cancer.

Zatonski et al. (1991) reported on a case–control study conducted in southwest Poland on the association of diet with pancreatic cancer. The study was conducted between 1985 and 1988 and involved 110 cases and 195 controls from the Opole Vlovodeship region of Poland. Dietary data were obtained by trained interviewers using a questionnaire that included 80 food items. The data from the diet history were converted into estimated daily intakes for various nutrients, including vitamins A, C and E and fiber.

The study revealed an inverse association with vitamin C intake with relative risks of 1.10, 0.30 and 0.37 for the upper quartiles of intake compared with the lowest (p = < 0.01). A strong positive association was observed with the intake of cholesterol with RR of 1.90, 3.77 and 4.31 for the three upper quartiles compared with the lowest (p = 0.01). Only weak inverse associations were noted for fiber and vitamin A. Vitamin E was apparently without effect. Overall the results of the study supports the potential importance of dietary factors in the cause of pancreatic cancer.

In Canada, pancreatic cancer ranks fourth among causes of death from cancer in both sexes. Ghadirian and associates (1991) conducted a population-based case–control study of dietary risk factors for pancreatic cancer. During 1984–1988, 179 cases (97 males and 82 females in the Greater Montreal area) with a clinical or histological diagnosis of cancer of the pancreas were studied. A total of 239 population-based control subjects (123 males and 116 females) were interviewed. All of the information used was obtained by intensive interviews with the use of a demographic questionnaire and a detailed food frequency history questionnaire. An average of 2.5 hours was spent completing an interview.

The results indicated an increased risk of pancreatic cancer with an increased intake of fat. The OR for the highest quartile of intake to the lowest quartile was 2.24 (95 percent CI = 0.74–6.73). The risk of pancreatic cancer appeared to increase with increasing intake of cholesterol. A reduced OR was associated with an increased intake of vitamin C, but the reduction was not statistically significant. The mean daily intake of vitamin C was calculated to be 150 mg for the cases and 192 mg for the controls. In general, the results of the study indicate a role for nutritional factors in the cause of pancreatic cancer.

In Australia, cancer of the pancreas accounts for nearly 5 percent of all deaths due to cancer. Baghurst et al. (1991) reported on a population-based case–control study conducted in Adelaide, South Australia, to investigate associations of diet with pancreatic cancer. The study, conducted in 1984–1987, included 104 cases of cancer of the pancreas and 253 community controls. An equal number of males and females was studied. A quantitative food frequency questionnaire was used to obtain information about the usual food and nutrient intake of the cases approximately 12 months prior to diagnosis of cancer. The questionnaire contained a list of 179 foods.

Fruits and several vegetables were consumed more by the controls than by the cases. Comparing the lowest quartile of intake of cholesterol to the highest quartile of intake, an RR of 3.19 was observed (95 percent CI = 1.58–6.47; p = 0.0002). The risk of pancreatic cancer was decreased with an increased intake of vitamin C, β-carotene and vitamin E. For vitamin C, the RR for the highest quartile of intake compared to the lowest intake was 0.46 (95 percent CI = 0.23–0.94; p = 0.025). The study suggests that several anti-oxidant nutrients in the diet may participate in minimizing the risk of cancer of the pancreas.

The role of dietary factors in the etiology of pancreatic cancer also was assessed by Olsen et al. (1991). For this purpose, a case–control study was conducted in Minneapolis–St. Paul, Minnesota area. The cases represented 212 white males aged 40–84 years whose death certificate listed pancreatic cancer (exocrine only). White male controls (n = 212) were selected through random digit telephone dialing. Dietary information was obtained on the diet of the subjects 2 years prior to their death from family members. Similar information was obtained from the controls. A food frequency questionnaire designed specifically for the study was used.

A reduced risk of pancreatic cancer was associated with increased intakes of vitamin C and β-carotene. Significant negative trends (p < 0.05) were observed. Although the protective effects observed were not impressive, the study provides further evidence that diet may have a role in the prevention of pancreatic cancer.

Howe et al. (1992) reported on the combined results of five simultaneous population-based case–control studies of pancreatic cancer and diet. Reports have been previously published on several of the individual populations. The combined report represents findings on pancreatic cancer risk and diet on populations in Adelaide (Australia), Montreal and Toronto (Canada), Utrecht (The Netherlands), and Opole (Poland). The five studies were conducted simultaneously with the use of a common study protocol, and ascertained the usual dietary intake in study subjects, using a comprehensive diet history. Particular attention was given to intakes of carbohydrates, cholesterol, retinol, fruits, vegetables, fiber, β-carotene and vitamin C. The combined study provided dietary histories for 802 cases and 1669 controls. The data from the dietary questionnaire were converted to estimated daily intakes of various nutrients using food composition tables specific to the country in which the study had been conducted.

A consistent positive association was the increased risk of pancreatic cancer with an increased intake of cholesterol and carbohydrates. The RR for the highest versus lowest quintile of intake of cholesterol was 2.68 (95 percent CI = 1.72–4.17). In contrast, a consistent inverse relationship existed for dietary fiber and vitamin C. The RR for the highest versus the lowest quintile of intake of vitamin C was 0.53 (95 percent CI = 0.38–0.76; p = 0.0007). Sources of vitamin C in the diet were not provided, although it was indicated that this aspect would be considered in another report. The results of this case–control study provide strong support to the hypothesis that dietary factors may alter the risk of pancreatic cancer. Particularly noteworthy was the consistency and strength of the association of vitamin C with a reduced risk of pancreatic cancer.

F. Colorectal Cancer

Chinese Americans have colorectal rates 4–7 times greater than rates among the general population in the People's Republic of China. In order provide answers to these differences, Whittemore et al. (1990) conducted a population-based case-control study of colorectal cancer among Chinese men and women in western North America and the People's Republic of China (China). With the use of a common protocol, past lifestyle characteristics were studied in 905 cases (432 from China; 473 from Los Angeles, San Francisco and Vancouver) of colorectal cancer diagnosed during 1981–1986, and on 2488 controls. Dietary information was obtained with the use of a diet history questionnaire that included 84 food items with some modifications to reflect foods consumed in China.

The study focused on the intake of fat in the diet. Colorectal cancer risk was significantly associated with an increased intake of saturated fat. No mention was given to any association with vitamin C. Noted, however, were the statistically significant trends of decreased colorectal cancer risk associated with an increased consumption of vegetables among Chinese-American men and women (p < 0.001) and among men in China (p = 0.02). Frequency of fruit consumption was not associated with a decreased risk of colorectal cancer. This would suggest that vitamin C provides no protection against colorectal cancer.

Trock et al. (1990) reviewed the results of epidemiologic studies that were conducted from 1970 through 1988 concerning colorectal cancer and components in the diet, including fruit, grains, fiber and vegetables. The review considered 23 case–control studies, seven international correlation studies, eight within-county correlation studies, two cohort studies and three time–trend studies. The evaluations of these epidemiologic studies provide considerable evidence that a diet rich in fiber and vegetables was associated with a reduced risk of colon cancer. Risk estimates based on vegetable consumption (OR = 0.48) were comparable to those based on an estimate of fiber intake (OR = 0.58). The possibility remains that the effects of vegetables may be due to nonfiber components. Vitamin C intake appears not to be a protective agent against colon cancer.

G. Prostate Cancer

In Western societies, prostate cancer has one of the highest incidence rates of all cancers. Several additional studies on dietary factors and prostate cancer have been reported. West et al. (1991) conducted a population-based case–control study in Utah. The investigation involved 358 cases diagnosed with prostate cancer between 1984 and 1985, along with 679 matched controls. The use of a quantitative food frequency questionnaire provided information on the dietary intake of calories, fat, protein, vitamin A, β-carotene, vitamin C, zinc, selenium and cadmium. The most significant associations were observed for older males (> 67 years) with aggressive tumors. For these individuals, an increased intake of fat was associated with an increased risk of prostate cancer (OR = 2.9; 95 percent CI = 1.0–8.4). For all cases, little association was noted between prostate cancer and dietary intakes of vitamin C, β-carotene, vitamin A, zinc, selenium and cadmium.

Bravo et al. (1991) conducted a case–control study in Madrid, Spain, to investigate the influence of dietary factors on prostate cancer. The cases consisted of 90 men histologically diagnosed with prostate cancer during the period of 1983–1987. The controls were 180 men randomly selected and matched by age to the cancer patients. The results of the study indicated that a high intake of animal fat increased the risk of prostate cancer. No associations of vitamin C or vitamin A with the risk of prostate cancer were observed.

H. Cervical/Ovarian Cancer

Interest in the relation of diet to the risk of cervical cancer has resulted in a number of additional studies. Verreault and colleagues (1989) conducted a population-based case–control study to investigate the relation of diet, particularly of folic acid and the vitamins A, C and E, to the risk of invasive cervical cancer. For the study, 189 women diagnosed with cervical cancer between 1979 and 1983 were selected from three counties in the Seattle, Washington area. For controls, 227 age-matched women were selected from the same area. With the use of a food frequency questionnaire consisting of 66 food items, dietary information was obtained for the year preceding the diagnosis of cervical cancer.

More frequent consumption of dark green and yellow vegetables resulted in a 60 percent reduction in risk of cervical cancer. Frequent consumption of fruit juices was also associated with a 70 percent reduced risk of cervical cancer. When considered in the calculated average daily nutrient intakes, a high intake of carotene was associated with a reduction in the risk of cervical cancer, although marginal in significance. A high intake of vitamin E was also related to a lower risk of cervical cancer. For vitamin C, a strong inverse relationship existed between intake of the vitamin and the risk of cervical cancer. The RR was 0.5 for the fourth quartile of intake compared to an RR of 1.0 for the first quartile (95 percent CI = 0.2–1.0; p = 0.04). The study indicates that diet may influence the risk of cervical cancer with suggestions that vitamin C may be a protective component.

Slattery et al. (1990), in a population-based case–control study conducted in Utah, investigated the relationship of the dietary intake of vitamins A, C and E and selenium to the risk of cervical cancer. For the study, 266 cervical cancer cases and 408 population-based controls were entered between 1984 and 1987. The participants were Caucasian females from the Salt Lake area. Dietary information was obtained with the use of a comprehensive questionnaire that listed 183 food items. The food quantities recorded in the questionnaire were converted into nutrient measurements with use of food composition tables.

Protective effects against cervical cancer were observed for vitamins A, C and E and β–carotene. However, when the data were adjusted for age, education and cigarette use, the protective effects were reduced. For vitamin C, the OR was 0.55 (95 percent CI = 0.33–0.91); for vitamin A, the OR was 0.71 (95 percent CI = 0.43–1.20); for β-carotene the OR was 0.82 (95 percent CI = 0.49–1.37), for vitamin E, the OR was 0.60 (95 percent CI = 0.36–1.01), and for selenium, the OR was 0.70 (95 percent CI = 0.42–1.16). Women who smoked received the highest protective effect from a high intake of vitamin C. In general, the protective effects from high intakes of vitamin A, β-carotene and selenium were minimal. High intakes of vitamin C and vitamin E provided somewhat more protection.

In Latin America, cervical cancer remains a leading cause of morbidity and mortality. Herrero and associates (1991) conducted a large case–control study on the association of nutrient status and invasive cervical cancer. The study involved 748 cases and 1411 hospital and community controls from Mexico, Panama, Columbia and Costa Rica. The cases were diagnosed with cervical cancer between January 1986 and June 1987. Information was obtained on the frequency of consumption of 58 foods commonly eaten in the areas of the study. Daily intake of specific micronutrients was derived from the food frequencies and the use of USDA or Latin American Food Composition tables.

The results indicated a slightly lower risk for invasive cervical cancer with the highest quartiles of consumption of fruit and fruit juices. No protective effects were associated with the intakes of vegetables, legumes or animal products. The intake of vitamin C was higher in the controls than in the cases (p = 0.002). Higher intakes of vitamin C were associated with a decreased risk of invasive cervical cancer. The OR was 0.69 for the highest quartile of intake of vitamin C versus the lowest quartile of intake (p = 0.003). Decreased risk also was associated with increased intakes of β-carotene (OR = 0.68; p = 0.02) and of other carotenoids (OR = 0.61; p = 0.003). Because of some inadequacies in the dietary data and differences in the socioeconomic status between the population groups studied, a degree of bias may have occurred that could have influenced the observations. Nevertheless, the study provides support for a dietary protective effect of vitamin C, carotenoids and possibly other substances found in fruits and vegetables against the development of invasive cervical cancer.

Potischman et al. (1991) studied the serum levels in eight micronutrients in a subset of cases (387) and controls (670) from the subjects studied by Herrero et al. (1991) on invasive cervical cancer. The objective was to determine whether lower serum levels of selected micronutrients were associated with a higher risk of invasive cervical cancer. Unfortunately, serum samples were not obtained for vitamin C analyses. Such data would be useful in evaluating the putative protective effects of vitamin C against cervical cancer.

During 1982–1983, Ziegler et al. (1991) investigated the association of diet and the risk of in situ cervical cancer among white women in the U.S. For this purpose, a case–control study was conducted on women with incident in situ and invasive cervical cancer. The cases were selected from five areas; namely, Birmingham, Chicago, Denver, Miami and Philadelphia. The majority of the cases were from the Denver area. Controls were selected by random-digit dialing and matched to the cases based on age. The study involved 229 cases and 502 controls. Dietary information was obtained with the use of a food frequency questionnaire that listed 75 food items.

The study indicated weak inverse associations between the risk of in situ cervical cancer and the intake of vitamin C, folate, carotenoids and vegetables. The associations did not appear to be significant. Vitamin A and vegetable consumption were unrelated to risk. Only dark yellow-orange vegetable intake and the use of multivitamin preparations were strongly related to a reduced risk of in situ cervical cancer. The findings of this study are not in concurrence with several other epidemiologic investigations on cervical cancer.

Dysplasias or cervical intraepithelial neoplasias (CIN) have been hypothesized to be a forerunner of cervical cancer. Because of this association, results of several recent studies on diet and cervical dysplasia will be mentioned. Basu et al. (1991) investigated the association of plasma levels of vitamin C and β-carotene with cervical dysplasias. The group studied was relatively small, consisting of 75 women of whom 30 had no evidence of cervical intraepithelial neoplasia. The remaining 45 women were stratified as to mild dysplasia (n = 8), moderate dysplasia (n = 19) and severe dysplasia (n = 18). The mean plasma vitamin C, retinol and β-carotene levels between the dysplastic groups were comparable.

VanEenwyk et al. (1991; 1992) conducted a case–control study in Chicago to investigate the association between cervical intraepithelial neoplasia (CIN) and dietary intakes and serum levels of carotenoids, vitamin C and folate. For the study, 102 cases with confirmed CIN I, CIN II or CIN III were enrolled along with 102 matched controls. A food frequency questionnaire was used to obtain dietary intake information, which was converted to nutrient intakes. An inverse association was found between cervical dysplasia risk and dietary vitamin C with adjusted OR (95 percent CI) of 0.2 (0.0–0.7), 0.6 (0.2–1.6), and 0.6 (0.2–1.8) for those participants in quartiles 4, 3 and 2, respectively, compared to quartile I (lowest level of vitamin C intake). Increasing levels of serum and red cell folate were significantly associated with a decreased risk of cervical dysplasia. Relatively high correlations between folate and vitamin C measurements were observed.

Consequently, with the data available it was not feasible to delineate the relative importance of these two nutrients as possible preventive agents in the etiology of cervical dysplasia.

American Indian women in the southwestern U.S.A. have high rates of cervical cancer and cervical dysplasia in contrast to low rates of cancer in other body sites. Buckley and colleagues (1992) conducted a pilot case–control study of cervical dysplasia in Pueblo and Navajo women in the Albuquerque, New Mexico area. The study involved women who were evaluated for cervical dysplasia between 15 June and 20 December, 1990, at the Indian Health Service Hospital in Albuquerque. Women with a diagnosis of a normal cervical mucosa from a Pap smear served as controls. The study involved 42 cases and 58 controls. Dietary information was obtained by 24-hour recalls from which nutrient intakes were calculated with the use of the USDA Survey Nutrient Database. The results of this pilot study indicated that the risk of cervical dysplasia was reduced with increased intakes of vitamin C, folacin or vitamin E. Although this pilot study has many shortcomings, the results provide justification for a larger and more intensive investigation as to the role of vitamin C and other nutrients in the development of cervical dysplasia in southwestern American Indian women.

Carcinoma of the vulva is a rare gynecologic tumor with risk factors similar to those reported for cervical cancer. Sturgeon et al. (1991) reported on a case–control study that involved 201 patients with vulvar cancer from hospitals in Chicago and upstate New York, and 342 community controls. Information on diet was obtained with the use of a food frequency questionnaire that listed 61 food items. The study indicated that vulvar cancer was unrelated to the intake of dark green vegetables, citrus fruits, legumes, folate, vitamin A and vitamin C. Increased intake of dark yellow-orange vegetables was associated with a decreased risk of vulvar cancer (OR of 1.6; lowest vs. highest intake; p = 0.03). Intake of β-carotene was unrelated to risk. From preliminary analytical information on the carotenoids present in fruits and vegetables, the investigators suggested that α-carotene might be the protective component in dark yellow-orange vegetables.

I. Other Cancer Sites and Studies

Cancer of the gallbladder is a relatively rare neoplasm, accounting for about 1 percent of all cancer deaths. Gallbladder cancer is more common in American Indians and in certain populations in South America and Central Europe. Poland is one of the countries with the highest gallbladder cancer incidence and mortality in Europe.

Zatonski et al. (1992) conducted a population-based case–control study of gallbladder cancer in the southwest part of Poland. For the study, 73 cases and 186 controls were identified and interviewed. Questionnaires were used to obtain information on demographic and socioeconomic aspects, smoking, past medical history, alcohol consumption and on the frequency of intake of 80 food items. The diet questionnaire focused on the food intake during the period of 1–2 years before the onset of symptoms of gallbladder cancer.

The major determinant of subsequent gallbladder cancer was a past history of gallbladder disease (OR = 12.5; 95 percent CI = 5.8–26.6). With respect to dietary effects, vitamin C showed an inverse association that was significant for the three highest quartiles of consumption (OR = 0.29; 95 percent CI = 0.10–0.86). A similar inverse association was observed for vitamin E. The study has limitations because of the small number of cases involved and the reliability of information concerning the distant past, particularly with respect to dietary information. The study does suggest that diet may be involved in the etiology of gallbladder cancer.

Few studies have been conducted on the possible association of diet with the occurrence of lower urinary tract cancer. Nomura et al. (1991) conducted a dietary study on 195 male and 66 female cases of lower urinary tract cancer from Oahu, Hawaii. The cases were of Caucasian and Japanese ancestry with lower urinary tract cancer diagnosed between 1977 and 1986. For each case, two population-based controls from Oahu were recruited. Information was obtained on the frequency of intake of 29 food items 1 year prior to diagnosis of the cancer. The individual vitamin C and A intakes were computed with the use of food composition tables.

No definitive associations between diet and lower urinary tract cancer were observed. The results of the study suggested that an increased consumption of vitamin C and dark green vegetables may reduce the risk of lower urinary tract cancer. In women, but not in men, the highest quartile of vitamin C intake (dietary plus supplements) was associated with a reduced risk of lower urinary bladder cancer (OR = 0.4; 95 percent CI = 0.2–1.1; $p = 0.03$).

Negri and colleagues (1991) used data from an integrated series of case–control studies conducted in northern Italy between 1983 and 1990 to analyze possible relationships between cancer risk and frequency of consumption of fruit and green vegetables. A series of hospital-based case–control studies served as the source of the data. The study design was limited by the small number of indicator foods investigated. Data analyses were restricted to only two broad food groups; namely, fruit and green vegetables. No mention was made of vitamin C intakes. The study provided only general conclusions. Thus, the frequent intake of green vegetables was related to a reduction of risk of several common epithelial cancers (esophagus, liver and larynx). A higher intake of fruit was associated with a protective effect against cancers of the upper digestive tract (stomach), respiratory tract (oral cavity and pharynx, esophagus, and larynx), liver and pancreas.

Stahelin et al. (1991) reported on the relationship of plasma anti-oxidant vitamins (vitamins A, C and E and carotene) on subsequent cancer mortality in the 12-year follow-up of the prospective Basel, Switzerland study. The Basel study started in 1960 with over 6000 healthy subjects (4858 men and 1461 women) from the Basel area. Follow-up examinations were performed in 1965–1966 and again in 1971–1973. At the time of the 1971–1973 examination cycle, plasma samples were collected on 2974 of the men in the study. The determination of vitamin levels in these plasma samples served as the primary baseline information for relating cancer mortality during the subsequent 12 years. During this period, 553 men died, 204 whose deaths were attributed to cancer. The cancer deaths included 68 with bronchus cancer and 37 with gastrointestinal cancer (20 with stomach cancer and 17 with large bowel cancer, excluding cancer of the rectum).

The overall mortality from cancer was associated with low mean plasma levels of carotene ($p < 0.01$) and of vitamin C ($p < 0.01$). Subjects who died from stomach cancer had mean vitamin C and vitamin A levels lower than those of the survivors ($p < 0.005$). in older subjects, low plasma levels of vitamin C increased the risk of stomach cancer (RR = 2.38) and gastrointestinal cancer (RR = 2.46). The Basel prospective study is unique in that the results on cancer risks have been derived from plasma analyses for vitamin C and of several other vitamins rather than from estimates of dietary intakes as used in most other investigations. However, plasma vitamin C levels can be subject to fluctuations and may not always be representative of long-term vitamin C status.

Enstrom et al. (1992) examined the relation between vitamin C intake and mortality using data obtained in the First National Health and Nutrition Examination Survey Epidemiologic Follow-Up Study. The cohort was based on a representative sample of 11348 noninstitutionalized U.S. adults aged 25–74 years. Nutrition information was obtained on these subjects during 1971–1974. The subjects have been followed up for mortality through 1984. The causes of death (1809 deaths) were related to the dietary intake of vitamin C (including supplements) estimated from the initial survey.

When the relation of the standardized mortality ratio (SMR) for all causes of death to increasing vitamin C intake was examined, a strong inverse association for males and weak inverse association for females was noted. With the highest level of intake of vitamin C, males had an SMR (95 percent CI) of 0.65 (0.52–0.80) for all causes, 0.78 (0.50–1.17) for all cancers, and 0.58 (0.41–0.78) for all cardiovascular diseases. From regression analyses, the investigators noted that the inverse relation of total mortality to vitamin C intake was stronger and more consistent in the population studied than the relation of total mortality to serum cholesterol and dietary fat intake.

Chen (1991) provided preliminary data on an ecological survey that investigated diet and cancer mortality in China. Information was obtained on subjects from 65 rural counties of China with the use of a questionnaire that contained 285 questions on dietary practice, environmental factors and other life-style characteristics. Blood and urine specimens were obtained for assay of various nutrients. The preliminary evaluation of the data indicates a negative correlation between the plasma levels of vitamin C, retinol and selenium, and mortality from gastric and esophageal cancer.

Chen et al. (1992) provided additional information on the relation of diet to cancer mortality in the People's Republic of China. The focus was on the association of antioxidant status and the mortality rates for selected cancer sites (stomach, esophagus, lung, liver, colorectum, breast and cervix). On the basis of the mortality rates for these cancer sites, 65 mostly rural counties in China were selected to represent the full range of mortality rates. Within each county, two communes were randomly selected to give a total of 130 survey sites. From each of these sites, 25 males and 25 females (aged 35–64 yrs) were randomly selected. A food frequency questionnaire was used to obtain information on dietary intakes, smoking and alcohol consumption. Fasting blood specimens were obtained from the 50 randomly selected subJects from each of the 130 communes. Plasma and erythrocyte pools were made from the samples from the 25 subjects of the same sex and commune. Hence, individual erythrocyte and plasma analytical values were not obtained.

The plasma vitamin C levels were consistently and independently inversely correlated with mortality rates of most cancer sites in males, including esophageal, liver and lung (p < 0.001 to p < 0.05). The associations between vitamin C and these cancers were considerably stronger in males than in females and may relate to the higher rates of these cancers in males. Selenium had a protective effect against esophageal and stomach cancers, while β-carotene appeared to have a protective effect against stomach cancer independent of retinol. Although pooled plasma samples were used for the analyses, this is one of the few studies in which direct information on the status of vitamin C and other nutrients was available rather than the indirect information provided from food frequency questionnaires.

J. Other Reviews on Vitamin C and Cancer

Additional information on the relation of vitamin C and cancer may be obtained from the reports of Singh and Gaby (1991), Block (1991; 1992), Henson et al. (1991), Forman (1991) and Byers and Perry (1992). Citations to early studies on the relation of vitamin C and cancer are available in these reports.

The additional studies noted in this addendum provide further evidence to support an important role for vitamin C in reducing the risk of cancer, particularly that of stomach cancer. Epidemiological data suggest that vitamin C may have a protective effect against several other types of cancers. Some of these studies indicate, however, that in addition to vitamin C, other nutrients in the diet, including vitamin E, carotenoids and folacin, may participate in the protective effect. The importance of each as a protective factor is difficult to evaluate from epidemiologic data. Intervention trials may be necessary to assess the importance of the association of specific dietary components with a reduced risk of cancer.

K. Bibliography

Baghurst, P.A.; McMichael, A.J.; Slavotinek, A.H.; Baghurst, K.I.; Boyle, P. and Walker, A.M. 1991. A case–control study of diet and cancer of the pancreas. *Am. J. Epidemiol.* 134:167–179.

Basu, J.; Palan, P.R.; Vermund, S.H.; Goldberg, G.L.; Burk, R.D. and Ronney, S.L. 1991. Plasma ascorbic acid and beta-carotene levels in women evaluated for HPV infection, smoking, and cervix dysplasia. *Cancer Detect. Prev.* 12:165–170.

Block, G. 1991. Epidemiologic evidence regarding vitamin C and cancer. *Am. J. Clin. Nutr.* 54:1310S–1314S.

Block, G. 1992. Vitamin C status and cancer. Epidemiologic evidence of reduced risk. *Ann. NY Acd. Sci.* 669:280–292.

Boeing, H. and Frentzel-Beyme, R. 1991. Regional risk factors for stomach cancer in the FRG. *Envir. Health Persp.* 94:83–89.

Boeing, H.; Frentzel-Beyme, R.; Berger, M.; Berndt, V. Gores, W.; Korner, M.; Lohmeir, R.I; et al. 1991. Case–control study on stomach cancer in Germany. *Int. J. Cancer* 47:858–864.

Bravo, M.P.; Castelianos, E. and del Rey Calero, J. 1991. Dietary factors and prostatic cancer. *Urol. Int.* 46:163–166.

Buckley, D.I.; McPherson, R.S.; North, C.Q. and Becker, T.M. 1992. Dietary micronutrients and cervical dysplasia in southwestern American Indian women. *Nutr. Cancer* 17:179–185.

Bueno de Mesquita, H.B.; Maisonneuve, P.; Runia, S. and Moerman, C.J. 1991. Intakes of foods and nutrients and cancer of the exocrine pancreas: A population-based case–control study in The Netherlands. *Int. J. Cancer* 48:540–549.

Buiatti, E.; Palli, D.; Blanchi, S.i Decarli, A.; Amadorl, D.; Avellini, C.; Cipriani, F.; Cocco, P.; Giacosa, A. et al. 1991. A case–control study of gastric cancer and diet in Italy. III. Risk patterns by histologic type. *Int. J. Cancer* 48:369–374.

Byers, T. and Perry, G. 1992. Dietary carotenes, vitamin C, and vitamin E as protective antioxidants in human cancers. *Annu. Rev. Nutr.* 12:139–159.

Chen, J. 1991. Dietary practices and cancer prevention. *IARC Sci. Publ.* 105:18–21.

Chen, J.; Geissler, C.; Parpia, B.; Li, J. and Campbell, T.C. 1992. Antioxidant status and cancer mortality in China. *Int. J. Epidemiol.* 21:625–635.

Chow, W.-H.; Schuman, L.M.; McLaughlin, J.K.; Bjelke, E.; Gridley, G.; Wacholder, S.; Co Chien, H.T. and Blot, W.J. 1992. A cohort study of tobaco use, diet, occupation, and lung cancer mortality. *Cancer Causes Controls* 3:247–254.

Enstrom, J.E.; Kanim, L.E. and Klein, M.A. 1992. Vitamin C intake and mortality among a sample of the United States population. *Epidemiol.* 3:194–202.

Freudenheim, J.L.; Graham, S.; Byers, T.E.; Marshall, J.R.; Haughey, B.P.; Swanson, M.K. and Wilkinson, G. 1992. Diet, smoking, and alcohol in cancer of the larynx: A case–control study. *Nutr. Cancer* 17:33–45.

Forman, D. 1991. The etiology of gastric cancer. *IARC Sci. Publ.* 105:22–32.

Ghadirian, P.; Simard, A.; Baillargeon, J.; Maisonneuve, P. and Boyle, P. 1991. Nutritional factors and pancreatic cancer in the francophone community in Montreal, Canada. *Int. J. Cancer* 47:1–6.

Gridley, G.; McLaughlin, J.K.; Block, G.; Blot, W.J.; Winn, D.M.; Greenberg, R.S.; Schoenberg, J.B.; Preston-Martin, S.; Austin, D.F. and Fraumeni, J.F., Jr. 1990. Diet and oral and pharyngeal cancer among blacks. *Nutr. Cancer* 14:219–225.

Henson, D.E.; Block, G. and Levine, M. 1991. Ascorbic acid: Biologic functions and relation to cancer. *J. Natl. Cancer Inst.* 83:547–550.

Herrero, R.; Potischman, N.; Brinton, L.A.; Reeves, W.C.; Brenes, M.M.; Tenorio, F.; de Britton, R.C. and Gaitan, E. 1991. A case–control study of nutrient status and invasive cervical cancer. I. Dietary indicators. *Am. J. Epidemiol.* 134:1335–1346.

Howe, G.R.; Ghadirian, P.; Bueno de Mesquita, H.B.; Zatonski, W.A.; Baghurst, P.A.; Miller, A.B.; et al. 1992. A collaborative case–control study of nutrient intake and pancreatic cancer within the search program. *Int. J. Cancer* 51:365–372.

Jain, M.; Burch, J.D.; Howe, G.R.; Risch, H.A. and Miller, A.B. 1990. Dietary factors and risk of lung cancer: Results from a case–control study, Toronto, 1981–1985. *Int. J. Cancer* 45:287–293.

Kneller, R.W.; Guo, W.-D.; Hsing, A.W.; Chen, J.-S.; Blot, W.J.; Li, J.-Y.; Forman, D. and Fraumeni, J.F., Jr. 1992. Risk factors for stomach cancer in sixty-five Chinese counties. *Cancer Epidemiol, Biomark & Prevent* 1:113–118.

Morales, M. and Llopis, A. 1992. Breast cancer and diet in Spain. *J. Environ Pathol., Toxicol. Oncol.* 11:157–167.

Negri, E.; La Vecchia, C.; Franceschi, S.; D'Avanzo, B. and Parazzini, F. 1991. Vegetable and fruit consumption and cancer risk. *Int. J. Cancer* 48:350–354.

Nomura, A.M.Y.; Kolonel, L.N.; Hankin, J.H. and Yoshizawa, C.N. 1991. Dietary factors in cancer of the lower urinary tract. *Int. J. Cancer* 48:199–205.

Olsen, G.W.; Mandel, J.S.; Gibson, R.W.; Wattenberg, I.W. and Schuman, L.M. 1991. Nutrient and pancreatic cancer: A population-based case–control study. *Cancer Causes Control* 2:291–297.

Palli, D; Decarli, A.; Cipriani, F.; Avellini, C.; Cocco, P.; Falcini, F.; Puntoni, R.; Russo, A.; et al. 1992. A case–control study of cancers of the gastric cardia in Italy. *Br. J. Cancer* 65:263–266.

Potischman, N.; Herrero, R.; Brinton, L.A.; Reeves, W.C. Stacewicz-Sapuntzakis, M.; Jones, C.J.; et al. 1991. A case–control study of nutrient status and invasive cervical cancer. *Am. J. Epidemiol.* 134:1347–1355.

Richardson, S.; Gerber, M. and Cenee, S. 1991. The role of fat, animal protein and some vitamin consumption in breast cancer: A case–control study in southern France. *Int. J. Cancer* 48:1–9.

Singh, V.N. and Gaby, S.K. 1991. Premalignant lesions: Role of antioxidant vitamins and beta-carotene in risk reduction and prevention of malignant transformation. *Am. J. Clin. Nutr.* 53:386S–390S.

Slattery, M.L.; Abbott, T.M.; Overall, J.C.; Robison, L.M.; French, T.K.; Jolles, C.; Gardner, J.W. and West, D.W. 1990. Dietary vitamins A, C, and E and selenium as risk factors for cervical cancer. *Epidemiol.* 1:8–15.

Stahelin, H.B.; Gey, K.F.; Eichholzer, M.; Ludin, E.; Bernasconi, F.; Thurneysen, J. and Brubacher, G. 1991. Plasma antioxidant vitamins and subsequent cancer mortality in the 12-year follow-up of the Prospective Basel Study. *Am. J. Epidemiol.* 133:766–775.

Sturgeon, S.R.; Ziegler, R.G.; Brinton, L.A.; Nasca, P.C.; Mallin, K. and Gridley, G. 1991. Diet and the risk of vulvar cancer. *Ann. Epidemiol.* 1:427–437.

Trock, B.; Lanza, E. and Greenwald, P. 1990. Dietary fiber, vegetables, and colon cancer: Critical review and metaanalyses of the epidemiologic evidence. *J. Natl. Cancer Inst.* 82:650–661.

VanEenwyk, J.; Davis, F.G. and Bowen, P.E. 1991. Dietary and serum carotenoids and cervical intraepithelial neoplasia. *Int. J. Cancer Inst.* 84:34–38.

VanEenwyk, J.; Davis, F.G. and Colman, N. 1992. Folate, vitamin C, and cervical intraepithelial neoplasia. *Cancer Epidemiol. Biomark. Prevent.* 1:119–124.

Verreault, R.; Chu, J.; Mandelson, M. and Shy, K. 1989. A case–control study of diet and invasive cervical cancer. *Int. J. Cancer* 43:1050–1054.

West, D.W.; Slattery, M.L.; Robison, L.M.; French, T.K. and Mahoney, A.W. 1991. Adult dietary intake and prostate cancer risk in Utah: A case–control study with special emphasis on aggressive tumors. *Cancer Causes Control.* 2:85–94.

Whittemore, A.S.; Wu-Williams, A.H.; Lee, M.; Shu, Z.; Gallger, R.P.; Deng-ao, J.; Lun, Z.; et al. 1990. Diet, physical activity, and colorectal cancer among Chinese in North America and China. *J. Natl. Cancer Inst.* 82:915–926.

Yu, H.; Rohan, T.E.; Cook, M.G.; Howe, G.R. and Miller, A.B. 1992. Risk factors for fibroadenoma: A case-control study in Australia. *Am. J. Epidemiol.* 135:247–258.

Zaridze, D.; Lifanova, Y.; Maximovitch, D.; Day, N.E. and Duffer, S.W. 1991. Diet, alcohol consumption and reproductive factors in a case–control study of breast cancer in Moscow. *Int. J. Cancer* 48:493–501.

Zatonski, W.A.; LaVecchia, C.; Przewozniak, K.; Maisonneuve, P.; Lowenfels, A.B. and Boyle, P. 1992. Risk factors for gallbladder cancer: A Polish case–control study. *Int. J. Cancer* 51:707–711.

Zatonski, W.; Przewozniak, K.; Howe, G.R.; Maisonneuve, P.; Walker, A.M. and Boyle, P. 1991. Nutritional factors and pancreatic cancer: A case–control study from southwest Poland. *Int. J. Cancer* 48:390–394.

Zheng, W.; Blot, W.J.; Diamond, E.L.; Norkus, E.P.; Spate, V.; Moris, J.S. and Comstock, G.W. 1993. Serum micronutrients and the subsequent risk of oral and pharyngeal cancer. *Cancer Res.* 53:795–798.

Ziegler, R.G.; Jones, C.J.; Brinton, L.A.; Norman, S.A.; Mallin, K.; Levine, R.S.; et al. 1991. Diet and the risk of in situ cervical cancer among white women in the United States. *Cancer Causes Control* 2:17–29.

Chapter 4

Vitamin E and Cancer

Ching K. Chow, Ph.D.

I. Introduction

Cancer is the second leading cause of death in many Western countries. More than 800,000 new cases of cancer are diagnosed each year in the United States, and over 400,000 die of cancer annually (National Cancer Institute, 1990; National Center for Health Statistics, 1986; National Research Council, 1989a; U.S. Department of Health and Human Services, 1988). The cause and possible control of cancer has been intensely investigated. It has been recognized that environmental factors have strong influences on the incidence of human cancer. Many chemical and physical agents in the environment have been identified or are suspected as human carcinogens. These include many direct-acting carcinogens, pro-carcinogens, co-carcinogens, and promoters.

Cancer is not a single disease entity. A large number of chemical and physical agents can affect the development of cancer in many different ways. In spite of the multiplicity of causative factors, most cancers seem to arise by a stepwise evolution involving progressive genetic changes, cell proliferation, and clonal expansion (Mergens and Bhagavan, 1989; National Research Council, 1989a; Weinstein, 1988). The initial stage, initiation, occurs at the DNA level and involves an irreversible genetic alteration such as oncogene activation, tumor suppressor gene inactivation, DNA amplification, gene transposition, or chromosome translocation. This initiation event does not necessarily result in tumor development, rather, it is the first step in a multistage/multifactorial process involving initiation, promotion, and progression. The transition between stages is complex and is thought to involve environmental (exogenous) and autocrine (endogenous) factors. There is generally a long latent period between carcinogen exposure and tumor development. In humans, this period could be as long as 30 years. Thus, it is possible that the process of carcinogenesis could be reversed or slowed if the progressive stages of cancer development were understood.

Increasing evidence indicates that diet and or nutritional status may play an important role in the etiology of human cancer. Diet is a complex mixture of chemical entities that contains factors that may cause or promote cancer (enhancing factors) as well as factors that are antimutagenic or anticarcinogenic (inhibitory factors). Dietary components may directly interact with mutagens or carcinogens and influence metabolic activation and detoxification, as well as regulate DNA repair and expression. Many dietary components have also been shown to be capable of enhancing or diminishing the mutagenic and carcinogenic activity of other substances.

II. Vitamin E and Carcinogenesis

A. Nomenclature

Vitamin E is the term suggested for all tocol and tocotrienol derivatives qualitatively exhibiting the biological activity of α-tocopherol. "Tocopherols" is the generic description for all mono-, di-, and trimethyl tocols and tocotrienols and is not synonymous with the term "vitamin E." All eight naturally occurring tocopherol compounds isolated from plant sources have a 6-chromanol ring and a phytol side chain (Chow, 1985; Machlin, 1991). There are four each of tocols and tocotrienols that occur naturally, differing in the number and position of methyl groups on the chromanol ring. While vitamin E refers to at least eight tocopherol structures, α-tocopherol predominates in many species and, based on animal studies, is significantly more biologically active than any other form of tocopherol.

Tocopherols exist mainly in the free alcohol form and are widely distributed in a variety of plant life. In addition to naturally occurring isomers, several types of synthetic vitamin E are available commercially. Most synthetic tocopherols are esters, particularly the acetate form. The ester form is less susceptible to oxidation and more suitable for food and pharmaceutical applications than the free form. To distinguish it from the synthetic one, the naturally occurring stereoisomer of α-tocopherol, formerly known as d-α-tocopherol or α-tocopherol, has been designated as RRR-α-tocopherol. The totally synthetic α-tocopherol, previously known as dl-α-tocopherol, has been designated as all-rac-α-tocopherol. The natural form of tocopherol (RRR) is more active than the synthetic one (all racemic).

B. Human Requirements

The biological activity of various forms is expressed as units of activity, and the relative values in international units (IU/mg) are: dl-α-tocopheryl acetate (all racemic), 1.00; dl-α-tocopherol (all racemic), 1.10; d-α-tocopheryl acetate (RRR), 1.36; d-α-tocopherol (RRR), 1.49; dl-α-tocopheryl succinate (all racemic), 0.89; and d-α-tocopheryl succinate (RRR), 1.21. In the United States, the current recommended dietary allowance for vitamin E ranges from 4.5 IU (3 α-tocopherol equivalents or 3 mg d-α-tocopherol) in infants, 9.0–10.5 in children (10 years or under), 15.0 in males (>11 years), 12.0 in females (>11 years), 15.0 in pregnant females, to 18.0 in lactating females (National Research Council, 1989b). The majority of tocopherols consumed in the United States is not the α form (Chow, 1985). Gamma-tocopherol, with 10–35 percent of biological activity of α-tocopherol, accounts for over half of the estimated total tocopherol intake.

Dietary deficiency of vitamin E is rare in the United States as normal American diets provide adequate amounts of vitamin E. The intake of vitamin E generally parallels the intake of polyunsaturated fatty acids. Foods with a high polyunsaturated fatty acid content generally are rich sources of tocopherols (Chow, 1985; Machlin, 1991); however, the human requirement for vitamin E can change due to the consumption of fats and oils. Consequently, the dietary requirement for vitamin E is related to the degree of unsaturation of the fatty acids in tissue lipids, which can be altered by dietary lipids (Horwitt, 1974, 1991).

The intake of total tocopherols is, in general, proportional to the amount of vegetable oil consumed as vegetable oils are among the best sources of tocopherols. The normal intake of vitamin E in American diets ranges between 4 and 33 α-tocopherol equivalents (α-TE) daily in adults not taking vitamin E supplements, with average values between 11 and 13 α-TE (Machlin, 1989). This level of intake results in average plasma/serum levels in adults of approximately 9.5 μg/mL (Machlin, 1991).

C. Functions

Vitamin E was discovered approximately 70 years ago as a lipid-soluble dietary factor necessary for the prevention of fetal death and resorption in rats (Evans and Bishop, 1922). Subsequently a number of species-dependent manifestations of vitamin E deficiency, such as liver necrosis in rats and pigs, erythrocyte hemolysis in rats and chickens, and white muscle disease in calves, sheep, mice, and mink, have been documented (Machlin, 1991;

Scott, 1970). Because of the lack of a definite clinical deficiency syndrome attributable to vitamin E, the need or use of this vitamin in humans had been questioned.

The essentiality of vitamin E for humans was recognized in the late 1960s in connection with studies on premature infants in which hemolytic anemia was associated with vitamin E deficiency (Bieri and Farrell, 1976). While it is difficult to produce vitamin E deficiency under experimental conditions in adult humans, recent studies have shown that deficiencies or subclinical deficiencies such as neurologic abnormalities do occur in association with malabsorption syndromes of various etiologies (Bieri and Farrell, 1982; Machlin, 1991; Sokol, 1988, 1989). Although many biochemical abnormalities have been found to be associated with vitamin E deficiency, the mechanism by which vitamin E prevents various metabolic and pathological lesions has not yet been elucidated.

Vitamin E is the most important lipid-soluble antioxidant and free radical scavenger. The suggestion that the function of vitamin E may be related to its membrane stabilization property (Lucy, 1972) does not conflict with the free radical scavenging mechanism or antioxidant function of vitamin E (Tappel, 1972). Several non-antioxidant functions of vitamin E have also been suggested. Vitamin E, for example, has been reported to regulate the de novo synthesis of xanthine oxidase (Catignani et al., 1974), modulate the activities of protein kinase C (Packer, 1991) and microsomal enzymes (Chen et al., 1982; Chow and Gairola, 1984), and inhibit tumor cell proliferation (Prasad and Edward-Prasad, 1982; Boscoboinik et al., 1991). Also, vitamin E may regulate immune response or cell-mediated immunity by modulating generation of prostaglandins and other lipid peroxidation products (Meydani et al., 1990).

The functional interrelationships among vitamin E and other micronutrients, notably selenium and vitamin C, have long been recognized (Chow, 1979, 1988). Selenium has been shown to prevent or reduce the severity of several symptoms of vitamin E deficiency (Chow, 1985; Machlin, 1991; Scott, 1970). As an integral part of the enzymes glutathione (GSH) peroxidase (Rotruck et al., 1972) and phospholipid hydroperoxide GSH peroxidase (Ursini et al., 1985), selenium may complement the antioxidant function of vitamin E via the hydroperoxide reduction function and thus reduce the requirement for the vitamin.

In addition to being an important water-soluble free radical scavenger and reducing agent, vitamin C seems to have a synergistic effect on vitamin E. This effect has been attributed to the involvement of vitamin C in the regeneration or restoration of vitamin E after it exerts its antioxidant function (Niki et al., 1982; Packer et al., 1979; Wefers and Sies, 1988). Similarly, GSH, in association with an enzyme or enzyme system(s), may also be involved in the regeneration of vitamin E (Reddy et al., 1982; Wefers and Sies, 1988). Furthermore, a GSH-dependent dehydro-ascorbate reductase and a NADH-semi-dehydro-ascorbate reductase appear to be involved in the regeneration or restoration of vitamin C (Chow, 1988; Diliberto et al., 1982).

Experimental evidence for the vitamin E regeneration or restoration in vivo, however, remains to be provided (Chow, 1991). While the nature of the vitamin E regenerative process in vivo, if any, and the agent(s) responsible are not yet clear, it does provide a rational explanation for the fact that it is very difficult to deplete adult animals or human subjects of the vitamin (Horwitt, 1962). Also, the possible involvement of vitamin C, GSH and other reducing agents in the regeneration of vitamin E and its functional interaction with selenium indicate an interdependence among various antioxidant defense systems (Chow, 1988, 1991).

D. Possible Role for Vitamin E in Carcinogenesis

Free radical-initiated peroxidative damage to the cell has been implicated in the pathogenesis of many cell injury and disease states including cancer, cardiovascular disease, and autoimmune diseases (Esterbauer and Cheeseman, 1987; Freeman and Crapo, 1982;

Halliwell, 1987). Whether vitamin E, the most important biological antioxidant and free radical scavenger, can prevent or slow down carcinogenesis has received considerable research interest. Investigation into the influence of dietary vitamin E on the induction and development of cancer has produced a large amount of data. Cell culture and certain animal studies, although not conclusive, suggest that vitamin E may possess antitumor properties (Chen et al., 1988; Mergens and Bhagavan, 1989).

Vitamin E has been suggested to play a role in several stages of carcinogenesis. These include

a) inhibition or blockage of mutagen or carcinogen formation from precursors via direct chemical interaction,

b) prevention of mutagens or carcinogens from reaching or reacting with DNA by scavenging mutagens or by enhancing detoxification processes, and

c) prevention of cancer progression by the enhancement of normal immune responses.

III. Assessment of Vitamin E Status

In an epidemiological study, the intake of vitamin E is estimated based on information obtained from subject interview and questionnaire, and the nutritional status of vitamin E is assessed based on the concentration of tocopherols in body stores. Many sources of potential errors are associated with each type of nutritional epidemiological study. Until they are properly addressed, meaningful assessment of the relationship between nutrient and cancer risk can not be achieved. It should be noted that, due to the absence of vitamin E deficiency in the general population, any relationship between this nutrient and human cancer may be difficult to demonstrate. Also, most clinical intervention trials are actually pharmacologic interventions that are not entirely relevant to dietary considerations.

The major problems associated with the assessment of vitamin E intake and status in epidemiological studies of human cancer are briefly summarized below.

A. Biochemical Assessment

At present there is no suitable index which accurately reflects dietary intake or body stores of vitamin E. Several indices, such as tocopherol concentrations in plasma/serum, erythrocytes, platelets or tissues, degree of erythrocyte hemolysis, and amounts of lipid peroxidation products (e.g., ethane, pentane, and malonaldehyde) generated, have been used to assess the nutritional status of vitamin E. Direct measurement of tocopherol concentrations, especially in tissues, is a logical choice over the indirect methods. Analysis of adipose tissue and liver biopsy samples for tocopherols, for example, is conceivably a reliable index of body stores of vitamin E and thus long-term vitamin E status (Rautalahti et al., 1990). However, in addition to its invasive nature, ethical and other considerations, such as whether representative samples are used, render it impractical for large population studies.

Measurement of tocopherol concentrations in erythrocytes is a better indicator for vitamin E than that of plasma/serum. However, it has not been widely employed since it is technically more cumbersome and difficult to determine tocopherol in the erythrocytes than in serum/plasma. Platelets have been shown to be more sensitive for measuring dose response to dietary vitamin E when compared to plasma, erythrocytes, or lymphocytes (Lehmann, 1981). Also, platelet tocopherol concentrations are independent of serum lipid levels (Vatassery et al., 1983), an important advantage relative to serum or plasma tocopherol concentrations. However, it is cumbersome to isolate platelets, and the procedure requires a larger blood sample. Therefore, measurement of tocopherol concentrations in blood plasma/serum remains the most practical method for the assessment of the nutritional status of vitamin E by most investigators. The discussion here is limited to serum/plasma since all the studies reviewed here employed only these samples for assessing vitamin E status.

1. Sample Storage

Major problems associated with the measurement of serum/plasma levels of vitamin E in epidemiological studies are the length and conditions of sample storage, as well as the frequency and manner of sample handling. Tocopherol oxidation (destruction) is accelerated by exposure to light, heat, alkali, and the presence of iron and copper salts. As exemplified in the articles cited in this review, serum/plasma samples had been stored at temperature ranging from $-18°C$ to $-70°C$ for as long as 13 years. Wald et al. (1988) re-analyzed the vitamin E levels in those original serum samples still available and compared these values to those obtained in 1981 (Wald et al., 1984) to determine the effect of sample storage and handling on serum vitamin E level. They found the mean level of vitamin E declined from 6.45 mg/L to 3.1 mg/L during a 5-year storage period (from 1981 to 1986) at $-20°C$ and suggested that the values reported in their 1984 publication might have been artifacts of freezing and thawing. This stresses the importance of ensuring that samples used for prospective follow-up study be stored properly and that records, especially freezing and thawing, are kept to ensure the comparability of cases and controls.

2. Methodology

Methods employed for quantifying plasma/serum vitamin E can have significant effects on the values obtained. High performance liquid chromatography with either UV-visible or fluorescence detection is a far more specific and sensitive method than fluorometric or spectrophotometric determination. While the majority of recent studies used a high performance liquid chromatographic technique to measure serum or plasma tocopherols, usually only the levels of α-tocopherol were reported to represent the status of vitamin E. However, the contribution of non-α-tocopherols to the total vitamin E activity can be significant (Chow, 1985; Machlin, 1991).

3. Clinical Considerations

The ability to absorb nutrients, including vitamin E, may be impaired in subjects with gastrointestinal cancer, especially for those with pancreatic or intestinal cancers. Consequently, it should not be surprising that the levels of plasma/serum vitamin E are lower in patients with gastrointestinal cancer. Both disease symptoms and drug treatments are likely to affect digestion and absorption of nutrients, including vitamin E, in other types of cancer. Also, certain types of chemotherapies and drugs may interact with and alter the nutritional status of vitamin E, independent of dietary intake.

4. Role of Blood Lipid Levels

Vitamin E is transported in blood via lipoproteins. In humans, α-tocopherol is found in all lipoprotein fractions. Since vitamin E is found in chylomicrons, fasted serum samples eliminate this source of potential variation based on the time blood is drawn after the subject's last meal. The ratio of plasma tocopherol to total lipid is usually a more reliable criterion of vitamin E status than tocopherol alone (Machlin, 1991). Often the ratio of tocopherol to cholesterol or tocopherol to the sum of cholesterol and triglycerides is used as a more convenient index than total lipids. Stähelin et al. (1989) reported that the adjustment of fasted plasma values to the sum of cholesterol and triglycerides allowed a lipid-independent estimation of vitamin E status. Since vitamin E is carried in the lipid fraction of the blood and shows significant correlations with lipid levels, blood lipid levels should be taken into consideration.

5. Biological Variability

A great deal of genetic and environmentally derived diversity is found in serum vitamin E levels. Helzlsouer et al. (1989), for example, have shown that the serum levels in controls averaged 11.1 µg/mL with a range of 5.3 to 25.7 µg/mL (n = 70). Also, Tangney et al. (1987) reported that day-to-day intra-individual variations in serum vitamin E levels can constitute an important source of error if single samples of blood are used to categorize individuals. Knekt et al. (1988a) studied the relationship between serum α-tocopherol levels and many of its possible determinants in 301 adult Finnish men and women, ages 40–79 years. They found that the mean α-tocopherol level among men was 8.6 µg/mL and among women was 10.5 µg/mL, and that serum α-tocopherol levels varied with age, geographical area, type of population, occupation, socioeconomic status, and marital status. Furthermore, they found that serum α-tocopherol levels were positively correlated with serum cholesterol and serum vitamin A in both sexes and with body-mass index and serum selenium in men. They concluded that the level of serum α-tocopherol, which is associated with the dietary intake of vitamin E, is dependent upon living conditions.

In view of the variability of tocopherol content in blood serum/plasma, it is necessary to develop more reliable procedures for assessing long-term vitamin E intake status rather than continuing to rely on serum/plasma tocopherol analysis. As mentioned above, measurement of tocopherol content in tissues, such as adipose biopsy samples (Rautalahti et al., 1990), is conceivably a more reliable index of vitamin E status than that of serum/plasma. However, ethical and other considerations prevent the routine use of this technique for large population studies.

B. Dietary Assessment

Accurate dietary intake is difficult to assess. Unless properly controlled and complete, assessment of dietary nutrient intake has limited value.

1. Interview Methods

Measurement of dietary intake is inherently error prone. For example, individuals' long-term intake of a given diet, food, or nutrient is difficult to assess accurately because their diets may have varied substantially over time. Well-trained persons and well-prepared questionnaires are required to perform the task properly. Of particular concern in the dietary assessment of vitamin E is that the consumption of some of the richest sources of tocopherols, e.g., soybean, sunflower, and cottonseed oils and products made from them such as margarine, is difficult to quantify by dietary history interviews (Bertram, 1987). Also, increased use of fat substitutes may complicate the assessment of dietary intake of fats and vitamin E by conventional interviewing techniques. Potential sources of errors in the use of interviews for obtaining food/nutrient intake information include

a) estimation of only recent intake rather than earlier dietary intake which may be more relevant to disease etiology,

b) reliance on limited food lists, and

c) errors in subject estimation of food-intake frequency and size of food portion eaten.

Cooperation and compliance of subjects are needed in order to obtain reliable information concerning vitamin E intake and other relevant data. These constitute the biggest problems associated with intervention studies as there is no easy and reliable method for assessing whether subjects took vitamin E supplements as instructed.

2. Food Composition Tables

One approach to a more reliable measurement of dietary intake has been the use of food-frequency questionnaires (Willett et al., 1983). However, the accuracy of this type of information also depends on the reliability of information in the food composition data used. Tocopherol content of foods is highly variable depending upon genetic, seasonal, processing, storage, and other factors. Another concern is the reliability of information about tocopherol content of various foods. The majority of information concerning tocopherol contents of various foods was obtained in the past using colorimetric, rather than high performance liquid chromatographic techniques. Furthermore, food processing and storage and culinary practices can significantly influence the destruction of tocopherols present in the food.

Despite the inherent errors involved in dietary measurement, nutritional epidemiological studies can provide useful information when a quality dietary assessment method is used. However, it should be noted that vitamin E is functionally interrelated to a number of nutrients including polyunsaturated lipids, β-carotene, selenium, and ascorbic acid (Chow, 1988, 1991; Machlin, 1991). The variable nature of human requirements for vitamin E due to changes in consumption of fats and oils has been reported (Horwitt, 1974). Thus, to identify ultimately the cancer risk associated with low levels of vitamin E, the status of other interacting nutrients needs to be assessed in combination with vitamin E.

IV. Vitamin E and Human Cancer

In recent years, the possibility that a higher intake of micronutrients, including vitamin E, may reduce the risk of certain human cancers has received considerable attention. This review deals only with recent reports concerning the possible role of vitamin E in the etiology and prevention of human cancers.

Epidemiological study designs can be classified according to the method of obtaining data: simple observation (non-experimental studies) or observation after some type of intervention (experimental studies) (Rogers and Longnecker, 1988). Intervention studies (clinical trials) are, in theory, the best and least likely to be biased methods to assess diet and cancer relationships. However, clinical trials are frequently not feasible for practical, financial, and ethical reasons. Follow-up and case–control studies are the two non-experimental study designs most commonly used in nutritional epidemiology. Data obtained with geographic correlation studies are less powerful and less useful than other non-experimental studies (Rogers and Longnecker, 1988). A review of the extant literature since 1987, organized by organ site, on the relationship of vitamin E and cancer follows. Summaries of cited human studies may be found in Appendix Tables 1–7.

A. Head and Neck Cancer

Drozdz et al. (1989) fluorometrically measured serum samples for vitamins A and E from 22 newly diagnosed cases of larynx cancer, 16 patients with nonmalignant laryngeal diseases, and 16 patients with other nonmalignant diseases, including cardiovascular disease and hernia, in Poland. Fasted serum samples were stored at $-40°C$ for less than 2 weeks. The levels of vitamin A, but not vitamin E, were lower in cases than either control group. There were no community-based controls nor was the hospital control group matched with cases for age, sex, or socioeconomic factors.

Gridley et al. (1990) conducted a population-based multicenter case–control study to assess the relationship between diet and oral and pharyngeal cancer among Afro-Americans. Cases were 248 pathologically-confirmed-incident patients with oral and pharyngeal cancer from the population-based cancer registries of Atlanta, Georgia; New Jersey; Los Angeles, Santa Clara and San Mateo counties of California. Cancers of the tongue and pharynx and other oral cancers were included, but not cancers of the lip, salivary glands, or nasopharynx. Controls were chosen using random-digit-dialing (for those under age 65) and the Health Care Financing Administration roster (for those aged 65 years or older) and were matched on sex and age. Interviews were administered to obtain information on demographic variables, tobacco and alcohol use, diet, occupation, and medical history. Because of death or severe disability, next-of-kin interviews were obtained for 56 cases and 3 controls. Of the total subjects, 190 cases (142 males and 48 females) and 201 controls (139 males and 62 females) were included in the analysis. Information on portion size and nutrient indices were derived from the Second National Health and Nutrition Examination Survey (NHANES II) and from data of the U.S. Department of Agriculture. Food group and nutrient indices were categorized into quartiles based on sex-specific distributions of the control group. The association between dietary factors and oral cancer was assessed by the odds ratio as an estimate of relative risk. An increased intake of fruits and vegetables was found to be associated with decreased risk of oral cancer among both men and women. Risk was also found to decline in both sexes with an increase in consumption of vitamin C and fiber and in men only with increased consumption of carotene and vitamin E.

The role of nutrients and dietary factors in relation to esophageal cancer was examined in a large case–control study conducted in Calvados, France, a region having a relatively high incidence of the disease (Tuyns et al., 1987). A total of 743 cases (704 males and 39 females) and 1975 controls (922 males and 1053 females) were interviewed about their usual food intake. The consumption of 40 food items was recorded, and intake of nutrients was derived from these data using food-composition tables. Relative risks for each nutrient or food item and the corresponding chi-square for association and for trend were computed over four levels of consumption. Higher intakes of vitamins E and C, along with fresh meat, citrus fruits and oils, were found to be associated with a reduction in risk of esophageal cancer. On the other hand, higher intake of retinol was found to be associated with increased risk of the cancer.

Van Helden et al. (1987) examined the relationship between nutritional status of vitamin E and certain other nutrients and risk of esophageal cancer in certain population groups in South Africa. Healthy subjects, who lived in the given area for 10 years or longer, were selected from areas known for high, intermediate, or low incidence of esophageal cancer. Plasma samples were kept at $-20°C$ until analyzed.

In one study, the levels of serum vitamin E averaged 5.3 (n = 16), 4.3 (n = 21), and 3.8 (n = 18) μg/mL, respectively, for subjects from low-, intermediate-, and high-incidence areas. In another study conducted in a different region, the values were 8.7 (n = 24) and 6.1 (n = 27) μg/mL, respectively, for subjects in low- and high-incidence areas. The age of subjects (both sexes) ranged from 32–50 years. The results suggest that deficiency in vitamin E (vitamin A and B_{12} were also studied) may play a role in the etiology of esophageal cancer. Whether dietary intake contributed to the difference in the serum level was not determined. Also, the levels of serum vitamin E from this study are lower than average values reported elsewhere (Machlin, 1989). In addition to storage conditions, genetic and other variables may account partly for the low values.

B. Breast Cancer

Basu et al. (1989) measured the serum levels of vitamin E, vitamin A, β-carotene, and selenium in the sera of 30 breast cancer patients with advanced stage breast cancer with distal metastases, 29 patients with benign breast disease, and 30 healthy age-matched controls in Edmonton, Canada. All of the cancer patients were drug-free for 1 month prior to sampling. Serum samples were obtained from the National Cancer Institute serum bank. No significant differences were found for the levels of vitamins E and A, β-carotene, or selenium. All cancer patients were in advanced stages with metastases, which may have affected serum nutrient levels.

Gerber et al. (1989) estimated the intake of vitamin E, total lipids, total cholesterol, and fatty acids in 120 female patients, hospitalized with a first diagnosis of breast cancer and 109 female controls, admitted for neurologic syndromes of other than cardiovascular and tumoral origin or for lumbalgias or disc pathologies, in Montpellier, France. Subjects' ages ranged from 25 to 65 years. The dietary history questionnaire covered 55 key food items in lipid and vitamin consumption and general overall nutritional habits. The weekly food consumption was converted to intake of nutrients by means of food composition tables. In addition to the fasting serum levels of vitamin E, total cholesterol, triglycerides, and fatty acids of patients and controls were measured. The results showed that while vitamin E intake was not significantly different, plasma levels of vitamin E were significantly higher in cases than in controls even after adjustment for serum cholesterol levels. In addition, plasma levels of the lipid peroxidation product, malondialdehyde were significantly lower than in controls. Given the potential interaction between neurological disorders, their treatment and nutritional intake, the appropriateness of this control group must be questioned.

In a related study, Gerber et al. (1990) investigated the nutritional factors related to breast cancer using a hospital-based case–control study in Milan, Italy and Montpellier, France. Vitamins A and E, triglycerides, and cholesterol were measured in blood samples taken from interviewed subjects. Cases were 214 Italian and 103 French patients with primary carcinoma of the breast without metastasis. None of the cases had previously undergone therapy. Controls (215 in Milan and 103 in Montpellier) were hospital-based in both studies. No differences were found in vitamin A or E consumption in either population. Levels of serum cholesterol and plasma vitamin E were significantly higher in cases than in controls in both populations. The difference in plasma vitamin E was confirmed after adjustment for total cholesterol and triglycerides. Nutrient consumption and relevant blood markers were directly or partially correlated in both populations. The odds ratio values for the highest quartiles were 4.2 for plasma vitamin E, 0.56 for serum malondialdehyde, 1.9 for total lipids and 1.9 for cholesterol. As in the previous study there were no community-based controls. Furthermore, there were no comparisons reported between control groups to control for potential cultural differences. Partial data from this study have been published elsewhere (Gerber et al., 1988).

In another prospective study on breast cancer, Russell et al. (1988) collected blood samples from 5086 women, ages 6 to 88 years, resident in Guernsey, United Kingdom and stored them at −20°C until analyzed. During the subsequent 8-year period 30 women developed breast cancer. The levels of α–tocopherol and retinol from the sera of these women and 288 age-matched controls were then analyzed. No relationship was found between serum vitamin E (or retinol) level and subsequent development of breast cancer. While the follow-up time is long enough, the number of cases is relatively small in this study. Also, it is not known whether storage of samples at −20°C for 8 years will similarly affect the results of all serum samples. It is conceivable that the storage conditions contributed to the relatively low levels of vitamin E reported in controls and pre-cancer patients (6.2 µg/mL and 6.5 µg/mL, respectively).

Toniolo et al. (1989) studied the relationship between intake of vitamin E and risk of breast cancer in Italy. Cases were 250 breast cancer patients (free of metastases, except in regional lymph nodes). Controls were 499 women from the general population stratified by age and geographical area. All subjects interviewed were given food-frequency questionnaires structured by meals. Indigenous foods and recipes were added to the database. No significant difference in vitamin E intake was found between groups. Reduced risk was found to be associated with decreased intake of fat, especially saturated fat and animal protein.

Langeman et al. (1989) measured the levels of cholesterol, α-tocopherol, and γ-tocopherol in 64 breast tissue samples (neoplastic and non-neoplastic from the same patient) in Basel, Switzerland. Breast tissue samples were obtained from biopsies submitted for diagnosis. Tissue was stored at −80°C prior to analysis. The levels of α- and γ-tocopherols were not significantly different between neoplastic and non-neoplastic samples but were correlated with the percent fat in both types of tissue. The values of α-tocopherol ranged widely from 16 to 1439 (mean 288) nmol/g fresh weight in cancerous tissue and from 36 to 1439 (mean 275) nmol/g for non-neoplastic tissue. There were no data on dietary intake or other measures of nutritional status presented in this paper.

In a double-blind, placebo-controlled crossover trial conducted in Pretoria, South Africa, Meyer et al. (1990) examined the effect of vitamin E on the treatment of benign breast disease (fibrocystic disease) using mammography as an objective and sensitive parameter. The subjects were 105 women, ages 25 to 45, who had mammographic evidence of benign breast disease. They received dl-α-tocopheryl acetate (600 mg per day) or placebo for 3 months. Breast examinations and mammography were done after each 3-month treatment, at approximately the same phase of the patients' menstrual cycles. Although there were no differences in clinical exam scores, 37 (43 percent) out of 83 cases who completed the trial reported improvement and 16 versus 10 placebo cases had mammographic improvement after vitamin E. There was no report of dietary intake, supplement use, or biochemical measures of nutrient status. After 3 months of supplementation it was concluded that vitamin E had no beneficial effect on the treatment of benign breast disease. While the risk of breast cancer is increased in fibrocystic disease patients, it is not clear whether fibrocystic breast disease is a pre-cancerous state.

C. Lung Cancer

Kok et al. (1987) measured the baseline levels of serum retinol, vitamin E, and cholesterol in 10,532 subjects in Rotterdam, The Netherlands. In the subsequent 9 years, 114 subjects died of cancer. Deaths in the first year of follow-up were excluded, as were eligible cases for which baseline data were incomplete or serum samples unavailable, leaving 69 cases (18 cases of lung cancer) for statistical analysis. Baseline serum micronutrient levels in these subjects were compared with levels in 138 controls who were matched for sex, age, and smoking status. The levels of vitamin E, but not of retinol, selenium, or cholesterol, were significantly lower in all cases than in controls. Risk analyses according to quintile comparisons showed a strong negative trend for vitamin E, suggesting an increased risk of all cancer associated with lower serum levels of vitamin E. The authors indicated that this was an ongoing study, and not much experimental detail was provided.

In a case–control study, LeGardeur et al. (1990) measured the serum levels of vitamins E, C, and A, carotenoids, total cholesterol, and retinol-binding protein from 59 newly diagnosed cases of lung cancer and 59 matched hospital controls in New Orleans. Controls were selected in a next-patient-encountered manner from the same hospital and matched to the index case by race, sex, age, and parish of residency. In addition, 31 community-based controls matched to the hospital controls were included for comparison. Nonfasting blood samples were collected from all subjects. Cases and hospital controls were given a structured interview to ascertain smoking habits and dietary intake patterns. Community controls were not interviewed.

There were more smokers in cases than controls, and the relative risk for smoking increased with the number of pack years of cigarettes smoked. Cases had significantly lower serum vitamin E and carotenoids than the controls. Adjustment for serum cholesterol levels reduced the case–control difference for serum vitamin E and carotenoid levels. The results suggest that serum vitamin E is associated with risk of lung cancer. The number of subjects employed in this study is relatively small, and composition of the hospital control group (34 percent with either cardiovascular disease or endocrine/metabolic disorders) make interpretation of this data difficult. See comments in Appendix Table for other concerns about this study.

Whether or not serum vitamin E and selenium concentrations are related to the incidence of lung cancer was studied in Sapporo, Japan (Miyamoto et al., 1987). The subjects were 115 children of 55 randomly selected cancer patients with primary lung cancer (squamous cell carcinoma, adenocarcinoma, small cell carcinoma, large cell carcinoma, and undefined lung cancer). Blood samples were collected from patients (28 males and 9 females), family members (54 males and 61 females), and 56 age-matched controls (28 males and 28 females) with no cancer history among their second degree relatives. Sera were stored at $-70°C$ for less than 3 months prior to analysis.

Family members of cases were found to have a trend toward lower vitamin E levels. Serum vitamin E levels were significantly lower among family members of adenocarcinoma patients than the controls. Serum vitamin E levels were also significantly lower in lung cancer patients than in the controls. These findings suggest that there are familial factors in serum vitamin E among families of lung cancer patients. Similar results were found for serum selenium. The lower levels of serum vitamin E and selenium observed may also be related to common familial dietary habits and/or hereditary factors in metabolizing vitamin E and selenium. Although many factors can influence blood levels of vitamin E (see III. A.), the mean value of serum vitamin E (14.1 µg/mL) in controls is much higher than the average values reported elsewhere.

D. Gastrointestinal and Pancreatic Cancer

A case–control study in high- and low-risk areas was conducted to determine dietary factors and their contribution to the marked geographic variation in mortality from gastric cancer within Italy (Buiatti et al., 1990). Trained interviewers questioned 1016 gastric cancer patients and 1159 controls randomly selected from comparable sex and age strata of the same population. Usual frequency of intake and portion size in a 12-month period 2 years before the interview were assessed for 146 food and beverage items. Levels of α-tocopherol and other nutrients were estimated using food tables.

Risks of gastric cancer were found to vary significantly with estimated nutrient intake; however, risk was found to decrease in proportion to intake of α-tocopherol, β-carotene, ascorbic acid, and vegetable fat, and increase with increasing consumption of nitrites and protein. A 5-fold difference was found between those with a high intake of α-tocopherol/ascorbic acid and a low intake of protein/nitrite compounds when compared to those with a high intake of protein/nitrite compounds and a low intake of α-tocopherol/ascorbic acid. The study also showed that gastric cancer risk decreased with rising α-tocopherol intake in almost all ascorbic acid tertiles and vice versa. Similar results were found when they were calculated separately for males and females.

The findings of Buiatti et al. (1990) are consistent with the view that the ability of α-tocopherol and ascorbic acid to inhibit nitrosation may contribute to a reduced cancer risk of gastric cancer (Birt, 1986; Trickler and Shklar, 1987). This population study demonstrated an inverse relationship between the risk of gastric cancer and α-tocopherol intake. Further studies using biochemical assays and follow-up studies are needed to confirm the role of vitamin E in the prevention of gastric cancer in humans.

Charpiot et al. (1989) examined the possible link between the risk of digestive cancer and serum levels of α-tocopherol, retinol, retinol-binding protein, and prealbumin in 70 patients with digestive cancer, 34 patients with colonic polyps, and 78 controls of both sexes, ages 31 to 94 years, from Marseille, France. Serum samples were stored at −18°C prior to analysis. Relative to controls, a significant decrease in serum levels of α-tocopherol, retinol, retinol-binding protein, and prealbumin was found in patients with digestive cancer, but not in the polyp group. Since retinol-binding protein and prealbumin levels (possible indicators of protein malnutrition) were decreased, the decreased levels of vitamins A and E observed in digestive cancer patients may be the result of malabsorption. Moreover, since no documentation of nutrient intake or clinical nutritional status was included, the possibility of a generalized malnutrition could not be ruled out. Control subjects were not matched with cases nor were they a pure community-based control group; a portion of control subjects were hospitalized for elective surgery.

Knekt et al. (1988b) studied the association between levels of α-tocopherol and selenium in serum and subsequent risk of gastrointestinal cancer in a longitudinal case–control study based on 36,265 initially cancer-free Finnish men and women from 25 population groups, ages 15–99 years. Serum levels of α-tocopherol and selenium at entry into the study were measured in stored samples of 150 incident gastrointestinal cancer cases diagnosed during a 6–10 year follow-up and from 276 controls who were matched for sex, age, and place of residence.

Subjects with low serum levels of α-tocopherol or selenium had a higher subsequent risk of cancer of the upper gastrointestinal tract (esophagus and stomach). This association persisted among men after adjustment of various confounding factors and after excluding those with cancer diagnosed during the first 2 years of follow-up. The relative risk of cancer among those who fell in the lowest quintile of serum α-tocopherol was 2.2 compared with those in the higher quintiles. Serum levels of α-tocopherol or selenium in general were not inversely related to colorectal cancer risk. It should be noted that serum samples were stored at −20°C for an average of 13 years.

During a follow-up of 6 to 10 years, 453 cancers were diagnosed among 21,172 Finnish men (Knekt et al., 1988c). The serum levels of α-tocopherol were measured in stored serum samples from these men and 841 controls matched for municipality and age. The mean levels of serum α-tocopherol among all cancer cases and controls were 8.02 and 8.28 mg/L, respectively. Significantly lower α-tocopherol levels were found only in patients with pancreatic cancer. The relative risk of cancer in persons in the two highest quintiles of serum α-tocopherol was lower in comparison with those in the three lowest quintiles. The association was strongest for the combined group of cancers unrelated to smoking and varied between subgroups of the study population as well as between different cancers. The association persisted when adjusted for serum cholesterol, vitamin A, selenium, and various confounding factors.

When all 36,265 Finnish participants were considered together, cancer of all sites was diagnosed in 766 persons during the 8-year follow-up period (Knekt et al., 1991). The levels of serum α-tocopherol were determined from these cancer patients and 1419 matched control subjects. Individuals with low α-tocopherol had about a 1.5-fold risk of cancer compared with those with a higher level. The strength of the association between serum α-tocopherol level and cancer risk varied for different cancer sites and was strongest for some gastrointestinal cancers and for the combined group of cancers unrelated to smoking. The relative risk of cancer for those with a low level of serum α-tocopherol was greater than 2.0 compared to those with a higher level of serum α-tocopherol for different sites of gastrointestinal cancer (stomach, pancreas, and colorectum), with the exception of colorectal cancer among men. Since vitamin E deficiency is associated with malabsorption syndromes of various etiologies (Bieri and Farrell, 1976; Machlin, 1991), and gastrointestinal cancer can lead to malabsorption, the lower vitamin E status of patients with gastrointestinal cancer may be a consequence of the disease rather than the cause.

Burney et al. (1989) measured levels of α-tocopherol, selenium, total carotenoids, β-carotene, lycopene, retinol, and retinol-binding protein in frozen sera ($-70°C$) from 22 cases of cancer of the pancreas and 44 matched control subjects drawn from a larger pool of residents of Washington County, Maryland. In addition to matching for race and age, subjects were matched for the time between the last meal and blood sampling. The cases had a higher, though not statistically significant, mean level of serum vitamin E than the controls. Yet, the authors concluded that "low levels of serum vitamin E appear to have a protective effect, but a chance association between vitamin E and cancer of the pancreas could not reasonably be excluded." The authors also commented that the interpretation of the data is attenuated by the small sample size and long storage time.

E. Colorectal Cancer

DeCosse et al. (1989) studied the effects of wheat fiber and vitamins C and E on rectal polyps in patients with familial adenomatous polyposis in New York. The initial study population was comprised of 72 adult patients (average age 35 years) who had a total colectomy and ileorectal anastomosis at least 1 year before entry into the trial. After 3 months on placebo, 58 patients were randomly divided into groups and daily received either

a) 8 capsules of a lactose placebo and 2.2 g of a low-fiber supplement (control group, 10 males and 12 females);

b) 4 g of ascorbic acid, 400 mg of dl-α-tocopherol and 2.2 g of the low-fiber supplement (vitamin group, 5 males and 11 females); or

c) both vitamins plus 22.5 g of a high-fiber supplement (high-fiber group, 6 males and 14 females).

Over the 4 years of the trial, each participant underwent proctosigmoidoscopy every 3 months for a total of 18 examinations.

Data obtained suggested an inhibitory effect on benign large bowel neoplasia by high fiber intake, but not by vitamin supplementation. Since the high-fiber group also received vitamin supplements, the possibility of an interactive effect can not be excluded. Several issues confound the interpretation of this study:

1) vitamin status was not assessed biochemically at baseline or during the trial;

2) because of the combined use of vitamins, an analysis of independent effects or inter-actions of individual vitamins was not possible; and

3) there was no control of dietary intake or reporting of previous or concurrent vitamin supplementation.

Freudenheim et al. (1990) conducted a case–control study of diet and rectal cancer in three counties in western New York. Cases were single, primary adenocarcinomas age 40 years or older with no previous history of cancer; controls were matched to cases on age, sex, and neighborhood, and selected by a standardized protocol. A total of 277 case–control pairs of males and 145 case–control pairs of females were interviewed about usual quantity and frequency of consumption of 129 food items. Intake of vitamin E and other nutrients was determined using U.S. Department of Agriculture food compo-sition data and other food composition data. It was determined that higher vitamin E intake was not associated with lower risk of rectal cancer, while vitamin C, carotenoids, and fiber intake were. There were strong associations of risk with increased intakes of total kilocalories and fat and somewhat weaker associations with carbohydrates, protein, and iron. Increasing intake of retinol was found to be associated with increased risk in this study.

McKeown-Eyssen et al. (1988) conducted a double-blind randomized trial to exam-ine the effects of vitamins C and E on the rate of recurrence of colorectal polyps, a pre-sumed precursor for colorectal cancer. Two hundred male patients (age unknown) who had at least one polyp in the colon or rectum, identified by colonoscopic examination at two Toronto hospitals, were selected for the study. All participated in a brief dietary inquiry and were asked to discontinue their own vitamin supplement, if any, for the dura-tion of the study. Participants were randomized to receive a supplement of vitamin E (400 mg dl-α-tocopherol) and vitamin C (400 mg ascorbic acid) or lactose placebo over a peri-od of 2 years. A random urine sample was collected to assess the compliance with vita-min supplementation.

One hundred thirty-seven patients completed the study. Polyps were observed in the second colonoscopy in 41.4 percent of 70 subjects on vitamin supplements and in 50.7 percent of 67 subjects on placebos. Further examination of the pathology of polyps and analysis of polyp recurrence data suggests that any reduction in the rate of polyp recur-rence associated with vitamin supplementation is small. The effect of vitamin E per se could not be assessed because all experimental subjects received both vitamins C and E. Also, the compliance of patients with the vitamin supplementation is difficult to assess as there was no biochemical assessment of vitamin status either at baseline or during the trial.

F. Cervical /Ovarian Cancer

Cuzick et al. (1990) measured levels of vitamins A and E in sera of young women aged 16–40 participating in a case–control study of cervical intraepithelial neoplasia (CIN) carried out in London between 1984 and 1988. Cases were histologically classified from biopsy material as CIN I (n = 110), CIN II (n = 103), or CIN III (n = 284). Controls were randomly selected either among the patients of general practitioners (n = 206) or among women attending family planning clinics (n = 206). Women with CIN I lesions were sim-ilar to the controls with respect to most epidemiological factors whereas women with CIN III demonstrated all the major risk factors for invasive cervical cancer. Blood sam-ples were collected from 68 percent of the controls and 86 percent of the cases. Serum levels of vitamins A and E were measured on age-stratified random samples composed of 45 controls, 30 cases of CIN I and 40 cases of CIN III.

The mean values of vitamin E, but not vitamin A, decreased from controls to CIN I to CIN III. Also, there was a significant trend for the estimates of the odds ratio for the risk of CIN I and CIN III for quintiles of vitamin E, but not vitamin A. Adjustments for the confounding effects of sexual behavior, smoking habits, and use of oral contraceptives slightly strengthened the relationship with CIN III but had no effect on CIN I. The number of samples analyzed for serum vitamins A and E in each group is small. Also, no information regarding vitamin intake and supplementation of subjects was reported.

Heinonen et al. (1987) measured serum concentrations of retinol, α-tocopherol, and total carotene in 88 women with gynecological cancer (9 vulvar, 15 cervical, 36 endometrial, and 28 ovarian carcinomas) and 31 gynecological patients receiving treatment for abnormal bleeding, uterine fibromas or genital prolapse in Tampere, Finland. None of the patients received vitamin A or E supplementation, but no dietary intake data were collected. No significant differences were found in the serum levels of α-tocopherol between cancer cases and controls. There were no healthy community-based controls. Cases were in varying clinical conditions and were not matched with controls.

Palan et al. (1991) studied the relationship of plasma levels of α-tocopherol and β-carotene with incidence of uterine and cervical dysplasias and cancer in a cross-sectional sampling of 116 women in New York City. Of the 116 subjects, 36 had negative cytology, normal colposcopy, were not using oral contraceptives, and had no gynecologic dysfunction (control group, average age 28.4). Eighty women had abnormal cytology and were referred for colposcopy. Of these, 27 had no significant pathology (No CIN, age 25.1). Forty-three were histopathologically graded and stratified as CIN I and CIN II (n = 31, age 27.4) or CIN III and carcinoma-in-situ (n = 12, age 30.7). The remaining 10 patients had pathologic evidence of cervical cancer (age 43.2). A blood sample was obtained from each subject prior to any therapeutic intervention.

An inverse association between plasma levels of both α-tocopherol and β-carotene and increasingly severe graded cervical pathology was reported. The effect of vitamin E was independent of smoking status. The findings suggest that vitamin E may play a role in the pathogenesis of cervical intraepithelial lesions and cervical cancer. The number of subjects in each group, however, is relatively small, and groups were not matched properly. Also, the plasma levels (ranging from 4.1 mg/L in the cancer group to 6.56 mg/L for controls) of α-tocopherol are lower than reported elsewhere.

Verreault et al. (1989) conducted a population-based, case–control study to assess the relation of dietary intake of vitamin E, as well as vitamins A and C and folic acid, to the risk of cervical carcinoma. Cases were 189 women diagnosed with cervical carcinoma in the Seattle area. Controls were 227 subjects selected using random digit dialing. Dietary intake during the year preceding diagnosis was assessed by using a 66-item food-frequency questionnaire. Mean daily intakes of nutrients were computed using standard portion sizes. The contents of vitamin E and other nutrients were estimated from food-composition tables. After adjustment for known risk factors, estimated consumption of vitamin E was related to the risk of cervical cancer. High vitamin E intake was related to a reduced risk, and the risk for women in the highest quartile was only one-third for those in the first quartile. Intake of retinol and folic acid was not found to be related to the risk of cervical cancer. This is the first report suggesting a protective effect of dietary vitamin E against invasive cervical cancer.

In the same Finnish study reported earlier (Knekt et al., 1988a), 313 of 15,093 female participants were diagnosed with cancer during the 8-year follow-up period (Knekt, 1988). Serum α-tocopherol levels of these cases were compared with 578 controls, matched for municipality and age. An inverse relation was observed between α-tocopherol levels and risk for cancer, even if the cancer cases of the first 2 years of follow-up were excluded. Women in the 3 lowest quintiles for α-tocopherol levels compared to those with highest values had a 1.6-fold risk of cancer when adjusted for possible confounding factors. It was suggested that a low level of α-tocopherol in general strongly predicted epithelial cancers while carrying an only slightly elevated risk of cancers in reproductive organs exposed to estrogens.

G. Other Sites

Helzlsouer et al. (1989) studied the association between the development of bladder cancer and serum levels of α-tocopherol and other micronutrients in Washington County, Maryland. Serum samples from 25,802 participants, aged 11–98, were collected in 1974 and stored at –70°C. In the subsequent 12-year period, 35 cases of bladder cancer developed among the participants. Comparisons of earlier serum levels among cases and two age and race-matched controls for each case showed that selenium, but not α-tocopherol, was significantly lower among cases than controls.

In another analysis of the Washington County, Maryland study no significant associations were observed for serum tocopherol levels and risk of prostate cancer (Hsing et al., 1990). Cases were 103 men who developed prostate cancer during the subsequent 13 years and control subjects matched for age, sex (all male), and race (all Caucasian).

Stryker et al. (1990) examined the relationship between the risk of malignant melanoma and dietary intake and plasma levels of retinol, carotenes, and α-tocopherol. Cases (n = 204, 96 males and 108 females) and controls (n = 248, 96 males and 152 females) were patients age 18 years or older making their first visit to a Boston dermatology subspeciality clinic for pigmented lesions. Intakes of nutrients were estimated using a semiquantitative 116-item food-frequency questionnaire, a write-in section for other foods, and questions on the use of vitamin and mineral supplements, and on type of fats used for baking and frying.

The levels of plasma retinol, α-tocopherol, lycopene, α-carotene, and β-carotene were not different between cases and controls. Controls, however, had a significantly higher intake of vitamin E, not counting vitamin supplementation. No significantly different associations with malignant melanoma were observed for higher plasma levels of lycopene, retinol or α-carotene in logistic regression analyses after control for age, sex, plasma lipids, and known constitutional risk factors (hair color and ability to tan). Intake of vitamin E from food alone displayed a trend of decreasing risk with increasing intake (p = 0.003). The odds ratio comparing the highest with the lowest quintile of vitamin E intake from food was 0.7 (p = 0.4) for plasma α-tocopherol and total vitamin E intake. Controls were clinic-based and were not matched with cases.

Kanematsu et al. (1989) measured the levels of vitamin A and vitamin E in plasma and human hepatocellular carcinoma and adjacent liver parenchymal tissues from 26 patients (21 men and 5 women) with an average age of 57.4 years (ranging from 36 to 71 years) in Fukuoka, Japan. Tissue samples were obtained from resected specimens, and morphologically characterized by microscopic examination. Histological examination showed that 19 had cirrhosis, 4 had fibrosis, and 1 had chronic active hepatitis. The other two had no evidence of cirrhosis, fibrosis, or hepatitis. Samples were stored at –80°C prior to analysis. The level of vitamin A, but not vitamin E, was significantly decreased in hepatocellular carcinoma compared to normal liver tissues. Plasma levels of vitamin E (mean = 0.46 mg/dL) were lower than the normal values. However, no control samples were available for comparison.

H. Combined Site Studies

Rougereau et al. (1987) studied the relationship between fat-soluble vitamins and cancer localization in cancer patients in France. The subjects were hospitalized patients, 464 males and 604 females, ages 20 to 65 years. Controls were 527 healthy males and 653 females ages 20 to 53 years. Fasting blood samples were drawn before surgical treatment, chemo- or radiotherapy and were analyzed within 24 hours. Serum samples from 880 controls were also analyzed for the levels of vitamin A, β-carotene, α-tocopherol and carcinomedin (1-keto-24-methyl-25-hydroxycholecalciferol). A statistical multidimensional analysis of data led to five separate groups of cancer types. Within each group, alterations of vitamin spectra were the same as controls but were significantly different between groups. All these groups are statistically different from the reference group. There was an inverse association of vitamin E level with cancers of the lung, gastrointestinal tract, and nervous systems, but not for hormonally related cancers. The authors suggest that carcinogenesis may alter fat-soluble vitamin metabolism and that altered vitamin metabolism may be involved in the carcinogenic process.

Rougereau et al. (1988) subsequently examined and followed the serum levels of carcinomedin, vitamin A, β-carotene and α-tocopherol of 42 subjects with various cancers (stomach, esophagus, breast, ovaries, uterus, etc.) for up to 38 months. The patients of both sexes were between 38 and 66 years of age and were in varying therapeutic situations. The follow-up period extended from the initial clinical diagnosis of the tumor or from its preoperative stage up to the end of treatment, remission, or death. Controls were 23 cancer patients treated with chemotherapy and/or radiotherapy, for whom the investigators had no knowledge of the clinical data. Patients whose serum vitamin A and α-tocopherol concentrations remained within normal limits survived longer than those with lower concentrations. The number of subjects in this study is small and the subjects (including designated controls) were in varying clinical and therapeutic situations.

From the same Washington County, Maryland survey reported earlier (Burney et al., 1989; Hsing et al., 1990), prediagnostic serum samples from 436 cancer cases representing 9 primary sites and 765 matched control subjects were also analyzed for vitamin E levels (Comstock et al., 1991; Schober et al., 1987). Higher serum vitamin E levels were found to associate with a reduced risk of the cancer of the lung, but not of colon, rectum, pancreas, melanoma, basal cell of skin, breast, prostate, or bladder.

In a prospective follow-up study conducted in Basel, Switzerland, Gey et al. (1987) measured the plasma levels of vitamin E and several micronutrients in approximately 3000 healthy male volunteers (mean age 51 years). The plasma analyses were performed immediately to avoid vitamin E destruction due to storage. The mortality (268 subjects or 9 percent of the population) was registered during the subsequent 7 years. A comparison of the baseline level of case subjects with all survivors (n = 2707) was made. Cholesterol and triglyceride-standardized vitamin E at 30 μM (12.9 mg/L) was used as the lowest tertile of cancer cases to estimate the relative risk adjusted for age and smoking. The absolute baseline plasma level of age-standardized mean α-tocopherol was significantly lower in subjects who later died of all types of cancers and of combined gastrointestinal cancers.

Twelve years after blood samples were taken from 2974 healthy men in Basel, 553 of the subjects died. Among these, 204 died from cancer, including 68 with bronchus cancer and 37 with gastrointestinal cancer (Stähelin et al., 1989, 1991). A comparison of the mean vitamin E values among the different groups considered revealed no significant differences. By contrast, vitamin A, β-carotene, and vitamin C were found to be associated with cancer mortality. The use of different statistical models may be partly responsible for the differing results in the 7-year versus 12-year follow-up studies. Unlike most other studies, fasting plasma levels of vitamin E were analyzed soon after sample collection. Thus the problem of oxidative destruction of vitamin E associated with long-term storage was avoided.

To investigate whether vitamin E status is related to future incidence of cancers, Wald et al. (1987) conducted a prospective study in London. Blood samples were collected from about 22,000 men ages 35–64 and sera stored at –40°C. During the subsequent 3–10 years, 271 men were identified as having developed cancer. The concentration of vitamin E was measured in serum samples obtained from these cases and from 533 control subjects matched for age, smoking history, and serum storage duration.

The mean vitamin E level was not significantly different between the cancer subjects and controls. However, the mean level of vitamin E in the cancer subjects, diagnosed within a year from the date of blood collection, was significantly lower than controls. For subjects whose cancers were diagnosed one or more years after blood collection, the difference was not statistically significant either for all cancers or for cancers of six sites (lung, colon and rectum, stomach, bladder, central nervous system, and skin) considered separately. The authors concluded that the low vitamin E levels observed in these subjects were a metabolic consequence of tumor development, rather than a precursor, of the cancer.

Connett et al. (1989) evaluated the baseline serum levels of β-carotene, total carotenoid, vitamins A and E, and retinol-binding protein of 156 men who died of cancer and 311 controls individually matched for age, smoking status, randomization group, date of randomization, and clinical center. The subjects were from a non-blinded, randomized trial of 12,866 men at risk of coronary heart disease, aged 35 to 57 years at baseline. Blood specimens were stored at –50° to –70°C for over 4 years. Except for β-carotene, serum levels of retinols, α-tocopherol, and retinol-binding protein were not found to differ significantly between cases and controls and were not related to any cancer site.

V. Summary and Conclusions

Many recent studies have attempted to relate serum or plasma levels of vitamin E, as well as intake of vitamin E, to the subsequent development of various cancers. Some of the studies have found that low levels of serum/plasma vitamin E or low dietary intake of the vitamin correlated with elevated risk of certain cancers; others have found no such correlations. In general, there are more studies suggesting a positive correlation between higher risk of cancers and lower intake or serum/plasma levels of vitamin E than those that do not find this association. Although several studies reported higher blood levels of vitamin E in cases than controls (Burney et al., 1989; Gerber et al., 1989, 1990), there have been no reports of a correlation between higher intake of vitamin E and higher risk of cancer. Currently, eight clinical intervention trials for vitamin E are in progress (Knekt, 1991). The completion of these large-scale studies is needed before the effectiveness of vitamin E in chemopreventive trials can be generalized. To date, no information obtained from intervention studies designed specifically to study the efficacy of vitamin E is available.

It should be pointed out that assessment of serum/plasma levels of vitamin E in cancer patients, especially those with gastrointestinal cancer, is not a specific indicator of vitamin E intake, as the results obtained may be the consequence, rather than a contributing factor, of the disease. Also, measurement of plasma/serum tocopherol levels, which is used almost exclusively in nutritional epidemiological studies, is not a reliable means for assessing long-term vitamin E status. Furthermore, many factors, such as

a) handling and storage conditions and length of storage of plasma/serum samples,

b) control of blood lipids and use of fasted versus fed samples,

c) methods of vitamin E measurement,

d) interviewing techniques, and

e) quality of data in food-composition table regarding tocopherol content, can significantly compromise the accuracy and reliability of information obtained.

With regard to the relation of vitamin E and cancer risk, the Surgeon General's Report on Nutrition and Health (U.S. Department of Health and Human Services, 1988) concluded that "Although some studies suggest it has a protective effect, in human studies no link was reported between vitamin E levels and risk of cancer when incidence rates at all sites were combined." The Report of the Committee on Diet and Health (National Research Council, 1989a) concluded that "vitamin E intake is in itself not related to overall risk of cancer, but that low serum levels of vitamin E coupled with low selenium may increase the risk of at least some cancer such as breast and lung cancer." The latest information available still is not sufficient to make a definite conclusion concerning the relationship between vitamin E intake and risk of human cancers.

More studies, especially well-designed, large-scale observational studies and intervention trials using human populations in various circumstances, are needed to establish the possible anticarcinogenic effect of vitamin E in humans. Also, a better understanding of the mechanisms by which vitamin E protects against free-radical-induced lipid peroxidation tissue injury, as well as the possible role of vitamin E in malignant transformation, tumor cell proliferation, immune defense system competence, and precancerous lesions, is necessary to evaluate the possible role of vitamin E in preventing human cancer.

VI. Bibliography*

Basu, T.K.; Hill, G.B.; Ng, D.; Abdi, E.; Temple, N. 1989. Serum vitamins A and E, β-carotene, and selenium in patients with breast cancer. *J. Am. Coll. Nutr.* 8:524–529.

Bertram, J.S.; Kolonel, L.N.; Meyskens, F.L., Jr. 1987. Rationale and strategies for chemoprevention of cancer in humans. *Cancer Res.* 47:3012–3031.

Bieri, J.G.; Farrell, P.M. 1976. Vitamin E. *Vitam. Horm.* 34:31–75.

Birt, D.F. 1986. Update on the effects of vitamins A, C, and E and selenium on carcinogenesis. *Proc. Soc. Exp. Biol. Med.* 183:311–320.

Boscoboinik, D.; Szewczyk, A.; Hensey, C.; Azzi, A. 1991. Inhibition of cell proliferation by α-tocopherol. *J. Biol. Chem.* 266:6188–6194.

Buiatti, E.; Palli, D.; Decarli, A.; Amadori, D.; Avellini, C.; Bianchi, S.; Bonaguri, C.; Cipriani, F.; Cocco, P.; Giacosa, A.; Marubini, E.; Minacci, C.; Puntoni, R.; Russo, A.; Vindigni, C.; Fraumeni, J.F., Jr.; Blot, W.J. 1990. A case–control study of gastric cancer and diet in Italy. II. Association with nutrients. *Int. J. Cancer* 45:896–901.

Burney, P.G.J.; Comstock, G.W.; Morris, J.S. 1989. Serologic precursors of cancer: serum micronutrients and the subsequent risk of pancreatic cancer. *Am. J. Clin. Nutr.* 49:895–900.

Catignani, G.L.; Chytil, F.; Darby, W.J. 1974. Vitamin E deficiency: immunochemical evidence for increased accumulation of liver xanthine oxidase. *Proc. Nat. Acad. Sci.* 71:1966–1968.

Charpiot, P.; Calaf, R.; Di-Costanzo, J.; Romette, J.; Rotily, M.; Durbec, J.P.; Garcon, D. 1989. Vitamin A, vitamin E, retinol binding protein (RBP), and prealbumin in digestive cancers. *Int. J. Vitam. Nutr. Res.* 59:323–328.

---

*This bibliography contains all reference citations that are either in the text or the tables or both.

Chen, J.; Goetchius, M.P.; Campbell, T.C.; Combs, G.F., Jr. 1982. Effect of dietary selenium and vitamin E on hepatic mixed-function oxidase activities and in vivo covalent binding of aflatoxin B1 in rats. *J. Nutr.* 112:324–331.

Chen, L.H.; Boissonneault, G.A.; Glauert, H.P. 1988. Vitamin C, vitamin E and cancer (review). *Anticancer Res.* 8:739–748.

Chow, C.K. 1979. Nutritional influence on cellular antioxidant defense systems. *Am. J. Clin. Nutr.* 32:1066–1081.

Chow, C.K. 1985. Vitamin E and blood. *World Rev. Nutr. Diet.* 45:133–166.

Chow, C.K., editor. 1988. Interrelationships of cellular antioxidant defense systems. *Cellular antioxidant defense mechanisms.* Boca Raton: CRC Press. Vol. 2. p. 217–237.

Chow, C.K. 1991. Vitamin E and oxidative stress. *Free Radic. Biol. Med.* 11:215–232.

Chow, C.K.; Gairola, G.C. 1984. Influence of dietary vitamin E and selenium on metabolic activation of chemicals to mutagens. *J. Agric. Food Chem.* 32:443–447.

Comstock, G.W.; Helzlsouer, K.J.; Bush, T.L. 1991. Prediagnostic serum levels of carotenoids and vitamin E as related to subsequent cancer in Washington County, Maryland. *Am. J. Clin. Nutr.* 53:260S–264S.

Connett, J.E.; Kuller, L.H.; Kjelsberg, M.O.; Polk, B.F.; Collins, G.; Rider, A.; Hulley, S.B. 1989. Relationship between carotenoids and cancer: the Multiple Risk Intervention Trial (MRFIT) Study. *Cancer* 64:126–134.

Cuzick, J.; De Stavola, B.L.; Russell, M.J.; Thomas, B.S. 1990. Vitamin A, vitamin E and the risk of cervical intraepithelial neoplasia. *Br. J. Cancer* 62:651–652.

DeCosse, J.J.; Miller, H.H.; Lesser, M.L. 1989. Effect of wheat fiber and vitamins C and E on rectal polyps in patients with familial adenomatous polyposis. *J. Natl. Cancer Inst.* 81:1290–1297.

De Vries, N.; Snow, G.B. 1990. Relationships of vitamins A and E and beta-carotene serum levels to head and neck cancer patients with and without second primary tumors. *Eur. Arch. Otorhinolaryngol.* 247:368–370.

Diliberto, E.J., Jr.; Dean, G.; Carter, C.; Allen, P.L. 1982. Tissue, subcellular, and submitochondrial distributions of semidehydroascorbate reductase: possible role of semidehydroascorbate reductase in cofactor regeneration. *J. Neurochem.* 39:563–568.

Drozdz, M.; Gierek, T.; Jendryczko, A.; Pierkarska, J.; Pilch, J.; Polanska, D. 1989. Zinc, vitamins A and E, and retinol-binding protein in sera of patients with cancer of the larynx. *Neoplasma* 36:357–362.

Esterbauer, H.; Cheeseman, K.H.; editors. 1987. Lipid peroxidation. Part II. Pathological implications. *Chem. Phys. Lipids* 45:103–368.

Evans, H.M.; Bishop, K.S. 1922. On existence of hitherto unrecognized dietary factor essential for reproduction. *Science* 56:650–651.

Freeman, B.A.; Crapo, J.D. 1982. Biology of disease: free radicals and tissue injury. *Lab. Invest.* 47:412–426.

Freudenheim, J.L.; Graham, S.; Marshall, J.R.; Haughey, B.P.; Wilkinson, G. 1990. A case–control study of diet and rectal cancer in western New York. *Am. J. Epidemiol.* 131:612–624.

Gerber. M.; Cavallo, F.; Marubini, E.; Richardson, S.; Barbieri, A.; Capitelli, E.; Costa, A.; de Paulet, A.C.; de Paulet, P.C.; Decarli, A.; Pastorino, U.; Pujol, H. 1988. Liposoluble vitamins and lipid parameters in breast cancer: a joint study in northern Italy and southern France. *Int. J. Cancer* 42:489–494.

Gerber, M.; Richardson, S.; Cavallo, F.; Marubini, E.; de Paulet, P.C.; de Paulet, A.C.; Pujol, H. 1990. The role of diet history and biologic assays in the study of diet and breast cancer. *Tumori* 76:321–330.

Gerber, M.; Richardson, S.; De Paulet, P.C.; Pujol, H.; De Paulet, A.C. 1989. Relationship between vitamin E and polyunsaturated fatty acids in breast cancer: nutritional and metabolic aspects. *Cancer* 64:2347–2353.

Gey, K.F.; Brubacher, G.B.; Stähelin, H.B. 1987. Plasma levels of antioxidant vitamins in relation to ischemic heart disease and cancer. *Am. J. Clin. Nutr.* 45:1368–1377.

Gridley, G.; McLaughlin, J.K.; Block, G.; Blot, W.J.; Winn, D.M.; Greenberg, R.S.; Schoenberg, J.B.; Preston-Martin, S.; Austin, D.F.; Fraumeni, J.F., Jr. 1990. Diet and oral and pharyngeal cancer among blacks. *Nutr. Cancer* 14:219–225.

Halliwell, B. 1987. Oxidants and human disease: some new concepts. *FASEB J.* 1:358–364.

Heinonen, P.K.; Kuoppala, T.; Koskinen, T.; Punnonen, R. 1987. Serum vitamins A and E and carotene in patients with gynecologic cancer. *Arch. Gynecol. Obstet.* 241:151–156.

Helzlsouer, K.J.; Comstock, G.W.; Morris, J.S. 1989. Selenium, lycopene, α-tocopherol, β-carotene, retinol, and subsequent bladder cancer. *Cancer Res.* 49:6144–6148.

Horwitt, M.K. 1962. Interrelations between vitamin E and polyunsaturated fatty acids in adult men. *Vitam. Hormon.* 20:541–558.

Horwitt, M.K. 1974. Status of human requirement for vitamin E. *Am. J. Clin. Nutr.* 27:1182–1193.

Horwitt, M.K. 1991. Data supporting supplementation of humans with vitamin E. *J. Nutr.* 121:424–429.

Hsing, A.W.; Comstock, G.W.; Abbey, H.; Polk, B.F. 1990. Serologic precursors of cancer: retinol, carotenoids, and tocopherol and risk of prostate cancer. *J. Natl. Cancer Inst.* 82:941–946.

Kanematsu, T.; Kawano, T.; Takenaka, K.; Matsumata, T.; Sugimachi, K.; Kuwano, M. 1989. Levels of vitamin A and cellular retinol binding protein in human hepatocellular carcinoma and adjacent normal tissue. *Nutr. Cancer* 12:311–319.

Knekt, P. 1988. Serum vitamin E level and risk of female cancers. *Int. J. Epidemiol.* 17:281–286.

Knekt, P. 1991. Role of vitamin E in the prophyaxis of cancer. *Ann. Med.* 23:3–12.

Knekt, P.; Seppänen. R.; Aaran, R.-K. 1988a. Determinants of serum α-tocopherol in Finnish adults. *Prev. Med.* 17:725–735.

Knekt, P.; Aromaa, A.; Maatela, J.; Alfthan, G.; Aaran, R.-K.; Teppo, L.; Hakama, M. 1988b. Serum vitamin E, serum selenium and the risk of gastrointestinal cancer. *Int. J. Cancer* 42:846–850.

Knekt, P.; Aromaa, A.; Maatela, J.; Aaran, R.-K.; Nikkari, T.; Hakama, M.; Hakulinen, T.; Peto, R.; Saxén, E.; Teppo, L. 1988c. Serum vitamin E and risk of cancer among Finnish men during a 10-year follow-up. *Am. J. Epidemiol.* 127:28–41.

Knekt, P.; Aromaa, A.; Maatela, J.; Aaran, R.-K.; Nikkari, T.; Hakama, M.; Hakulinen, T.; Peto, R.; Teppo, L. 1991. Vitamin E and cancer prevention. *Am. J. Clin. Nutr.* 53:283S–286S.

Kok, F.J.; van Duijn, C.M.; Hofman, A.; Vermeeren, R.; de Bruijn, A.M.; Valkenburg, H.A. 1987. Micronutrients and the risk of lung cancer. *N. Engl. J. Med.* 316:1416.

Langemann, H.; Torhorst, J.; Kabiersch, A.; Krenger, W.; Honegger, C.G. 1989. Quantitative determination of water- and lipid-soluble antioxidants in neoplastic and non-neoplastic human breast tissue. *Int. J. Cancer* 43:1169–1173.

LeGardeur, B.Y.; Lopez-S., A.; Johnson, W.D. 1990. A case–control study of serum vitamins A, E, and C in lung cancer patients. *Nutr. Cancer* 14:133–140.

Lehmann, J. 1981. Comparative sensitivities of tocopherol levels of platelets, red blood cells, and plasma for estimating vitamin E nutritional status in the rat. *Am. J. Clin. Nutr.* 34:2104–2110.

Lucy, J.A. 1972. Part 1. Cellular biochemistry of vitamin E. Functional and structural aspects of biological membranes: a suggested structural role for vitamin E in the control of membrane permeability and stability. *Ann. N. Y. Acad. Sci.* 203:4–11.

Machlin, L.J. 1989. Use and safety of elevated dosages of vitamin E in adults. *Int. J. Vitam. Nutr. Res.* (Suppl. 30):56–68.

Machlin, L.J. 1991. Vitamin E. In: Machlin, L.J., ed. *Handbook of vitamins.* 2nd ed. New York: Marcel Dekker. p. 99–144.

McKeown-Eyssen, G.; Holloway, C.; Jazmaji, V.; Bright-See, E.; Dion, P.; Bruce, W.R. 1988. A randomized trial of vitamins C and E in the prevention of recurrence of colorectal polyps. *Cancer Res.* 48:4701–4705.

Mergens, W.J.; Bhagavan, H.N. 1989. α-Tocopherols (vitamin E). In: Moon, T.E.; Micozzi, M.S.; eds. *Nutrition and cancer prevention: investigating the role of micronutrients.* New York: Marcel Dekker, Inc. p. 305–340.

Meydani, S.N.; Barklund, M.P.; Liu, S.; Meydani, M.; Miller, R.A.; Cannon, J.G.; Morrow, F.D.; Rocklin, R.; Blumberg, J.B. 1990. Vitamin E supplementation enhances cell-mediated immunity in healthy elderly subjects. *Am. J. Clin. Nutr.* 52:557–563.

Meyer, E.C.; Sommers, D.K.; Reitz, C.J.; Mentis, H. 1990. Vitamin E and benign breast disease. *Surgery* 107:549–551.

Miyamoto, H.; Araya, Y.; Ito, M.; Isobe, H.; Dosaka, H.; Shimizu, T.; Kishi, F.; Yamamoto, I.; Honma, H.; Kawakami, Y. 1987. Serum selenium and vitamin E concentrations in families of lung cancer patients. *Cancer* 60:1159–1162.

National Cancer Institute. 1990. *Cancer statistics review 1973–1987.* DHHS Publ. No. (NIH) 90-2789. Available from: U.S. Government Printing Office, Washington, DC.

National Center for Health Statistics. 1986. *Vital statistics of the United States, 1982.* Vol. 2. Mortality. Part A. Department of Health and Human Services Publication No. (PHS) 86-1122 Available from: U.S. Government Printing Office, Washington, DC.

National Research Council, Committee on Diet, Nutrition and Cancer. 1989a. *Diet and health: implications for reducing chronic disease risk.* Washington, DC: National Academy Press.

National Research Council, Food and Nutrition Board. 1989b. *Recommended dietary allowances.* 10th ed. Washington, DC: National Academy Press. p. 150–158.

Niki, E.; Tsuchiya, J.; Tanimura, R.; Kamiya, Y. 1982. Regeneration of vitamin E from α-chromanoxyl radical by glutathione and vitamin C. *Chem. Lett.* (June):789–792.

Packer, J.E.; Slater, T.F.; Willson, R.L. 1979. Direct observation of a free radical interaction between vitamin E and vitamin C. *Nature* 278:737–738.

Packer, L. 1991. Protective role of vitamin E in biological systems. *Am. J. Clin. Nutr.* 53:1050S–1055S.

Palan, P.R.; Mikhail, M.S.; Basu, J.; Romney, S.L. 1991. Plasma levels of antioxidant β-carotene and α-tocopherol in uterine cervix dysplasias and cancer. *Nutr. Cancer* 15:13–20.

Prasad, K.N.; Edwards-Prasad, J. 1982. Effects of tocopherol (vitamin E) acid succinate on morphological alterations and growth inhibition in melanoma cells in culture. *Cancer Res.* 42:550–555.

Rautalahti, M.; Albanes, D.; Hyvönen, L.; Piironen, V. 1990. Effect of sampling site on retinol, carotenoid, tocopherol, and tocotrienol concentration of adipose tissue of human breast with cancer. *Ann. Nutr. Metab.* 34:37–41.

Reddy, C.C.; Scholz, R.W.; Thomas, C.E.; Massaro, E.J. 1982. Vitamin E dependent reduced glutathione inhibition of rat liver microsomal lipid peroxidation. *Life Sci.* 31:571–576.

Rogers, A.E.; Longnecker, M.P. 1988. Biology of disease—dietary and nutritional influences on cancer: a review of epidemiologic and experimental data. *Lab. Invest.* 59:729–759.

Rotruck, J.T. 1972. Selenium: biochemical role as a component of glutathione peroxidase. *Science* 179:588–590.

Rougereau, A.; Person, O.; Rougereau, G. 1987. Fat soluble vitamins and cancer localization associated to an abnormal ketone derivative of D3 vitamin: carcinomedin. *Int. J. Vitam. Nutr. Res.* 57:367–373.

Rougereau, A.; Person, O.; Rougereau, G.; Sallerin, T.; Hellegouarch, R. 1988. Serum levels of carcinomedin (1-keto-24-methyl-25-hydroxycholecalciferol) as as indicator of the progression of cancer: preliminary results of a prospective study. *Int. J. Vitam. Nutr. Res.* 58:381–386.

Russell, M.J.; Thomas, B.S.; Bulbrook, R.D. 1988. A prospective study of the relationship between serum vitamins A and E and risk of breast cancer. *Br. J. Cancer* 57:213–215.

Schober, S.E.; Comstock, G.W.; Helsing, K.J.; Salkeld, R.M.; Morris, J.S.; Rider, A.A.; Brookmeyer, R. 1987. Serologic precursors of cancer. I. Prediagnostic serum nutrients and colon cancer risk. *Am. J. Epidemiol.* 126:1033–1041.

Scott, M.L. 1970. Studies on vitamin E and related factors in nutrition and metabolism. In: Deluca, H.F.; Suttie, J.W.; eds. *The fat-soluble vitamins*. Madison, WI: University of Wisconsin Press. p. 355–368.

Sokol, R.J. 1988. Vitamin E deficiency and neurologic disease. *Ann. Rev. Nutr.* 8:351–373.

Sokol, R.J. 1989. Vitamin E and neurologic function in man. *Free Radic. Biol. Med.* 6:189–207.

Stähelin, H.B.; Gey, K.F.; Eichholzer, M.; Lüdin, E.; Bernasconi, F.; Thurneysen, J.; Brubacher, G. 1991. Plasma antioxidant vitamins and subsequent cancer mortality in the 12 year follow-up of the prospective Basel Study. *Am. J. Epidemiol.* 133:766–775.

Stähelin, H.B.; Gey, K.F.; Eichholzer, M.; Lüdin, E.; Brubacher, G. 1989. Cancer mortality and vitamin E status. *Ann. N. Y. Acad. Sci.* 570:391–399.

Stryker, W.S.; Stampfer, M.J.; Stein, E.A.; Kaplan, L.; Louis, T.A.; Sober, A.; Willett, W.C. 1990. Diet, plasma levels of beta-carotene and alpha-tocopherol, and risk of malignant melanoma. *Am. J. Epidemiol.* 131:597–611.

Tangney, C.C.; Shekelle, R.B.; Raynor, W.; Gale, M.; Betz, E.P. 1987. Intra- and interindividual variation in measurements of β-carotene, retinol, and tocopherols in diet and plasma. *Am. J. Clin. Nutr.* 45:764–769.

Tappel, A.L. 1972. Vitamin E and free radical peroxidation of lipids. *Ann. N. Y. Acad. Sci.* 203:12–28.

Toniolo, P.; Riboli, E.; Protta, F.; Charrel, M.; Cappa, A.P.M. 1989. Calorie-providing nutrients and risk of breast cancer. *J. Natl. Cancer Inst.* 81:278–286.

Trickler, D.; Shklar G. 1987. Prevention by vitamin E of experimental oral carcinogenesis. *J. Natl. Cancer Inst.* 78:165–169.

Tuyns, A.J.; Riboli, E.; Doornbos, G.; Péquignot, G. 1987. Diet and esophageal cancer in Calvados (France). *Nutr. Cancer* 9:81–92.

U.S. Department of Health and Human Services. 1988. *The Surgeon General's report on nutrition and health*. Available from: U.S. Government Printing Office, Washington, DC.

Ursini, F.; Maiorino, M.; Gregolin, C. 1985. The selenoenzyme phospholipid hydroperoxide glutathione peroxidase. *Biochim. Biophys. Acta* 839:62–70.

Van Helden, P.D.; Beyers, A.D.; Bester, A.J.; Jaskiewicz, K. 1987. Esophageal cancer: vitamin and lipotrope deficiencies in an at-risk South African population. *Nutr. Cancer* 10:247–255.

Vatassery, G.T.; Krezowski, A.M.; Eckfeldt, J.H. 1983. Vitamin E concentrations in human blood plasma and platelets. *Am. J. Clin. Nutr.* 37:1020–1024.

Verreault, R.; Chu, J.; Mandelson, M.; Shy, K. 1989. A case–control study of diet and invasive cervical cancer. *Int. J. Cancer* 43:1050–1054.

Wald, N.J.; Boreham, J.; Hayward, J.L.; Bulbrook, R.D. 1984. Plasma retinol, β-carotene and vitamin E levels in relation to the future risk of breast cancer. *Br. J. Cancer* 49:321–324.

Wald, N.J.; Nicolaides-Bouman, A.; Hudson, G.A. 1988. Plasma retinol, beta-carotene and vitamin E levels in relation to the future risk of breast cancer. *Br. J. Cancer* 57:235.

Wald, N.J.; Thompson, S.G.; Densem, J.W.; Boreham, J.; Bailey, A. 1987. Serum vitamin E and subsequent risk of cancer. *Br. J. Cancer* 56:69–72.

Wefers, H.; Sies, H. 1988. The protection by ascorbate and glutathione against microsomal lipid peroxidation is dependent on vitamin E. *Eur. J. Biochem.* 174:353–357.

Weinstein, I.B. 1988. The origins of human cancer: molecular mechanisms of carcinogenesis and their implications for cancer prevention and treatment. *Cancer Res.* 48:4135–4143.

Willett, W.C.; Stampfer, M.J.; Underwood, B.A.; Speizer, F.E.; Rosner, B.; Hennekens, C.H. 1983. Validation of a dietary questionnaire with plasma carotenoid and α-tocopherol levels. *Am. J. Clin. Nutr.* 38:631–639.

Appendix

Criteria for Inclusion of Articles in Appendix Tables

Articles in peer-reviewed journals related to the topic of this review were selected primarily on the basis of date and content. In general, papers appearing in 1987 or thereafter were included, provided that they presented original data from studies in humans. Certain items tabulated for the sake of completeness may not have been cited in the body of the text if their weight or relevance did not add significantly to development of the author's argument. Reviews have not been listed except as they included new data or useful meta-analyses.

APPENDIX TABLE 1   Vitamin E and Head and Neck Cancer

Study	Type/Location	Subject Number and Description	Methods
de Vries et al., 1990	Cross-sectional Netherlands	71 cases of *squamous cell cancer of the head and neck* (HNC-I), with only a single tumor. 17 cases HNC with at least 1 additional tumor (HNC-II).	Serum levels of vitamin A, vitamin E, and β-carotene were measured.
Drozdz et al., 1989	Case–control Poland	22 newly diagnosed cases of *larynx cancer*. 16 patients with nonmalignant laryngeal disease. 16 patients with other nonmalignant diseases including CVD or hernia.	Overnight-fasted serum samples were collected and stored at –40°C for no more than 2 wk. Serum vitamins A and E were measured fluorometrically.
Gridley et al., 1990	Case–control Four regions: New Jersey, Atlanta, Los Angeles, Santa Clara and San Mateo, California	190 cases of *oral (and pharyngeal) cancer* (142♂, 48♀) including cancers of tongue and pharynx and other oral cancers, excluding cancers of the lip, salivary gland, or nasopharynx. 201 population-based controls (139 ♂, 62 ♀) matched for age and sex. All subjects were Afro-Americans.	All subjects (or next-of-kin in those cases who were too ill) were given a structured interview to get data on tobacco and alcohol use, diet (61-item food-frequency questionnaire), medical history, occupation, and demographics. Reference period for food was normal intake during adulthood. Intakes were adjusted for seasonal variations in availability. Vitamin supplement usage was collected but did not affect outcomes.
Tuyns et al., 1987	Case–control France	743 cases (704♂ and 39♀) of *esophageal cancer*. 1975 controls from the same geographical region.	All subjects interviewed about usual food intake with 40-item food-frequency questionnaire. Risk analysis was done heavy vs light consumers adjusted for age, two levels of alcohol and tobacco consumption, and residence (rural vs urban).
van Helden et al., 1987	Cross-sectional South Africa	Study I 63 subjects from 3 incidence areas, high, intermediate, low based on incidence of *esophageal cancer* (EC). Study II 77 subjects from 2 incidence areas.	Study I Healthy subjects from 3 rural areas, high, intermediate, low based on incidence of EC. Samples collected during dry season. Study II Healthy subjects from 2 areas high and low incidence of EC. Samples collected during wet season. Blood samples were collected from individuals with no overt clinical signs of deficiency. Serum frozen at –20°C. All samples were treated uniformly in terms of duration of storage. Vitamin E measured by HLPC.

Results	Comments
Statistically significant differences between groups for serum vitamin A and vitamin E levels (HNC-I > HNC-II). No difference between groups for β-carotene.	No diet, no documentation of disease history, no supplementation data, no control group. No description of analytical methods, no time period for sampling to analysis. No demographics, no control for smoking, alcohol, or any other confounding risk factors.
There was no difference in levels of vitamin E in any of the group comparisons. Mean levels of vitamin A were lower in cases than either control groups.	Inappropriate control groups. No diet data or report on supplement use. No matching of groups for age, sex, SES.
↓ risk in ♂ associated with carotene and vitamin E. ↑ intake of fruits and vegetables was associated with a decreased risk for oral cancer across sexes, although effect was stronger for ♂. Similar decline in risk associated with vitamin C and fiber.	No biochemistry, reliance of retrospective diet data, no data on time period between diagnosis and participation (cases obtained from a cancer registry). The study not designed to address specific nutrients. Mean or median intakes for nutrients not reported. No direct comparison to Caucasian population sample.
Significant association between vitamin E intake and relative risk. Higher intakes associated with significantly decreased risk. Cases consumed fewer proteins of animal origin and more proteins of vegetable origin and had a higher intake of sugars and starches of vegetable origin. Cases had a lower P:S ratio—oils associated with decreased risk, butter associated with increased risk.	No biochemistry. No control for time between diagnosis and study. No documentation of medications or other treatment. No data on medical or family health history. Hard to determine environmental from genetic effects.
Study I Levels of vitamin A and E and red cell folate were significantly different. For each nutrient the highest concentrations were found in the low risk group. All concentrations were without exception in the lower range of clinically acceptable levels. This was especially true for vitamin E.	No diet data, no matching for age, sex or demographics. No data on tobacco use, medical or family health history, occupation, or other potential environmental or genetic factors.
Study II Significant differences between high and low incidence groups for vitamins A, E, and B12 and red cell folate. Mean level of vitamin E was lowest.	

APPENDIX TABLE 2 Vitamin E and Breast Cancer

Study	Type/Location	Subject Number and Description	Methods
Basu et al., 1989	Case–control Canada	89 subjects: 30 w/advanced stage *breast cancer* (BC) w/distal metastases, 29 with benign breast disease, 30 healthy age-matched controls.	All of the BC patients were drug-free for 1 mo prior to sampling. Serum samples were obtained from NCI serum bank. Analysts were blinded as to subject category. Vitamin E measured by HPLC with reverse phase column and UV detection.
Gerber et al., 1989	Case–control France	120 cases of *breast cancer*. 109 controls hospitalized for non-malignant and non-CVD related neurological disorders. Recruitment over a 4-yr period (1982–1986).	Subjects given a structured interview containing SES data, menopausal status, reproductive and health history, and food-frequency questionnaire (for 55 items). Subjects were asked about duration of nutritional habits and changes, if any, of the diet in the previous yr. Fasting blood samples were drawn the day after admission to hospital and stored at −18°C for unknown duration. Vitamin E measured by HPLC
Gerber et al., 1990	Case–control Milan, Italy Montpelier, France	317 cases of primary non-metastasizing breast cancer (214 Italy, 103 France). 318 hospital-based controls (215 Italy, 103 France).	Blood sampling and interview same as Gerber et al., 1989. Additional assays for retinol, β-carotene, vitamin C and riboflavin. The Italian sample was asked about all foods eaten; whereas the French group was only asked about key lipid- and vitamin-rich foods. Reference period was the previous yr unless diet had changed, in which case subjects were asked about the previous 12 mo.
Meyer et al., 1990	Intervention (randomized double-blind placebo-controlled crossover design) South Africa	105 cases with mammographic evidence of *benign breast disease* (31.5% had benign tumors, 23.8% had ductal hyperplasia, 19.1% had benign tumors and fibroadenosis, and 16.2% had fibrocystic disease).	Data collected on menstrual and reproductive history, dietary and smoking habits, and family history of breast disease. Cases received either 600 mg α-tocopherol acetate or placebo for 3 mo, returned for exam and switched. Exams done by same examiner.
Russell et al., 1988	Case–control England	30 cases of *breast cancer* (BC). 288 controls matched for age and menopausal status. Subjects selected from a pool of samples from 5086 volunteer ♀ collected over an 8-yr period (1977–1985).	Serum samples collected and stored at −20°C until analyzed by HPLC.
Toniolo et al., 1989	Case–control Italy	250 cases of *breast cancer* (free of metastases, except in regional lymph nodes. Controls were 499 ♀ from general population stratified by age (± 10 yr) and geographical area.	All subjects interviewed (unblinded) were given modified food-frequency questionnaire structured by meals. Indigenous foods and recipes were added to the database. General demographic data was obtained from electoral rolls. Interview data included SES data, health and reproductive history.

Results	Comments
No significant difference between groups for vitamin E. Levels of all nutrients studied (vitamin E, A, β-carotene, and selenium) were lower in the BC group than in controls, although not significantly.	Although BC group was drug free there was no mention of supplements in any group. Age was the only matching variable. No dietary intake data or nutritional history. No clinical nutrition data. All BC patients were in advanced stage and metastasizing therefore effects may have been secondary to disease.
No significant differences in intake between groups. Plasma total cholesterol (TC) and vitamin E were higher in cases than controls. Differences in vitamin E were greater in premenopausal women as was the ratio vitamin E/TC (which was not significant in postmenopausal patients). Plasma vitamin E was significantly correlated with safflower oil intake in all subjects. Dietary vitamin E (adjusted for age and TC) was significantly associated with plasma vitamin E in both groups. Other significant findings relate to evidence of lower lipid peroxidation in cases than controls.	Possibly inappropriate control group (all were suffering neurological or spinal problems; no medication history was reported). Although stage of disease was known there was no analysis using this variable. Duration of sample storage not given. Relevant time frame for dietary information was not clear and retrospective.
No difference in lipid-soluble vitamin intake between groups. There was a higher serum level of cholesterol and plasma vitamin E in cases compared to controls of both groups. A significant difference was found in total fat and cholesterol between cases and controls of both groups; in the French groups there was a difference in saturated and mono-unsaturated fat intake. Increased risk associated with dietary cholesterol, total dietary lipids, plasma vitamin E, and serum zinc (only measured in Italian sample).	No community-based controls. No comparison of controls to each other or to community standards. Blood levels were correlated with past intake (data based on long retrospective period). Differences in quantification of diet records between 2 study sites. Blood assays were blinded and all vitamin assays were performed at the same lab. Storage time was not given.
83 cases completed the trial. 37 reported subjective improvement while on vitamin E, 19 while on placebo. No difference in clinical exam scores. 16 cases in vitamin E group showed mammographic improvements compared to 10 in placebo.	No baseline or trial diet data reported, no reported previous supplement use, no biochemical data, and no matching for age, or demographics. While the number of cases showing subjective and clinical improvement were greater while on vitamin E, it did not approach statistical significance due to small sample size. Whether those who did worse while on placebo got better on vitamin E or vice versa was not discussed.
No differences between controls and BC cases for vitamins E, A, or RBP.	No diet or supplement usage data nor matching for smoking or SES. No risk analysis only descriptive statistics. Long storage time at –20˚C.
No difference in vitamin E intake between groups. Reduced risk was associated with decreased intakes of fat especially saturated fat and animal protein.	Not blinded, no biochemistry, long period of time between diagnosis or treatment and study (on average 7.8 mo after diagnosis). Retrospective diet data not necessarily indicative of diets prior to diagnosis. Smoking histories not reported.

APPENDIX TABLE 3   Vitamin E and Lung Cancer

Study	Type/Location	Subject Number and Description	Methods
Kok et al., 1987	Nested case–control Netherlands	69 cases of cancer death; 18 cases of *lung cancer*. 138 controls matched for age, sex, and smoking status. Subjects selected from a cohort of 10,532 subjects.	Baseline blood samples analyzed for serum α-tocopherol, β-carotene, retinol, selenium, and cholesterol.
LeGardeur et al., 1990	Case–control Louisiana	59 cases of newly diagnosed *lung cancer* (LC). 59 hospitalized controls (HC) matched for sex, race, age (within 5 yr), and county of residence. 31 community controls (CC) non-hospitalized matched to hospital controls for age, race, and sex.	Non-fasting blood samples collected from all subjects. Hospitalized cases and controls were given a structured interview about smoking habits and dietary intake. Community controls were not interviewed. Serum analyses were performed within a mo of blood collection. Vitamin E was measured colorimetrically.
Miyamoto et al., 1987	Cross-sectional Japan	115 children of 55 patients with primary *lung cancer* (CLC). 56 age-matched controls with no cancer (NLC) among relatives. 37 lung cancer patients (LC) who had not received any treatment.	Venous blood samples collected and stored at −70°C; all samples analyzed within 3 mo of collection. Vitamin E determined by high speed liquid chromatography.

Results	Comments
There was no effect of vitamin E levels on risk of lung cancer; however vitamin E levels were inversely associated with risk of all cancers. Lung cancer cases had a 9% lower level of vitamin E than controls; however, this difference was not statistically significant. There were no associations between levels of other nutrients and cancer either total or lung.	Little detail of methodology given as this report is a letter to the editor. Small sample size, especially of the lung cancer cases. No diet data.
Mean serum levels of carotenoids, vitamin E, and total cholesterol for LC cases were significantly lower than HC. Although reported as no difference, HC subjects had significantly lower levels of vitamin C and vitamin E than CC. Cholesterol-adjusted serum levels of vitamin E were still significantly lower in LC cases than HC.	No diet data reported. No questionnaire data for CC group. The CC group was compared to HC group to test for appropriateness of HC as controls for LC group. Text reported no difference. Data in table indicated significant differences in the major dependent variables vitamin C and E. LC and HC group were not matched for smoking history. In addition the nature of the illnesses (e.g., 20% CHD, 14% metabolic endocrine or nutritional disorders) of the HC group also made it an inappropriate control. No comparisons between CC group and LC cases, although the LC cases did have lower levels of vitamin E and C and retinol and carotenoids. Given the inappropriateness of the controls and poor matching, the use of a paired t-test must be questioned. Poorly designed study.
Serum α-tocopherol levels were significantly lower in CLC group than NLC group. The difference was more pronounced in children of adenocarcinoma patients. The LC group had lower levels than either the NLC or CLC groups. There was no association between sex or smoking habits and serum vitamin E.	No diet data or reference to supplement use. No matching for SES factors. Samples not fasted.

APPENDIX TABLE 4   Vitamin E and Gastrointestinal and Pancreatic Cancer

Study	Type/Location	Subject Number and Description	Methods
Buiatti et al., 1990	Case–control Italy	1016 patients with *gastric cancer* (GC). 1159 age- and sex-matched controls randomly selected from same area.	Subjects given a questionnaire covering demographics, SES, smoking, medical, occupational, family, and dietary history. Food frequency covered the 2 yr prior to the interview.
Burney et al., 1989	Case–control Maryland	22 cases of *pancreatic cancer* (PC); 44 controls matched for race, sex, and hr between the blood sampling and last meal. The 2 control subjects nearest in age to a case were selected.	Subjects were drawn from the larger pool of residents who had given blood samples during the period of Sept.–Nov. 1974. Samples were frozen at −70°C until assayed for retinol, total carotenoids, β-carotene, lycopene, and α-tocopherol by HPLC.
Charpiot et al., 1989	Case–control France	208 subjects. 70 cases with *digestive cancer* (DC). 34 patients with colonic polyps. 78 healthy controls.	12-hr fasted blood samples were drawn from hospitalized cases before chemical, surgical, or radiological therapy. Samples were drawn from polyp and control groups just after hospitalization. Retinol and vitamin E assayed via HPLC. Other measures included RBP and prealbumin (TTR).
Knekt et al., 1988b	Case–control Finland	150 cases with primary *gastrointestinal cancer* (esophagus, stomach, duodenum, colon, and rectum). 276 controls matched for age, sex, and place of residence. Subjects drawn from a pool of 36,263 survey participants. Cases identified over a variable time period of 5–9 yr.	Baseline questionnaire included info about occupation, drug use, medical history, and smoking habits. Body-mass index was used to describe obesity. Serum samples were collected and stored at −20°C for between 11–15 yr before analysis of selenium, vitamin E, and vitamin A. α-tocopherol was quantified by HPLC.

Results	Comments
Increased GC risk with increasing intakes of protein, starch, and nitrites. No change in risk trend related to intake of fat, carbohydrates, cholesterol, fiber, calcium, alcohol, retinol, and nitrates. Lower GC risk with vitamins C and E and β-carotene. Risk decreased proportionally with increased intakes of vitamins C and E but not retinol or β-carotene. In a stepwise multiple regression protein, vitamins E and C were selected for the final model.	No clinical nutrition data reported, the study relied on retrospective data, neither duration of illness nor severity were documented. Reliance on various different databases from different countries for dietary analysis. Use of vitamin supplements was surveyed in an earlier pilot study and found not to be a contributing factor in this population. Most of the dietary vitamin consumed by these groups was associated with olive oil (28% of control intake).
No differences between groups for smoking history, education, or marital status.	No diet or supplement use data, no medical history, or information about time of onset of PC.
There were no significant differences in any measures except lycopene and selenium which were both lower in cases.	Storage of serum for 12 yr can result in invalid results.
There was a protective although not statistically significant effect of low levels of vitamin E.	
Retinol, RBP, TTR, and vitamin E were significantly lower in cases than controls. There were no differences between polyp group and controls. Lower carrier proteins presumed to be indicative of protein malnutrition.	Stage or type of cancer not documented. No dietary intake data or supplement use reported. Aside from a statement about a lack of "denutrition" in the control groups, there was no documentation about clinical nutrition status. Sample storage time was not given. There was no matching for sex, or SES.
Mean vitamin E and selenium were lower in cases than controls, especially when data was partitioned by location in GI tract.	No diet data, supplement use data, or matching for SES or seasonal variations in food supply and time of blood sampling.
Upper GI cancers (stomach and esophagus) were associated with lower vitamin E and Se levels with case ♂ being significantly lower than control ♂ for Se.	Long storage time.
There were no interactions between serum Se and serum vitamin E and cancer.	Aside from removing those who were diagnosed within 2 yr of sampling, there was no control for time to diagnosis of cancer.
High Se levels were protective against upper GI cancer at both high and low levels of vitamin E. The relative risk for upper GI cancer adjusted for cholesterol and smoking was higher for both low vitamin E and Se.	
In general, there was no association between serum Se and vitamin E and colorectal cancer. However, colorectal cancer risk was higher for ♀ with low vitamin E levels.	

APPENDIX TABLE 5   Vitamin E and Colorectal Cancer

Study	Type/Location	Subject Number and Description	Methods
DeCosse et al., 1989	Intervention-randomized, double-blind, placebo-controlled New York, NY	58 patients with *familial adenomatous polyposis* drawn from an initial pool of 72 who had total colectomy and ileorectal anastomosis 1 yr prior to the study.	*Control group*: 8 caps placebo (lactose)/d + 2.2 g of low fiber. *Vitamin group*: 4 g vitamin C/d + 400 mg vitamin E/d + 2.2 g of low fiber. *Fiber group*: both vitamins + 22.5 g of high fiber/d. 3-mo placebo period, 4-yr trial. All groups received 30 mg vitamin C, 2,000 IU vitamin A and equivalent amounts of several other vitamins and minerals (about 30% RDA). Patients had 18 examinations over test period, and completed a 3-d diet diary and a food-frequency questionnaire for each visit.
Freudenheim et al., 1990	Case–control New York, NY	422 cases of *rectal cancer* (277 ♂, 145♀). 422 sex-, race-, age- (± 5 yr), neighborhood-matched controls.	Subjects given a 2.5 hr interview with a food frequency-questionnaire. Reference period previous year for controls and for cases 1 yr prior to the onset of symptoms. Other information included smoking and alcohol use, occupational and health histories, seasonality of intake, preparation, and food storage.
McKeown-Eyssen et al., 1988	Intervention (randomized double-blind trial) Toronto, Canada	185 cases with at least 1 polyp in the colon or rectum. 96 received vitamins. 89 received placebo. All subjects were presumed to be polyp free at start of the trial.	Data included a 9-item food-frequency questionnaire, demographics, smoking status, bowel habits, previous polyp history, and vitamin supplement use. Subjects randomized to 400 mg vitamins E and C or lactose placebo over 2-yr period and re-examined (blinded). Compliance tested with random urine samples.

Results	Comments
Subject groups were comparable in demographics, median time since colectomy, median intake of fiber at baseline, and prior supplementation with vitamins C and E. There were no discernable effects for the vitamins. The high fiber group had the stronger benefit especially during the middle years of the trial. Compliance for all groups decreased over the course of the trial.	No blood levels of the vitamins were reported for baseline or during the trial. No data of dietary vitamin intakes at baseline or during trial were reported. Because of combined use of vitamins, an analysis of independent effects or interactions of individual vitamins was not possible.
No association between intake of vitamin E and risk. Decreased risk with increasing intake of carotenoids, vitamin C, and dietary fiber from vegetables. Increased risk with increasing intakes of calories, fat, carbohydrate, and iron.	Reliance on retrospective food frequency interviews. No data on use of supplements or stage of disease (except that "only relatively alert, healthy subjects could tolerate the 2.5 hr. interview"). Well conceived study.
The 2 groups were matched for all parameters except that the vitamin group had more members who used vitamin C supplements prior to trial. There were no differences in food-frequency items. 137 subjects (75%) completed the trial. Polyps found in 41.4% of vitamin group and 50.7% of placebo.	No biochemical data either at baseline or after trial. Insufficient power due to small sample size. Because of the design, the study could not distinguish differences in effect of individual vitamins.

APPENDIX TABLE 6   Vitamin E and Cervical/Ovarian Cancer

Study	Type/Location	Subject Number and Description	Methods
Cuzick et al., 1990	Case–control London	45 controls 30 cases of *Cervical Intraepithelial neoplasia* I (CIN I) 40 cases CIN III Subjects chosen from a pool of 110 CIN I, 284 CIN III, and 833 controls involved in a larger study. Serum samples were randomly selected from an age-stratified sample.	Sera were analyzed blindly for vitamins A and E by HPLC. Samples were stored for an unspecified period at an unspecified temperature.
Heinonen et al., 1987	Case–control Finland	88 cases of *gynecologic cancer* (9 vulvar, 15 cervical, 36 endometrial, 28 ovarian) of various clinical stages. 31 controls receiving treatment for abnormal bleeding, uterine fibromas, or genital prolapse.	Blood samples were collected the day before surgery or treatment in all subjects and stored at $-70°C$. α-tocopherol, total carotenes, and retinol were measured by HPLC.
Palan et al., 1991	Cross-sectional New York, NY	10 cases of *cervical cancer*. 36 controls with no problems. 27 with abnormal cytology but no cancer (No CIN). 43 were graded histopathologically (CIN I–III).	Samples collected prior to treatment. β-carotene, retinol, and α-tocopherol were measured immediately by HPLC.
Verreault et al., 1989	Case–control Washington (state)	189 cases of *cervical cancer*. 227 controls selected by random digit dialing. Age stratified ($\pm$ 10 yr).	Subjects were given a 35-minute structured inter-view with questions about demographics, health and reproductive history, smoking history, height and weight (self-reported), and sexual activity. 66-item food-frequency questionnaire. Questions about vitamin supplement use. Data analysis adjustment variables were education, smoking, frequency of PAP smears, use of contraceptives, age at first intercourse, number of lifetime sexual partners, and previous history of cervico-vaginal infections.

Results	Comments
The mean levels of serum vitamin E showed a significant decreasing trend lower in cases (CIN III and I) than controls and III were less than I. Significant trends were found in vitamin E levels for both CIN I and III with higher levels being protective. This trend was strengthened when adjustments were made for smoking, sexual behavior, and use of oral contraceptives.	No diet data or reported use of supplements. No matching for SES.
No significant differences were found in the serum levels of the vitamins and carotene in patients with vulvar, cervical, or endometrial cancer compared to the controls. Cases with ovarian cancer had a significantly lower mean serum level of retinol than the controls, while carotene and vitamin E levels were similar in both groups.	No community-based controls. No diet. Groups were not matched for age, or other potential risk factors, i.e., smoking, demographics. Fasting status of subjects was not documented.
Mean levels of vitamins A and E were significantly reduced in all cases of dysplasia and cancer. Inverse association between nutrient levels and severity of dysplasia.	No diet, no supplement data, no demographics, no SES, small sample size. Control group may have been self-selected and more health conscious.
High vitamin E intake was significantly associated with lower risk. Use of vitamin A and E supplements was associated with slight reduction in risk. After adjustment for known risk factors, frequent consumption of dark green or yellow vegetables and fruit juices was related to lower risk. There was a significant inverse relationship between vitamin C intake and risk.	Use of retrospective diet assessment (referring to a period several yr prior to interview). The average delay between the reference date (time of telephone contact) and interview was 2.8 yr in cases and 2.7 yr in controls). No biochemical data.

APPENDIX TABLE 7   Vitamin E and Cancer—Other Sites

Study	Type/Location	Subject Number and Description	Methods
Helzlsouer et al., 1989	Case–control Maryland	35 cases of *bladder cancer*. 70 controls (2/case) matched for nearest age, sex, race, and within 2-hr interval of blood sampling and last meal. Sample pool was 20,305 residents of Washington Co., MD. Cases were identified over an 11-yr period (1975–1986).	Serum samples were collected in 1974 and stored at −70°C as part of a blood-banking project for cancer research. All participants were given a questionnaire that included demographics, smoking history, medication use, and vitamin supplement use (with special reference to the 48 hr period prior to blood sampling). Serum retinol, carotenoids, and vitamin E measured by HPLC.
Hsing et al., 1990	Case–control Maryland	103 cases *prostate cancer*. 103 controls matched for race (all white), age, and sex (all ♂). Subjects drawn from same pool as Helzlsouer et al., 1989 (see above).	Same as Helzlsouer et al., 1989 (see above) except that 30 cases and 30 control samples were analyzed at a different lab as part of a pilot study. The remaining 140 samples (70/70) were analyzed as above. Interlaboratory variations ranged from 3% for retinol to 11% for β-carotene. None reported for α-tocopherol.
Stryker et al., 1990	Case–control Boston	204 cases of *malignant melanoma*. 248 control patients who were making first visit to clinic.	Data collected about diet (116-item food-frequency questionnaire), use of vitamin and mineral supplements, type of fats used for cooking, medical history, constitutional and life style factors, demographic data, pigmentation characteristics, and past medical history. Fasting serum samples collected and stored at −70°C for up to 6 mo. Vitamin E was measured by HPLC.
Kanematsu et al., 1989	Cross-sectional Japan	26 patients (21 ♂ and 5 ♀) consecutively admitted for hepatic resection. 10 cases of human hepatocellular carcinoma (HCC). 19 patients had cirrhosis, 4 had fibrosis, 1 had chronic active hepatitis, and 1 had none of these conditions.	Fasting AM blood samples were drawn and assessed for plasma levels of vitamin A (retinol) and E (presumably α-tocopherol), retinol binding protein (RBP), and prealbumin (PA). Tissue concentrations of vitamins A and E were measured in resection samples. In HCC samples comparisons were made between malignant hepatic tumor and adjacent "normal" parenchymal tissue.

Results	Comments
Cases had lower mean nutrient levels of all nutrients than controls. There was a significant association between vitamin E levels and supplement use, but not for any other nutrient. There were no significant differences in prediagnostic levels of any nutrients except selenium which was lower in cases. There was no difference in risk by tertiles for any serum nutrient level except selenium. Serum α-tocopherol levels were non-significantly lower in cases.	Controls were more likely to have used supplements. There was no analysis of the vitamin E and selenium relationship. Similarly, there was no testing for interactions between any of the nutrients studied. Aside from supplement data, no dietary data was collected. Long storage time between collection and analysis. Overall sample pool characteristics were biased towards middle-aged, white, better educated, married ♀.
No differences or associations in vitamin E levels between cases and controls.	See Helzlsouer et al., 1989 above.
No differences in descriptive or risk trend analyses between groups. Some of the higher levels of α-tocopherol were associated with a decreased risk of melanoma (non-significantly). Intake of vitamin E from food alone was significantly associated with a trend of decreased risk with increased intake.	Possibly inappropriate controls as all subjects were patients in skin clinic. Controls may have been more health conscious. Analyses were adjusted for age and sex but no control for SES. Subjects in case group included patients who knew their diagnosis before the study began.
No difference in vitamin E or cellular RBP levels. Statistically significant difference in levels of retinol between tumor and adjacent "normal" cells. There was no correlation between blood and tissue vitamin A levels. Low levels of retinol in tumor tissue not related to availability of cellular RBP.	Not a nutrition study—no diet, no control comparisons. No comparisons reported between HCC cases and those without cancer. Within-subject comparisons are of questionable value because of the appropriateness of the adjacent tissue in cancer patients as a control specimen.

APPENDIX TABLE 8   Vitamin E and Cancer—Combined Site Studies

Study	Type/Location	Subject Number and Description	Methods
Comstock et al., 1991	Case–control Maryland	436 cases with cancer (distribution of cases over various sites). 765 controls matched by age, race, sex, mo blood was donated, and time since last meal. Subjects were selected from a pool of 25,620 residents who donated blood samples during a 4-mo period in 1974.	Serum was stored at –73°C, thawed, and refrozen after aliquoting. Carotenoids and vitamin E assayed by HPLC. Sample sets included cases before and after diagnosis and 2 matched controls.
Connett et al., 1989	Nested case–control Minnesota	156 cases of cancer deaths. 311 controls matched for age, smoking status, randomization group, date of randomization, and clinical center. Subjects drawn from a pool of 12,866 subjects at high risk for coronary heart disease involved in an intervention trial (MRFIT).	Subject selection was by risk status for CHD: smoking, diastolic BP, serum cholesterol at initial screening. Subjects then seen twice. Blood collected at second visit and stored at –50°C to –70°C. Matched triads were analyzed within 3 mo of each other. Average duration of sample storage was not reported. The cancer cases (deaths) occurred over a 10-yr period (1973–1983). On the third visit all subjects completed a 24-hr dietary recall. Serum vitamin analyses were by HPLC.
Gey et al., 1987	Prospective cohort study Basel, Switzerland	3000 healthy ♂. 268 deaths over 7-yr period. 2707 controls (survivors). 38% of total deaths (102) were from cancer.	Samples collected over a 2-yr period (1971–1973). Plasma analyzed immediately (no storage). Comparisons were adjusted for age and cigarette smoking.
Knekt et al., 1988c	Case–control Finland	453 cases of *cancer of all sites*. 841 controls drawn from the same municipality as cases and matched for age, time of baseline exam, and duration of sample storage time. Subjects selected from a cohort of 21,172 ♂ involved in a longitudinal study.	All subjects answered baseline questions about occupation, use of drugs, previous and current illnesses, and smoking habits. All subjects were asked not to eat, drink, or void for at least 4 hr prior to the initial exam. Serum samples were analyzed for content of α-tocopherol, retinol, β-carotene, retinol-binding protein, and selenium. Serum cholesterol and hematocrit were also determined. Subjects were also asked about supplement use.
Knekt et al., 1991	Case–control Finland	766 cases of *cancer of all sites*. 1419 controls matched for age, sex, and duration of storage. Subjects from same pool as Knekt et al., 1988 (see above).	Same as above.
Stähelin et al., 1989	Case–control Basel, Switzerland	204 cases of death from all cancer. Controls were from the remainder of the sample pool of 2974 ♂.	Fasted serum samples were collected and immediately analyzed. Descriptive statistics included analysis of covariance for age and smoking. Risk analysis used the lower quartile as high-risk group. Adjustments also made for cholesterol and triglycerides to derive a lipid-independent estimate of vitamin levels.
Wald et al., 1987	Case–control London, England	271 cases of cancer. 533 controls with no cancer matched for age, duration of storage of serum sample, smoking status and habits (type), and duration of smoking habit. Subjects derived from pool of 22,000 ♂ aged 35–64 who donated serum during period 1975–1982.	Serum collected and stored at –40°C. Vitamin E measured by HPLC. Samples were tested in 4 series: 2 in 1981, 1 in 1983 and 1 in 1985. Cases always run with same matched-control pair.

Results	Comments
Cases were distributed as follows: 103 prostate, 99 lung cancer, 72 colon cancer, 34 rectum cancer, 22 pancreatic, 30 breast cancer, 35 bladder, 21 basal cell and 20 melanoma.	No diet history, intake or supplement use data were reported.

Cases were distributed as follows: 103 prostate, 99 lung cancer, 72 colon cancer, 34 rectum cancer, 22 pancreatic, 30 breast cancer, 35 bladder, 21 basal cell and 20 melanoma.

Prediagnostic serum vitamin E was lower in cases than controls for colon, rectum, lung, prostate, and bladder cancers. Only lung cancer showed a significant dose-response trend in a protective direction. The odds ratios for 4 different cell types of lung cancer were all increased for low serum vitamin E, although not significantly (presumably due to small n's).

Serum levels of α-tocopherol were not related to cancer of any site.

No diet history, intake or supplement use data were reported.
Samples were stored for about 15 yr prior to analysis.
Samples were thawed and refrozen prior to analysis.
All subjects drawn from a pool from the same geographical location.
No matching for SES.

This was a prospective cohort study of CHD from which data on cancer was extracted.
All subjects were at risk for CHD, 63% were smokers, therefore the generalizability of these results is suspect. There was a potential impact of storage time on outcomes.
Questionable reliability of a single 24-hr dietary recall. Many of the "controls" may have been in early stages of cancer (7 died of cancer after the cutoff date for inclusion).

Descriptive statistics demonstrated significantly lower levels of vitamin E in cancer group as a whole when compared with survivors.
Significantly lower absolute levels of vitamin E in combined gastrointestinal cancer group than in survivors. Trend analysis indicated that lower levels of vitamin E (and β-carotene, vitamin A) were associated with increased risk of death from all cancer.

High serum α-tocopherol was associated with a ↓ risk for cancer. The association was strongest for the combined groups of cancers unrelated to smoking (all cancers other than lip, oral cavity, and pharynx, respiratory organs, and urinary bladder).

No diet data, no control for seasonal variations in intake of antioxidant-rich foods, supplement use, or medications at time of sampling.

No diet data or matching for SES.
Long storage time.
Aside from removing those who were diagnosed within 2 yr of sampling, there was no control for time to diagnosis of cancer.

Mean serum vitamin E levels were significantly lower in cases than controls. Subjects with low level of vitamin E had about 1.5-fold risk of cancer compared to controls. There was no association with lip, oral and pharynx, lung, or bladder cancers, or hormone-related cancers (breast, ovary, endometrium, and prostate). ♀ with low vitamin E and low Se had a 3x higher risk of hormone-related cancer.

Same as above.

There were no differences between groups for serum vitamin E levels. Vitamin A, C, and β-carotene were associated with cancer mortality either by site or with overall cancer mortality. In risk analysis only for bronchial cancer was there an insignificant tendency toward increased risk for low vitamin E levels.
Subjects with low cholesterol levels were found to be at significantly increased risk for cancer death.

No diet, no supplement use data, no matching for SES.
See comment for Gey et al. (1987) above.

No difference in mean levels between cases and matched controls. The mean levels of vitamin E of cases diagnosed <1 yr after blood collection was significantly lower than controls. For cases diagnosed >1 yr after collection there were no significant differences between total cases or cases by site.

No diet nor supplement use data.
No matching for SES.
No data on health history of controls.
Statistical analyses based on paired t-test of differences in levels between cases and controls. This may not be an appropriate test for between-subject differences in a heterogeneous population sample.

Vitamin E and Cancer: An Update

Ching K. Chow, Ph.D.

I. Introduction

The report "Vitamin E and Cancer" was originally prepared by the Life Sciences Research Office, Federation of American Societies for Experimental Biology, for the Food and Drug Administration in 1991, as monograph 8C of Nutrient–Disease Relationships. Since then, a number of articles relating to this subject area have appeared. This update reviews recent journal articles on the relationship between vitamin E intake and human cancer risk. Review articles are not included unless they contain new data or useful meta-analyses. While efforts have been made to include all pertinent articles, some may still be missed.

II. Vitamin E and Human Cancer

To make an easier comparison with the original report, this section (and the accompanying Table Update) is organized according to the types of cancer.

A. Head and Neck Cancer

Four of six recent reports suggested a beneficial effect of increased vitamin E intake in reducing the risk of head/neck cancer. In an intervention trial carried out in Houston, Texas, Benner et al. (1993) treated 45 patients, who had symptomatic leukoplakia or dysplasia, with α-tocopherol, 400 IU twice daily, and followed them for 24 weeks to assess the toxicity and response. They found that 20 of the 43 patients who completed 24 weeks of treatment had clinical responses and 9 had histological responses in reducing premalignant leukoplakia lesions. Histological response was defined as reversal of dysplasia and reversion to normal epithelium, and clinical response was disappearance or decrease of the lesion. This study was designed specifically to evaluate the efficacy of vitamin E treatment. However, there were no placebo controls.

In a hospital-based case–control study conducted in four U.S. cities, Barone et al. (1992) obtained information on dietary intake, vitamin supplement and other data using a standardized questionnaire from 290 male oral cancer cases and 133 esophageal cancer cases and from two matched controls for each case. They observed that use of vitamin E supplements appeared to exert a protective effect among oral cancer cases, and supplemental use of both vitamins C and E had protective effects among esophageal cancer cases. The number of vitamin E supplement users, however, was relatively small (21 in oral cavity cancer cases and 66 in controls, 7 in esophageal cancer cases and 32 in controls).

Zheng et al. (1993) conducted a nested case–control study within a cohort of 25802 adults, who donated blood in 1974, in Washington County, Maryland. The serum levels of nutrients in 28 individuals, who developed oral and pharyngeal cancer during 1975–1990, were compared to those of 112 matched controls. Serum samples were analyzed for α-tocopherol after being stored at –70°C for approximately 16 years. A reduced risk of pharyngeal cancer was found to be associated with high serum levels of α-tocopherol. However, high risk was also found to correlate with higher serum levels of γ-tocopherol. Since γ-tocopherol accounts for only a small portion of total vitamin E activity, this association is not likely to be important.

In a population-based case–control study conducted during 1984–1985 in New Jersey; Atlanta, Georgia; Los Angeles, California and Santa Clara and San Mateo counties, California, Gridley et al. (1992) obtained information on dietary intake and vitamin supplements from 1114 pathologically confirmed incident cases of oral and pharyngeal cancer and 1268 matched controls. There was no association between intake of multivitamin products, but users of supplements of individual vitamins, including vitamins A, B, C and E, were at lower risk of oral and pharyngeal cancer. After adjustment for use of other supplements, vitamin E was the only supplement that remained associated with a significant reduction of cancer risk. This epidemiology study demonstrated an association between a reduced oral cancer risk and vitamin use. Information on the dosage of vitamin supplements, however, was not ascertained. Use of vitamin supplements was defined as having been taken on a regular basis for 6 months or longer.

Two case–control studies reported no significant association between vitamin E intake and risk of head/neck cancer. In a study involving 35 early diagnosed esophageal cancer cases and 35 matched controls conducted in Hyderabad, India, Prasad et al. (1992) analyzed blood levels of α-tocopherol and several other nutrients, and found that the relative risk was significantly higher for those with low blood levels of retinol and zinc. The blood levels of α-tocopherol were lower in the cases than the controls. However, the difference was not statistically significant. The controls were recruited from attendants accompanying the patients or from patients suffering from minor ailments (noncancerous).

In another case–control study conducted among white men in three counties of western New York from 1975 to 1985, Freudenheim et al. (1992) interviewed 250 pathologically confirmed laryngeal cancer cases and 250 matched controls to determine usual diet and lifetime use of tobacco and alcohol. No significant relationship was found between the development of laryngeal cancer and intake of vitamins E and C. Carotenoids were negatively associated with the cancer risk, whereas higher dietary fat was associated with increased risk. Interestingly, higher intake of total calories, protein or retinol was also found to be associated with increased risk.

B. Breast Cancer

Most recent studies suggest an absence of association between vitamin E intake and risk of breast cancer. Richardson et al. (1991) conducted a hospital-based case–control study of 924 patients (409 cases and 515 controls) in Montpelier, France, to investigate the role of consumption of fat, animal protein and vitamins on breast-cancer risk. Control subjects were patients admitted for neurological, neurosurgical disorders or general surgery. Increased consumption of fat, but not animal protein, was found to be significantly associated with increased risk of breast cancer. There was no evidence of risk reduction with increased consumption of vegetables, β-carotene or vitamin E.

In a nested case–control study carried out in Toronto, Canada, Rohan et al. (1993) followed a cohort of 56837 women enrolled in the Canadian National Breast Screening Study from 1982–1987. Based on self-administered dietary history questionnaires obtained from 519 incident, histologically confirmed cases of breast cancer cases and 1182 matched controls, they found that higher intakes of fiber, pasta, cereal and vegetables rich in vitamins A and C, β-carotene and vitamin C were associated with a reduced risk of breast cancer. Vitamin E intake was not found to be associated with an altered risk of breast cancer.

In a case–control study, London et al. (1992) investigated the relationship between serum levels of retinol, carotenoids and tocopherols as well as intakes of retinol, carotene and vitamin E and the risks of breast cancer and proliferative benign breast disease (BBD) of postmenopausal women in the Boston area. Serum nutrient data were obtained from 377 women with newly diagnosed stage I or II breast cancer and 173 women with proliferative BBD, and 403 controls who were evaluated at the same institutions but did not require a breast biopsy or whose biopsy revealed nonproliferative BBD. No significant association was observed between serum levels of α-tocopherol, γ-tocopherol, retinol, β-carotene and risk of proliferative benign breast disease. The risk of breast cancer was decreased among women in the highest quintile of vitamin E intake from food sources only, but less so for total vitamin E intake, including supplements.

In a prospective study to determine whether dietary habits are associated with disease-free survival in patients with breast cancer who have undergone treatment, Holm et al. (1993) interviewed 240 women, 50–65 years old, who had surgery for pathological stage I–II breast cancer between 1983 and 1986 in the Stockholm region within 4 months of breast cancer diagnosis. During the 4-year follow-up period, 52 patients had treatment failure. Thirty estrogen-receptor-rich patients who had treatment failure reported higher intakes of total fat, saturated fatty acids and polyunsaturated fatty acids than did the 119 estrogen-receptor-rich patients who did not have treatment failure. For treatment failure within the first 2 years, the multiple odds ratio (OR) was increased with an increase in vitamin E intake. No association between dietary habits and treatment failure was found for women with estrogen receptor-poor cancers.

Gerber et al. (1991) conducted a hospital-based case–control study in Montpelier, France, to determine the relationship between the blood and cellular levels of vitamin E and several nutrients and the risk of breast cancer. Blood levels of selenium, zinc, copper and vitamins E and C were measured in 48 cases and 50 controls. The blood and cellular levels of these antioxidants were found to be overall higher in breast cancer cases than that of the controls, and the differences were significant for serum zinc and plasma and leukocyte vitamin E. The results were slightly modified when vitamin pill users were excluded from case and control samples.

C. Lung Cancer

Both of the recent reports suggest that a reduced lung cancer risk may be associated with increased vitamin E intake. In a case–control study to determine the risk of developing lung cancer, Tominaga et al. (1992) measured the serum levels of vitamins A and E, carotene and selenium in 31 newly diagnosed lung cancer patients and 31 matched controls from outpatients with no cancer in Utsunomia, Japan. A highly significant inverse association was found between serum levels of vitamins A and E and the risk of lung cancer. The relative risk (RR) for the low versus high tertile were 5.94 for serum vitamin A and 8.44 for serum vitamin E. The RR for lung cancer was also high when three or all four micronutrient levels in the lowest tertile were evaluated.

Knekt (1993) conducted a cohort study and a nested case–control study among 29994 men, aged 15 and over, who participated in a multiphasic screening examination in various parts of Finland during 1968–1972. In the cohort study on dietary intake, 121 lung cancer cases occurred among 5254 individuals during the 19-year follow-up period. In the case–control study on serum vitamin E, cases were 144 subjects, who developed lung cancer during 1968 and 1977, among a cancer-free population of 21172 men. A total of 270 matched controls was selected by pair matching from the same population. Serum samples were stored at –20 C for about 15 years prior to analysis for α-tocopherol. A significant inverse association was found between vitamin E status and lung cancer incidence among nonsmokers but not smokers in both studies. The RR of lung cancer between the lowest and highest tertiles of serum levels of vitamin E was 6.6 among nonsmokers and 0.8 among smokers. Nonsmokers with simultaneously low serum levels of vitamin E and other micronutrients (β-carotene, retinol, vitamin C and selenium) had a 12-fold greater risk of lung cancer than those with more satisfactory levels. Smokers with low serum levels of the micronutrients had a threefold greater risk of lung cancer compared to smokers with higher levels. Similarly, in the cohort study for dietary intake, the RR of lung cancer between the lowest and highest tertiles of vitamin E intake were 3.3 and 0.8 for smokers and nonsmokers, respectively. Different dietary habits between smokers and nonsmokers seem to contribute to the differences in relative risks observed.

D. Gastrointestinal and Pancreatic Cancer

The only recent report dealing with the relationship between vitamin E status and risk of gastrointestinal and pancreatic cancer is included in the section of the combined site study. In the cancer follow-up study of the Finnish Mobile Clinic Health Examination Survey, Knekt (1992) found that the levels of serum vitamin E were inversely correlated with the incidence of pancreas and stomach cancer. However, the lower levels of serum vitamin E observed in the cancer cases are not surprising because the absorption of vitamin E in patients with gastrointestinal or pancreatic cancer might have been impaired.

E. Colorectal Cancer

In an attempt to evaluate the association between serum vitamin E concentration and risk of colorectal cancer risk in greater detail, Longnecker et al. (1992) pooled and analyzed the original data from five prospective studies published previously (Knekt et al., 1988b; Nomura et al., 1985; Schober et al., 1987; Stahelin et al., 1984; Wald et al., 1987). Subjects were categorized according to study-specific quartiles of serum α-tocopherol levels within the study. The pooled analysis included a total of 289 cases of colorectal cancer and 1267 matched controls. For cancers of the colon and rectum combined, the matched OR for the highest quartile of serum α-tocopherol concentration compared with the lowest was 0.6. Adjustment for serum cholesterol level attenuated the OR to 0.7.

Both of the recent intervention studies to examine the efficacy of vitamins A, C and E were conducted in Italy. Paganelli et al. (1992) treated 23 randomly selected patients, aged 40–80 who entered in the study after complete endoscopic removal of adenoma, with a daily supplement of vitamins A, C and E or placebo for 6 months. Six biopsy specimens from 20 patients treated with vitamin supplements and 21 treated with placebo were taken from normal appearing rectal mucosa before treatment and after 3 and 6 months to study cell proliferation. Abnormal expansion of the proliferative compartment was decreased progressively from baseline values ($p < 0.05$ after 3 months, and < 0.01 after 6 months) in patients receiving vitamin supplements. No statistically significant change in cell kinetics was observed in the placebo group.

Similarly, Roncucci et al. (1993) treated 70 patients, who had at least one suspected adenoma in the large bowel identified and removed, with a daily supplement of vitamins A, C and E, 61 patients with lactulose and 78 patients with placebo. Subjects were followed at regular intervals for an average of 18 months. Polyps recurring before 1 year from index colonscopy were considered missed by the endoscopist. Among the 209 subjects evaluated, the recurrence of adenoma were 5.7, 14.7 and 35.9 percent in the vitamin, lactulose and placebo group, respectively. The fraction of subjects remaining free of adenomas was significantly different among the three groups.

The results obtained from those two intervention studies are suggestive that vitamins A, C and E have a chemopreventive value. However, since patients received a mixture of vitamins A, C and E, it is not known whether treatment with vitamin E alone has the same effect or not.

F. Cervical/Ovarian Cancer

The findings from the recent reports dealing with the relationship of vitamin E intake and cervical/ovarian cancer are also mixed. In a case–control study conducted in the southwestern U.S. to examine the relationship of dietary intake of vitamin C, folacin, vitamin E, carotenoids and retinol with cervical cytological abnormalities, Buckley et al. (1992) obtained dietary intake information from 42 dysplasia patients and 58 matched controls from American Indian women who have higher rates of cervical cancer and cervical dysplasia in contrast to low rates of cancers for other sites. Based on information obtained from 24-hr dietary recalls, women with low intake of vitamins E and C and folacin were found to be at increased risk of having cervical dysplasia, although the mean differences between cases and controls were not statistically significant.

In another case–control study conducted in Birmingham, Alabama, between 1985 and 1988, Barone et al. (1993) assessed the diets of 103 cases who had endometrial cancer and 236 matched controls. Logistic regression was used to evaluate the effect of diet on endometrial cancer after adjustment for total calories, age, race, education, smoking status and health status. A significant association was found between higher intake of carotene and protein and lower incidence of endometrial cancer. More frequent consumption of several vegetables and dairy products was associated with a statistically significant decreased risk of endometrial cancer. However, intake of animal and vegetable fats and vitamins C, D and E was not significantly associated with endometrial cancer.

In another case–control study to evaluate whether lower levels of serum micronutrients are associated with a higher risk of invasive cervical cancer, Potischman et al. (1991) analyzed micronutrient levels in sera of 387 cervical cancer cases and 670 controls from four Latin American countries. Serum levels of retinol, α-tocopherol, cryptoxanthin, lutin, lycopene or α-carotene were not significantly different between cases and controls. After adjustment for confounding factors, a trend of decreasing risk was found to be associated with higher levels of β-carotene, while increased risk was associated with increased γ-tocopherol levels. Blood and dietary information of this study was published separately (Herrero et al., 1991); but no information on vitamin E intake was included.

G. Cancer of Other Sites

In a case–control study to assess the association between bladder cancer and dietary factors Vena et al. (1992) used an interview-based dietary history questionnaire to estimate dietary intake from 351 white males, who had confirmed carcinoma of bladder, and 855 matched controls drawn from the same western New York population. An increase of bladder cancer was found to be significantly associated with higher intake of calories, fat, carbohydrates, sodium and proteins. However, no significant differences between cases and controls were seen for intake of vitamins A, C and E, niacin, thiamin, riboflavin or calcium.

Similarly, Riboli et al. (1991) carried out a multicenter case–control study on bladder cancer and diet in five regions of Spain. Usual dietary habits from 432 male cases and 792 controls were investigated by means of an interview-based dietary history questionnaire. Bladder cancer cases were selected from 12 hospitals in the study areas. Each case was matched by two controls, one identified in the same hospital and one drawn from population lists. Relative risk for specific foods and nutrients were adjusted for tobacco smoking and energy intake. Significantly higher risk of bladder cancer was found to be associated with higher intake of saturated fat. Intake of vitamin E was related slightly to a reduced risk which was not modified by adjustment for fat. No association was found between bladder cancer risk and intake of retinol or carotene.

H. Cancer of Combined Sites

Shibata et al. (1992) conducted a large prospective study involving a cohort of 11580 upper-middle class residents in a retirement community near Los Angeles. The participants, initially free from cancer, were surveyed for food consumption and use of vitamin supplements, and were followed from 1981 to 1989. A total of 1335 incident cancer cases of all sites were diagnosed during this period. After adjustment for age and smoking, no evidence of a protective effect was found for any dietary variables in men. However, a significant inverse association was observed between vitamin C supplement use and bladder cancer risk. In women, supplemental use of vitamins A and C had a protective effect on colon cancer risk. In addition, β-carotene intake and supplemental use of vitamins A, C and E were associated with a nonsignificant reduction of lung cancer risk in women.

Chen et al. (1992) carried out an ecological study in 65 mostly rural counties in China to investigate the relationship between sex-specific rates for selected cancer sites (including esophagus, stomach, liver, lung, colorectal, breast and cervix) and a variety of biochemical indicators of anti-oxidant status, and oxidative stress. Within each county two communes were randomly selected to give a total of 130 survey sites. Information on dietary intake and health status and fasted blood samples were collected from 50 randomly selected adults (25 males and 25 females) aged 35–64 years at each of the survey sites. Mortality rates by age and sex for each cancer site were obtained in a retrospective survey of causes of death in 1973–1975. Site-specific cancer mortality rates for each county were calculated for all ages up to 64. Plasma levels of α-tocopherol were found to be positively correlated with the cancer mortality rates of liver and lung in males, but not in females. None of the associations between α-tocopherol and cancer mortality rates were significant after adjusting for plasma total cholesterol levels. Ascorbic acid was most negatively associated with most cancers, selenium with esophageal and stomach cancers and β-carotene with stomach cancer. The number of subjects in several types of cancer was rather small.

Based on a comprehensive survey investigating several sites of cancer in the cancer follow-up of the Finnish Mobile Clinic Examination Survey, Knekt (1992) carried out a nested case–control study and a follow-up study in various parts of in Finland. The nested case–control study was based on the 766 cancer cases that occurred during a 10-year follow-up period among 32265 persons initially free from cancer. Serum levels of α-tocopherol, β-carotene and retinol from the cancer cases and 1419 matched controls were measured after storing at –20C for about 15 years. The association between serum levels of α-tocopherol and cancer incidence was estimated for 19 cancer sites. Serum α-tocopherol levels were found to be lower among cancer cases than among controls for melanoma, larynx, esophagus, pancreas, cervix, endometrium, nervous system, stomach, prostate, colorectal, lung, skin and kidney, as well as the category of cancers of all sites. However, the association was statistically significant only in melanoma, pancreas, stomach and all sites. The cohort follow-up study was carried out for the persons participating in the dietary history study. During the 20-year follow-up, 121 lung cancer cases occurred among the 5254 participating men who were initially free from cancer.

Significant inverse gradients were found between intake of β-carotene, α-tocopherol and vitamin C and the incidence of lung cancer among nonsmokers but not smokers.

III. Comments

Methodological difficulties in assessing intake and status of vitamin E continue to be a potential source of error. Many studies relied solely on information obtained from self-administered food frequency questionnaires or interviews to estimate vitamin E intake. The adequacy of questionnaires employed as well as the skill and experience of persons responsible are very critical in obtaining reliable information. Also, the tocopherol content of vegetable oils varies greatly depending upon species, harvest time, oil-processing and storage conditions. In addition, the intake and contribution of non-α-tocopherols to total vitamin E activity need to be properly addressed. Furthermore, the question concerning the completeness and accuracy of tocopherol content data available in food composition tables remains to be dealt with.

Most of the recent studies measured the serum/plasma levels of vitamin E (mainly α-tocopherol) by more accurate high-performance liquid chromatographic procedures. While plasma/serum vitamin E level is a good indicator for recent intake, it is not necessarily a suitable indicator for tissue status or long-term intake. Factors such as whether fasted blood samples are obtained, health status of the subjects and sample storage conditions and duration can significantly influence the plasma/serum levels of the vitamin E obtained. For example, patients with gastrointestinal disorders are expected to have lower levels of serum/plasma vitamin E due to the impairment of absorption. However, repeatable and reliable information on vitamin E intake can be obtained. Knekt and associate (1988a, 1993), for example, examined the short-term and long-term repeatabilities of serum level and of daily consumption of vitamin E by repeating the serum determinations and dietary interviews 4–8 months and 4–7 years after the baseline examination. They found that the interclass correlation coefficient for short-term repeatability was 0.52 for the serum determinations and 0.78 for the dietary interview, and the corresponding coefficients for long-term repeatability were 0.65 and 0.34, respectively.

It has long been expected that a number of well-designed large-scale intervention studies, including several National Cancer Institute supported chemoprevention trials, started in recent years will provide a definite answer or shed more light concerning the efficacy of anti-oxidants in cancer prevention. However, only a few of those intervention studies are designed specifically to examine the efficacy of vitamin E. Therefore, even as information from those studies becomes available, a definite conclusion concerning the association between vitamin E intake and cancer risk may or may not be reached. One of the difficulties lies with the definition concerning the protective effect against cancer risk or lack thereof. Should absence of a protective effect against cancer risk in any site be regarded as evidence of its ineffectiveness, or should any protective effect be considered as an evidence of its effectiveness?

In summary, most of the recent studies dealing with head/neck, lung and colorectal cancer suggest a protective effect of vitamin E against cancer risk. Also, the results obtained from the majority of recent studies suggest no association between vitamin E status and the risk of breast, bladder and cervical cancer. The information available to date still is not sufficient to make a definite conclusion concerning the relationship between vitamin E intake and cancer risk.

Bibliography

Barbone, F.; Austin, H. and Partridge, E.E. 1993. Diet and endometrial cancer: A case–control study. *Am. J. Epidemiol.* 137:393–403.

Barone, J.; Taioli, E.; Hebert, J.R. and Wynder, E.L. 1992. Vitamin supplement use and risk for oral and esophageal cancer. *Nutr. Cancer* 18:31–41.

Benner, S.E.; Winn, R.J.; Lippman, S.M.; Poland, J.; Hansen, K.S.; Luna, M.A. and Hong, W.K. 1993. Regression of oral leukoplakia with α-tocopherol: A community clinical oncology program chemoprevention study. *J. Natl. Cancer Inst.* 85:44–47.

Buckley, D.I.; McPherson, R.S.; North, C.Q. and Becker, T.M. 1992. Dietary micronutrients and cervical dysplasia in southwestern American Indian Women. *Nutr. Cancer* 17:179–185.

Chen, J.; Geissler, C.; Parpia, B.; Li, J. and Campbell, T.C. 1992. Antioxidant status and cancer mortality in China. *Int. J. Epidemiol.* 21:625–635.

Freudenheim, J.L.; Graham, S.; Byers, T.E.; Marshall, J.R.; Haughey, B.P.; Swanson, M.K. and Wilkson, G. 1992. Diet, smoking, and alcohol in cancer of the larynx: A case–control study. *Nutr. Cancer* 17:33–45.

Gerber, M.; Richardson, S.; Salkeld, R. and Chappuis, P. 1991. Antioxidants in female breast cancer patients. *Cancer Invest.* 9:421–428.

Gridley, G.; McLaughlin, J.K.; Block, G.; Blot, W.J.; Gluch, M. and Fraumeni, J.F. 1992. Vitamin supplement use and reduced risk of oral and pharyngeal cancer. *Am. J. Epidemiol.* 135:1083–1092.

Herrero, R.; Potischman, N.; Brinton, L.A.; Reeves, W.C.; Brenes, M.M.; Tenorio, F., deBritton, R.C. and Gaitan, E. 1991. A case–control study of nutrient status and invasive cervical cancer. *Am. J. Epidemiol.* 134:1335–1346.

Holm, L.-E.; Nordevang, E.; Hjalmar, M.-L.; Lidbrink, E., Callmer, E. and Nilsson, B. 1993. Treatment failure and dietary habits in women with breast cancer. *J. Natl. Cancer Inst.* 85:32–36.

Kabat, G.C.; Augustive, A. and Hebert, J.R. 1988. Smoking and adult leukemia. *J. Clin. Epidemiol.* 41:907–914.

Knekt, P. 1992. Vitamin E and cancer: Epidemiology. *Ann. NY Acad. Sci.* 669:269–279.

Knekt, P. 1993. Vitamin E and smoking and the risk of lung cancer. *Ann. NY Acad. Sci.* 686:280–288.

Knekt, P.A.; Aromaa, A.; Maatela, J., Aaran, R.-K.; Nikkari, T.; Hakama, M., Hakulinen, T.; Peto, R.; Saxen. E. and Teppo, L. 1988a. Serum vitamin E and risk of cancer among Finnish men during a 10-year follow-up. *Am. J. Epidemiol.* 127:28–41.

*Knekt, P.; Aromaa, A.; Maatela, J.; Alfthan, G.; Aaran, R.-K.; Teppo, L. and Hakama, M. 1988b. Serum vitamin E, serum selenium and the risk of gastrointestinal cancer. *Int. J. Cancer* 42:846–850.

London, S.J.; Stein, E.A.; Henderson, I.C.; Stampfer, M.J.; Wood W.C.; Remine, S.; Dmochowski, J.R.; Robert, N.J. and Willett, W.C. 1992. Carotenoids, retinol, and vitamin E and risk of proliferative benign breast disease and breast cancer. *Cancer Causes Control* 3:503–512.

Longnecker, M.P.; Martin-Moreno, J.-M.; Knekt, P.; Nomura, A.M.Y.; Schober, S.E.; Stahelin, H.B.; Wald, N.J.; Gey, K.F. and Willett, W.C. 1992. Serum α-tocopherol concentration in relation to subsequent colorectal cancer: Pooled data from five cohorts. *J. Natl. Cancer Inst.* 84:430–435.

Nomura, A.M.Y.; Stemmermann, G.N.; Heibrun, L.K.; Salkeld, R.M. and Viulleumier, J.P. 1985. Vitamin levels and the risk of specific sites in men of Japanese ancestry in Hawaii. *Cancer Res.* 45:2369–2372.

Paganelli, G.M.; Biasco, G.; Brandi, G.; Santucci, R.; Gizzi, G.; Villani, V.; Cianci, M.; Miglioli, M. and Barbara, L. 1992. Effect of vitamins A, C, and E supplementation on rectal cell proliferation in patients with colorectal adenomas. *J. Natl. Cancer Inst.* 84:47–51.

Potischman, N.; Herrero, R.; Brinton, L.A.; Reeves, W.C.; Stacewicz-Sapuntzakis, M.; Jones, C.J.; Brenes, M.M.; Tenorio, F.; de Britton, R.C. and Gaitan, E. 1991. A case–control study of nutrient status and invasive cervical cancer. *Am. J. Eoidemiolog.* 134:1347–1355.

Prasad, M.P.R.; Krishna, T.P.; Pastricha, S.; Krishnaswamy, K. and Quereshi, M.A. 1992. Esophageal cancer and diet—a case–control study. *Nutr. Cancer* 18:85–93.

Riboli, E.; Gonzalez, C.A.; Lopez-Abente, G.; Errezola, M.; Izarzugaza, I. Esxolar, A.; Nebot, M.; Hemon, B. and Agudo, A. 1991. Diet and bladder cancer in Spain: A multi-center case–control study. *Int. J. Cancer* 49:214–219.

Richardson, S.; Gerber, M. and Centee, S. 1991. The role of fat, animal protein and some vitamin consumption in breast cancers: A case–control study in southern France. *Int. J. Cancer* 48:1–9.

Rohan, T.E.; Howe, G.R.; Friedenreich, C.M.; Jain, M. and Miller, A.B. 1993. Dietary fiber, vitamins A, C, and E, and risk of breast cancer: A cohort study. *Cancer Causes Control* 4:29–37.

Roncucci, L.; Di Donato, P.; Carati, L.; Ferrari, A.; Perini, M.; Bertoni, G.; Bedogni, G.; Paris, B.; Svanoni, F.; Girola, M. and Ponz de Leon, M. 1993. Antioxidant vitamins or lactulose for the prevention of the recurrence of colorectal adenomas. *Dis. Colon Rectum.* 36:227–234.

*Schober, S.E.; Comstock, G.W.; Helsing, K.J.; Salkeld, R.M.; Morris, J.S.; Rider, A.A. and Brookmeyer, R. 1987. Serologic precursors of cancer. 1. Prediagnostic serum nutrients and colon cancer risk. *Am. J. Epidemiol.* 126:1033–1041.

Shibata, A.; Pagnanini-Hill, A.; Ross, R.K. and Henderson, B.E. 1992. Intake of vegetables, fruits, beta-carotene, vitamin C and vitamin supplements and cancer among the elderly: A prospective study. *Brit. J. Cancer* 66:673–679.

*Stahelin, H.B.; Bosel, F.; Buess, E. and Brubacher, G. 1984. Vitamins and plasma lipids: Prospective Basel study. *J. Natl . Cancer Inst.* 73:1463–1468.

Tominaga, K.; Saito, Y.; Mori, K.; Miyazawa, N.; Yokoi, K.; Koyama, Y.; Shimamura, K.; Imura, J. and Nagai, M. 1992. An evaluation of serum microelement concentrations in lung cancer and matched non-cancer patients to determine the risk of developing lung cancer: A preliminary study. *Jap. J. Clin. Oncol.* 22:96–101.

Vena, J.E.; Graham, S.; Freudenheim, Mashall, J.; Zielezny, M., Swanson, M. and Sufrin, G. 1992. Diet in the epidemiology of bladder cancer in western New York. *Nutr. Cancer* 18:255–264.

Wald, N.J.; Thompson, S.G.; Densem, J.W.; Boreham, J. and Bailey, A. 1987. Serum vitamin E and subsequent risk of cancer. *Brit. J. Cancer* 56:69–72.

Zheng, W.; Blot, W.J.; Diamond, E.L.; Norkus, E.P.; Spate, V.; Mossis, J.S. and Comstock, G.W. 1993. Serum micronutrients and the subsequent risk of oral and pharyngeal cancer. *Cancer Res.* 53:795–798.

*Appeared in the original report.

TABLE UPDATE   Vitamin E and Cancer

A. Head and Neck Cancer

Study	Type/Location	Subject Number and Description	Methods
Benner, S.E. et al., 1993	Intervention study; Houston, Texas	43 patients (24 males and 19 females; 41 white and 2 black; mean age 55.6) with bidimensionally measurable symptomatic leukoplakia or leukoplakia with dysplasia.	Subjects were treated with α-tocopherol (400 IU) twice daily for 24 weeks. Participants were seen in follow-up visits at 6, 12 and 24 weeks to assess toxicity and to repeat lesion measurements. Serum α-tocopherol levels were determined fluorometrically at baseline and at the 6- and 24-week visits.
Barone, J. et al., 1992	Hospital-based case–control study; New York	Cases were 290 male histologically confirmed oral cancer and 133 males with esophageal cancer. Controls were 580 sex-, race-, age-, hospital- and time-of-admission-matched patients. Control diagnoses include non-neoplastic diseases, benign neoplasms and cancers believed not to be related to the use of tobacco and alcohol products. Subjects were part of a tobacco-related case–control cancer study involving eight hospitals in four U.S. cities (Kabat et al., 1988).	Information on demographic characteristics, dietary intake, vitamin supplements, cigarette use and alcohol intake was collected using a standardized questionnaire administered at the time of hospitalization.
Zheng, W. et al., 1993	Nested case–control study; Washington County, Maryland	Cases were 28 subjects, who were diagnosed with primary oral and pharyngeal cancer during the period of 1975–1990, from a total of 25802 individuals who donated blood in 1974. Four sex-, race-, age- and status-of-blood-collection-matched controls for each case were selected from those in the same cohort who were alive and free of diagnosed cancer (except for skin cancer) at the date the case was diagnosed.	The serum levels of retinol, tocopherols, selenium and carotenoids were analyzed. At the time of blood collection, information on demographic characteristics, smoking history and use of medication during the 48 hr prior to blood collection was also obtained.
Gridley, G. et al., 1992	Population-based case–control study; New Jersey, Atlanta, Los Angeles and Santa Clara and San Mateo counties, California.	1114 pathologically confirmed incident cases of oral and pharyngeal cancer and 1268 age-, race- and sex-matched controls. Cancer of the tongue, pharynx and other oral cancers were included as cases, but cancers of the lip, salivary gland or nasopharynx were excluded. The study was conducted during 1984–1985.	Information on demographic variables, tobacco and alcohol use, diet intake (and vitamin supplement), occupation and medical history were obtained via interviews, usually in the home.
Prasad, M.P.R. et al., 1992	Case–control study; Hyderabad, India	35 (23 males average age 58 years old and 12 females average age 51 years old) early diagnosed esophageal cancer cases and 35 age-, sex-, socioeconomic-status-, family-size- and smoking- and drinking-habits-matched controls.	Random blood samples were drawn for measuring the levels of α-tocopherol, retinol, hemoglobin, albumin, folate, iron, copper, magnesium and zinc, and status of thiamin and riboflavin. Dietary consumption pattern over the last 6 months was assessed by an oral questionnaire.
Freudenheim, J.L. et al., 1992	Case–control study, three counties of western New York	250 white male incident, pathologically confirmed, laryngeal cancer cases and 250 race-, age-, sex- and neighborhoodmatched controls. The study was conducted between 1975 and 1985 from a total of 938 eligible cases.	Information on dietary intake, alcohol use and lifetime exposure to cigarettes, cigars and pipes was obtained by an in-depth food frequency questionnaire.

A. Head and Neck Cancer

Results	Comments
46% (20/43) of the patients had clinical responses and 21% (9/43) had histologic responses. Mean serum α-tocopherol levels were 16.1 µg/mL at baseline and 34.3 µg/mL after 24 weeks of treatment.	Study was designed specifically to evaluate the efficacy of vitamin E treatment, but there were no placebo controls; information on vitamin E intake was not obtained.
Among oral cancer cases use of vitamin E supplements, and among esophageal cancer cases supplemental use of vitamins E and C were associated with a reduced OR of cancer. When stratified by smoking status, the protective effect of vitamin C use in esophageal cancer was significant only among current smokers, as was vitamin E use.	The number of subjects who took vitamin E supplements was small (approximately 7% of all the cases and 11% of all the controls); no blood levels of nutrients were measured.
Serum levels of carotenoids, particular β-carotene, were lower among subjects who developed oral and pharyngeal cancer. High serum levels of α-tocopherol also were related to a low oral cancer risk in later years, but the risks were elevated significantly with increasing serum levels of γ-tocopherol and selenium.	The number of cases was small; no information on vitamin intake or supplements was obtained; serum samples were stored at –70C for about 16 years.
There was no association between cancer risk and intake of multivitamin products, but users of supplements of individual vitamins, including vitamins A, B, C and E, were at lower risk after controlling for the effect of tobacco, alcohol and other risk factors for these cancers. After further adjustment for use of other supplements, vitamin E was the only supplement that remained associated with a significant reduction in cancer risk.	Reliance on information obtained via interviews; information on supplement dose was not ascertained; blood levels of nutrients were not measured.
RR of esophageal cancer was significantly higher for patients with low plasma levels of retinol and zinc. The status of vitamin E was not significantly associated with the risk of esophageal cancer.	The number of subjects was small; blood levels of vitamin E were measured by a spectrophotometric procedure; intake of vitamin E was not estimated.
Carotenoids were inversely associated with risk among the lightest smokers, whereas dietary fat was positively associated with risk among the heaviest smokers. Total calories, protein and retinoids were associated with increased risk, and there was no relationship between laryngeal cancer and vitamins C and E, carbohydrate or dietary fiber.	No blood levels of nutrients were measured; reliance on food frequency interviews; no data on supplement use.

(continued)

TABLE UPDATE   *(continued)*

		B. Breast Cancer	
Study	Type/Location	Subject Number and Description	Methods
Richardson, S. et al., 1991	Hospital-based case–control study; Montpelier, France	Cases were 409 women aged 28–66 with histologically confirmed primary carcinoma of the breast and had not undergone any therapy. Controls were 515 women in the same age group admitted for the first time for neuro-logical or neurosurgical disorders or hospitalized for general surgery. Patients with neoplastic or cardiovas-cular diseases were excluded.	Information on food and alcohol consumption and dietary habits was obtained using a dietary history questionnaire administered during interview.
Rohan, T.E. et al., 1993	Case–control study; Toronto, Canada	519 incident, histologically confirmed cases of breast cancer identified between 1982 and 1987, and 1182 age-, screening-center- and date-of-enrollment-matched controls who had not developed breast cancer at the end of the follow-up period. Subjects were from a cohort of 56837 women who enrolled in the Canadian National Breast Screening Study before 1982 and had completed questionnaires.	Intake of fiber, β-carotene and vitamins A, C and E was estimated based on information obtained from self-administered dietary questionnaires. Information on the use of vitamin supplements was also obtained.
London, S.J. et al., 1992	Case–control study; Boston MA	Cases were 377 postmenopausal women newly diagnosed with stage I or II breast cancer. Controls were 403 women who were evaluated at the same institutions but did not require a breast biopsy or whose biopsy revealed normal tissue or nonprolifer-ative benign breast disease (BBD). Subjects with a prior history of cancer (exclusive of nonmelanoma skin can-cer) were excluded.	Subjects were asked to complete a questionnaire regarding history and breast cancer risk factors and a semiquantitative food frequency questionnaire. Serum samples were analyzed for the levels of retinol, β-carotene, α-carotene, lycopene, α-toco-pherol and γ-tocopherol by HPLC. Intakes of retinol, carotene and vitamin E were estimated based on food composition tables. Information on vitamin supplements were also obtained.
Holm, L.E. et al., 1993	Prospective study; Stockholm, Sweden	240 women, 50–65 years old, who had pathological stage I (39%) or stage II (60%) breast cancer. 149 patients were classified as estrogen receptor rich and 71 as estrogen receptor poor (20 had no data). 209 of the subjects were postmenopausal.	Subjects were interviewed for their dietary habits (including frequency of food consumption) during the past year in patient's home within 4 months of breast cancer diagnosis, and were treated (radiother-apy, chemotherapy and/or tamoxifen) and followed for at least 4 years or until death if it occurred during this period.
Gerber, M. et al., 1991	Hospital-based case–control study; Montpelier, France	Cases were 48 French women aged 25–65 years with diagnosed breast cancer at stages T1, N0, N1 or N2, without metastasis. Controls were 50 women hospitalized in neurology or neurosurgery wards for early symp-toms of diseases other than cancer or cardiovascular conditions.	Information on the socioeconomic situation, nutri-tion, reproductive, familial and medical history was obtained via a questionnaire. Fasted blood samples were obtained on the day after admission. Serum samples were measured for selenium, zinc and vita-mins C and E. Leukocyte levels of vitamins C and E and red cell levels of vitamin E were also measured.

B. Breast Cancer

Results	Comments
Increased consumption of fat, but not animal protein, vegetable or vitamin E, was associated with increased risk of breast cancer.	Reliance on information obtained by interviews; controls were patients of various diagnoses; no blood levels of vitamin E were measured.
Higher intake of fiber was associated with lower risk of breast cancer. Inverse relationship with breast-cancer risk was observed in association with consumption of pasta, cereals and vegetables rich in vitamins A and C. Statistically nonsignificant reductions in risk were observed with increasing intake of dietary retinol, β-carotene and vitamin C. Vitamin E intake was not associated with altered risk of cancer.	Reliance on self-administered dietary questionnaires; no blood levels of nutrients were measured.
No significant association was observed between serum levels of retinol, β-carotene, α-carotene, lycopene, α-tocopherol and γ-tocopherol and risk of proliferative BBD or breast cancer. The risk of breast cancer was decreased among women in the highest quintile of vitamin E intake from food sources only, but less so for total vitamin E intake including supplements.	Controls were patients of various diagnoses, 313 cases and 349 controls completed food frequency questionnaires; serum samples were stored at –70C for up to 9 months.
Fifty-two patients had treatment failure during follow-up; 5 had a new cancer of the contralateral breast, 18 had local recurrences and 29 had distant metastases. The 30 patients with estrogen receptor-rich tumors who had treatment failure reported higher intakes of total fat than did the 119 patients who did not have treatment failure. For treatment failure within the first 2 years, the multiple OR was 1.19 for each 1 mg increase in vitamin E intake per 10 MJ of energy. No association between dietary habits and treatment failure was found for women with estrogen receptor-poor cancers.	Reliance on information obtained from interviews; no appropriate controls; no blood levels of vitamin E were measured.
The levels of serum zinc and plasma and leukocyte vitamin E were significantly higher in cases than in controls. The difference was borderline significant for leukocyte vitamin C. The results were slightly modified when vitamin pill users were excluded from case and control samples.	Sample size was small; controls were not properly matched with cases; 10 cases and 13 controls took unspecified types/amounts of vitamin supplements; serum samples were stored at –18C for an unspecified time.

(continued)

TABLE UPDATE   (*continued*)

C. Lung Cancer

Study	Type/Location	Subject Number and Description	Methods
Tominaga, K. et al ., 1992	Case–control study; Utsunomiya, Japan	31 newly diagnosed lung cancer cases and matched outpatient controls.	Serum levels of vitamins A and E, carotene and selenium were determined.
Knekt, P., 1993	Cohort and nested case–control studies; various parts of Finland.	Cohort study: 121 lung cancer cases occurred among 5254 individuals initially free from cancer during a 19-year followup; case–control study: 144 lung cancer cases occurred among 21172 men initially free of cancer and 270 sex-, age- and date-of-blood collection-matched controls.	Information on smoking status and food consumption during the previous year was obtained. Also, serum samples were taken from 21387 participants. The stored serum α-tocopherol, β-carotene and retinol levels were determined 15 years later. Association between serum vitamin E and subsequent lung cancer risk was followed for up to 19 years.

D. Gastrointestinal and Pancreatic Cancer (see H. Combined Site Study [Knekt, 1992])

E. Colorectal Cancer

Study	Type/Location	Subject Number and Description	Methods
Longnecker, M.P. et al., 1992	Prospective case–control study; Helsinki, Hawaii, Maryland, Basel and London	289 cases of colorectal cancer and 1267 matched controls. Subjects were pooled from five prospective studies (Knekt et al., 1988; Nomura et al., 1985; Schober et al., 1987; Stahelin et al., 1984 and Wald et al., 1987).	Data reported in five studies were pooled and analyzed to evaluate the association between serum vitamin E concentration and risk of colorectal cancer. Subjects were categorized according to study-specific quartiles of serum α-tocopherol levels within the study.
Paganelli, G.M. et al., 1992	Intervention study, Bologna, Italy	Subjects were 46 patients (27 males and 19 females, aged 40–80) who completed endoscopic removal of adenomas.	Twenty-three patients (15 male and 8 female, average age 63.7 years old) were randomly assigned to receive vitamins A (30,000 IU axerophthol palmitate), C (1,000 mg ascorbic acid) and E (70 mg d,l-α-tocopherol acetate) daily for 6 months. Twenty-three patients (12 males and 11 females, average age 64.1 years) were randomly assigned to receive an indistinguishable placebo. Six biopsy specimens from each patient were taken from normal appearing rectal mucosa before and after 3 and 6 months of treatment for determining rectal cell proliferation using autoradiographic technique. All subjects were asked to maintain their dietary habits during the treatment period.
Roncucci, L. et al., 1993	Intervention study; Modena, Italy	209 patients (130 males and 79 females, average age 59.2 years) with at least one suspected adenoma in the large bowel identified and removed during 1985 and 1990.	After polypectomy, subjects were randomized into three groups of 70, 61 and 78, and were given daily doses of I) 30,000 IU vitamin A, 1 g vitamin C and 70 mg vitamin E, II) 20 g lactulose and III) placebo, respectively, for up to 36 months. After the initial examination and removal of polyps, endoscopic surveillance was planned after 6–8, 12–18 and 24–36 months to assess the recurrence rate of adenomatous polyps. Subjects were encouraged to continue their usual diets and lifestyles.

C. Lung Cancer

Results	Comments
A significant inverse association was found between serum vitamins A and E and lung cancer. The RR for the low verse high tertiles were, respectively, 5.9 and 8.4 for vitamin A and vitamin E. The RR of lung cancer was also high when 3 or all 4 micronutrient levels in the lowest tertile were evaluated.	Sample size was small; no information on untake of vitamins A and E was obtained.
There was a significant inverse association between vitamin E status and lung cancer occurrence among nonsmokers but not smokers in both studies. The RR of lung cancer between the lowest and highest tertiles of serum vitamin E was 6.6 among smokers and 0.8 among smokers. The RR of lung cancer between the lowest and highest tertiles of vitamin E intake was 3.3 among nonsmokers and 0.8 among smokers.	Well-designed studies; serum samples for the case–control study were stored at –20C for about 15 years prior to analysis.

D. Gastrointestinal and Pancreatic Cancer (see H. Combined Site Study [Knekt, 1992])

E. Colorectal Cancer

For cancers of the colon and rectum combined, the matched OR for the highest quartile of serum α-tocopherol concentration compared with the lowest was 0.6. Adjustment for serum cholesterol level attenuated the OR to 0.7.	Data were pooled from five different studies conducted in five different locations; the duration and conditions for storage of blood specimens varied considerably from study to study; incident cases of colorectal cancer were used as the endpoint for four studies, the other one used death from colorectal cancer as the endpoint.
In patients (n = 20) receiving vitamins, the abnormal expansion of the proliferative compartment decreased progressively from baseline values, with increasing statistical significance (p < 0.05 after 3 months, P < 0.01 after 6 months). No significant difference in cell kinetics was found in the placebo group (n = 21).	Sensitive and specific method was employed to assess the efficacy of vitamin treatment; subjects were randomly assigned to receive vitamins A, C and E or placebo; no blood/tissue levels of vitamins were measured.
The recurrence of adenomas was 5.7, 14.7 and 35.9%, respectively, for Groups I, II and III. The number of subjects remaining free of adenomas was significantly different among the three groups.	Subjects in Group I received a mixture of vitamins A, C and E; control subjects (Group III) were not matched with the treated subjects; no information on dietary intake and blood levels of vitamins A, C and E were obtained.

(continued)

TABLE UPDATE   (*continued*)

F. Cervical/Ovarian Cancer

Study	Type/Location	Subject Number and Description	Methods
Buckley, D.I. et al., 1992	Case–control study; Albuquerque, New Mexico	Cases were 42 American Indian women, aged 18–67 years (average age 34.9), with slight, moderate or severe dysplasia diagnosed within the past year. Controls were 58 race-, sex- and age-matched women (average age 27.7) who had a diagnosis of normal cervical mucosa within the past year.	Dietary intake information was obtained by a 24-hr recall, and nutrient intake was estimated using food and nutrient composition data.
Barbone, F. et al., 1993	Case–control study; Birmingham, Alabama	103 cases with histologically confirmed adenocarcinoma and 236 age- and race-matched controls. The controls were selected from women with an intact uterus. Study was conducted between 1985 and 1988.	A food frequency questionnaire was used to obtain dietary habits during the year preceding their illness (cases) or in the year preceding their interview (controls). Nutrient intake was computed on the basis of the frequency of consumption of each unit of food and of the nutrient content of the specified portions. Information on vitamin supplements was also collected.
Potischman, N. et al., 1991	Case–control study; Colombia, Costa Rica, Panama and Mexico.	387 stage I or II invasive cervical cancer cases were recruited from hospitals over a period of 18 months, and 670 age-matched controls were randomly selected from admission lists of general hospitals, excluding patients with psychiatric disorder or diseases of neoplastic-, endocrine-, nutritional-, selected-circulatory-, gynecologic- and smoking-related diagnoses.	Subjects were interviewed for food consumption frequency, demographic, socioeconomic, reproductive, occupational and medical history, as well as on sexual, hygiene and contraceptive practices. Blood samples were collected from cases before treatment, and from community and hospital controls in hospital or at home. Serum samples were analyzed for carotenoids, retinol and tocopherols.

G. Other Sites

Study	Type/Location	Subject Number and Description	Methods
Vena, J.E. et al., 1992	Case–control; Buffalo, Niagara Falls and Rochester, New York	Cases were 351 white males, 35–90 years of age, with histologically confirmed transitional cell carcinoma of the bladder. Controls were 855 race, age, sex and neighborhood of residence matched. Subjects were identified between 1979 and 1985 from hospital pathology records.	Nutrient intake was estimated by comprehensive interviews with the use of a detailed food frequency questionnaire and of published food composition data.
Riboli, E. et al., 1991	Multicenter case–control study; Barcelona, Cadiz, Guipuzcoa, Madrid and Vizcaya, Spain	Cases were 432 male bladder cancer patients (<80 years), who had been diagnosed or treated during 1985–1986. Controls were 792 age-, sex- and area-of-residence-matched patients whose main diagnosis excluded chronic respiratory diseases, coronary heart disease, infections of the urinary tract, haematuria and cancer of the respiratory tract. Among them were 360 sets with 1 case and 2 controls (one from the same hospital and the other from the municipal registers or census files) and 72 sets with 1 case and 1 control.	Information on tobacco smoking and occupational history, dietary habits (including the types of vegetables, fruit, oil and other fats consumed), lifetime use of analgesic drugs and the past urinary infections was obtained by an interview-based dietary history questionnaire.

F. Cervical/Ovarian Cancer

Results	Comments
Although mean differences between cases and controls were not statistically significant, women with low intake of vitamins C and E and folacin were at increased risk of having cervical dysplasia when the data were analyzed as stratified for level of intake (low vs. high intake OR were 3.0 for vitamin C, 3.3 for folacin and 1.7 for vitamin E).	No blood levels of nutrients were obtained; reliance on a single 24-hr recall; the mean age difference between cases and controls was large.
The association of higher carotene intake and lower incidence of endometrial cancer was statistically significant. There was no significant relation between endometrial cancer and the intake of vitamins C, D and E.	Reliance on food frequency questionnaire; no blood levels of nutrients were measured.
Cases did not differ significantly from controls in mean serum levels of retinol, cryptoxanthin, lycopene, α-carotene, lutin or α-tocopherol. Increased risk was associated with decreased β-carotene and increased γ-tocopherol levels.	Controls were hospital patients of various diagnoses. Serum samples were collected from four Latin American countries and were stored at –70C for different time periods prior to analysis in the U.S.; blood samples were collected without regard for time of day or fasting status; no information on vitamin supplements was obtained.

G. Other Sites

Results	Comments
An increased risk of bladder cancer was associated with higher intake of calories, fat, carbohydrates, sodium and proteins. Increased carotenoid consumption was associated with a decreased risk of bladder cancer for those under 65 years. No significant differences between cases and controls were seen for intake of vitamins A, C, D and E, niacin, thiamin, riboflavin and calcium.	Reliance on interviews; no information on the levels of blood nutrients and the use of vitamin supplements.
Higher risk of bladder cancer was associated with higher intake of saturated fat. Higher intake of vitamin E was associated with a slightly reduced risk which was not modified by adjustment for fat. No association was found with intake of retinol or carotene.	Reliance on information obtained from interviews; no vitamin use or blood levels of nutrients were determined; subjects were identified from the registers of 12 hospitals located in five study areas.

(continued)

TABLE UPDATE   *(continued)*

		H. Combined Sites Studies	
Study	Type/Location	Subject Number and Description	Methods
Shibata, A. et al., 1992	Prospective study; Los Angeles	11580 residents of a retirement community of almost entirely Caucasian and of the upper-middle socioeconomic class, initially free of cancer, were followed from 1981 to 1989. A total of 1335 incident cancer cases were diagnosed during the period.	Information on demographic, socioeconomical status, medical history, personal habits, use of cigarettes and vitamin supplements and frequencies of food consumption was obtained via questionnaires. Follow-up was maintained by annual mailing to all participants for up to 9 years.
Chen J. et al., 1992	Ecological study; 65 counties, China.	Based on the mortality rates for seven major cancer sites, 3250 male and 3250 female adults aged 35–64 years were randomly selected from a total of 130 survey sites (2 communes in each of 65 counties).	Information on dietary habits, blood and urine, as well as questionnaire data on frequency of food intake, cigarette and alcohol consumption and other lifestyle characteristics were collected from 50 randomly selected individuals (25 male and 25 female) at each of the 130 survey sites. Plasma levels of β-carotene, retinol and α-tocopherol were measured by HPLC.
Knekt, P., 1992	a) Nested case–control study and b) cohort follow-up study, Finland	a) case–control study: 766 cancer cases of all sites and 1419 sex-, age- (15 and over) and date-of-blood-collection-matched controls. Subjects were from a total of 40201 Finnish Mobile Clinic Health Examination Survey conducted during 1968–1972; b) cohort study: 5254 men initially free from cancer participated in the dietary history study. During the 20 year follow-up, 121 of those subjects developed lung cancer.	The nested case–control study was based on the cancer cases occurring during 1968 and 1977 in the subsample with stored serum samples. The serum α-tocopherol, β-carotene and retinol levels were determined about 15 years after the baseline examination using HPLC. The association between serum vitamin E and cancer incidence was estimated for 19 different cancer sites. In the cohort study, dietary history was obtained from participating men, and their intake of vitamin C, α-tocopherol, β-carotene, retinol and selenium was computed, based on food composition tables. The incidence of lung cancer among subjects was followed for up to 20 years.

Abbreviations: OR—odds ratio; RR—relative risk.

H. Combined Sites Studies

Results	Comments
After adjustment for age and smoking, no protective effect was found for any of the dietary variables in men. However, an inverse association was observed between vitamin C supplement use and bladder cancer risk. In women, reduced cancer risks of all sites combined and of the colon were noted for combined intake of all vegetables and fruits, fruit intake alone and dietary vitamin C. Supplemental use of vitamins A and C showed a protective effect on colon cancer risk in women. Beta-carotene intake and supplemental use of vitamins A, C and E were associated with a non-significant reduction of lung cancer risk in women.	Reliance on questionnaires returned by subjects via mail; the questionnaire was designed specifically to measure intake of foods rich in carotenoids and vitamins A and C. No blood levels of vitamins were measured.
County-level cumulative sex- and site-specific mortality rates for all types of cancer were 11.2% for males and 6.7% for females. Plasma levels of α-tocopherol were positively correlated with the cancer mortality rates of liver and lung in males but not in females. None of the associations between α-tocopherol and cancer mortality rates were significant after adjusting for plasma total cholesterol levels. Beta-carotene (stomach of males and females) and ascorbic acid (all causes, esophageal, stomach, liver and lung of males) were negatively correlated with cancer mortality rates. Selenium was found to correlate negatively with esophageal and stomach cancers of males and females. The plasma levels of retinol were not significantly correlated with the cancer mortality rates of any sites.	The number of subjects in several types of cancer was small, no intake data of micronutrients were employed for the analysis.
The mean level of serum α-tocopherol was lower among cancer cases than among corresponding controls for most of the sites studied, and was significantly inversely related to the subsequent occurrence of cancer at all sites, and cancers of pancreas, stomach and melanoma. The differences on the other 15 sites were not significant. The dietary study revealed significant inverse gradients between intake of β-carotene, α-tocopherol and vitamin C and the incidence of lung cancer among nonsmokers, but not smokers.	Well-designed studies; portions of the results from this study appeared in Knekt (1993); serum samples were stored at $-20°C$ for about 15 years.

Chapter 5

Lipids and Cancer

Kenneth K. Carroll, Ph.D.

I. Introduction

A. Background

In 1982, the National Research Council's Committee on Diet, Nutrition, and Cancer (NRC) concluded "that of all the dietary components it studied, the combined epidemiological and experimental evidence is most suggestive for a causal relationship between fat intake and the occurrence of cancer" (National Research Council, 1982). This conclusion was based primarily on the strong positive correlation between dietary fat and cancers of the breast, colon, prostate and a number of other sites observed in intercountry studies and on the results of numerous experiments on animals showing that those fed high-fat diets develop cancer more readily than those fed low-fat diets, especially in the breast and colon. The evidence from studies on experimental animals indicated that dietary fat had a promoting effect on tumorigenesis (Carroll, 1975).

The Surgeon General's Report on Nutrition and Health (U.S. Department of Health and Human Services, 1988) concluded that "Despite some inconsistencies in the data relating dietary fat to cancer causation … the weights of the studies to date are strongly suggestive of the role for dietary fat in the etiology of some types of cancer." The report of the NRC Committee on Diet and Health (National Research Council, 1989) summarized the conclusions by saying that the weight of evidence indicates that high-fat diets are associated with higher risk of several cancers, especially of the colon, prostate, and breast. Some inconsistencies in the data were also noted in this report.

B. Scope of Work

The purpose of the present article is to provide an up-to-date assessment of the role of dietary lipids in cancer, taking into account papers that have appeared since the above reports were published. Emphasis will be given to studies on humans, and experiments on animals will only be considered when they seem particularly pertinent to the discussion. Human studies reviewed in this report are summarized by organ site in the Appendix Table.

II. Epidemiological Evidence

The following kinds of studies have been used to provide information on the role of dietary lipids in cancer:

- Intercountry and intracountry correlations
- Studies on migrants
- Time-trend studies
- Cohort studies

- Case–control studies
- Intervention studies

The strengths and weaknesses of these different kinds of studies will be considered in turn.

A. Intercountry and Intracountry Correlations

Intercountry correlations normally compare age-adjusted cancer incidence or mortality in different countries with availability of dietary fat in those countries. The cancer incidence data are collected by cancer registries (e.g., Whelan et al., 1990) and are not necessarily representative of cancer incidence in the country as a whole when the population base for the registry does not cover the entire country. Cancer mortality data are collected by the World Health Organization (e.g., World Health Organization, 1990) and the accuracy of such data probably varies considerably from one country to another. Dietary fat intakes are based on disappearance data collected by the Food and Agriculture Organization of the United Nations (e.g., Food and Agriculture Organization of the United Nations, 1980) and overestimate actual intake since much food is wasted and not actually eaten, e.g., cooking oil.

In early plots of cancer incidence or mortality against dietary fat, intake was usually expressed as g/person/d (Armstrong and Doll, 1975; Carroll, 1975; Carroll and Khor, 1975). A better approach is to plot dietary fat as percent of total calories (Carroll, 1986a). This provides more realistic values but also tends to overestimate, since the fat in food is more likely to be lost or discarded to a greater extent than carbohydrate or protein, which are the other main sources of dietary calories.

Cancer is thought to develop over a relatively long period of time, thus cancer incidence and mortality should probably be compared with dietary fat intake over a period of preceding years when it may be influencing the carcinogenic process. In practice, this does not seem to be a serious consideration because cancer incidence and mortality and the level of dietary fat in any particular country change rather slowly with time. Other limitations of ecologic studies include: the difficulty of isolating effects of one particular dietary factor, the inability to control for other confounding factors related to living standard and life style, and the high potential for sources of error in the collection of data on diet and on cancer incidence and mortality. In spite of these various uncertainties and inaccuracies, plots of cancer incidence or mortality at sites such as the breast and colon have consistently shown strong positive correlations with dietary fat in these intercountry comparisons (see Figures 1a and 1b).

Even in countries where cancer is most prevalent, any particular type of cancer occurs only in a minority of the population. (For example, recent statistics indicate that one out of nine women is expected to develop breast cancer in the United States.) Thus, if a high-fat diet is acting to promote breast cancer, a large proportion of the female population is protected either by its innate genetic makeup or has not been exposed to adequate initiating stimuli for breast cancer to develop or it is protected by other exogenous factors (e.g., dietary factors).

In comparing the large populations involved in intercountry studies, it seems possible that these genetic and initiating factors may largely cancel out. Although most of the population in any country will not develop cancer under the existing environmental conditions, a segment that is genetically more susceptible may develop cancer under one set of conditions but not under another (Figure 2). It is thus possible to observe environmental effects on cancer even in populations with large genetic diversity.

Breast

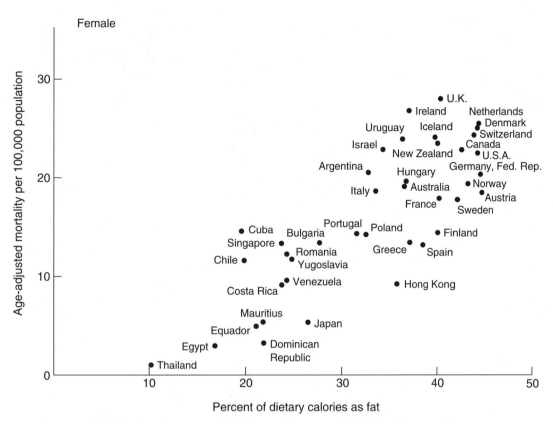

Figure 1a.   Positive correlation between percentage of dietary calories as fat and age-adjusted mortality from breast cancer (Carroll, 1991). (Used with permission.)

In addition to intercountry correlations, there have been a number of studies on subgroups within countries whose diet and lifestyle differ from those of the majority of the population. An example is the Seventh-Day Adventists who have somewhat lower incidence of cancer at several different sites than other Americans (Phillips et al., 1980). Comparisons of different ethnic groups or different regional populations within countries have not shown a consistent relationship between dietary fat and cancer (Vogel and McPherson, 1989) but this may be because the effects of smaller differences in dietary fat intake are obscured by other factors that influence carcinogenesis. Such studies may nevertheless help to provide clues to the role of diet in cancer (Willett, 1990a).

B. Migrant Studies

Studies on migrants have provided the strongest evidence that the geographical differences in cancer incidence and mortality observed in intercountry studies are related to environmental rather than genetic factors (McMichael and Giles, 1988; Prentice et al., 1988). The results of these studies have shown that the pattern of cancer in migrants changes from that in their country of origin and approaches that of their newly adopted country. The rate of change varies for cancer at different organ sites (for example, colon

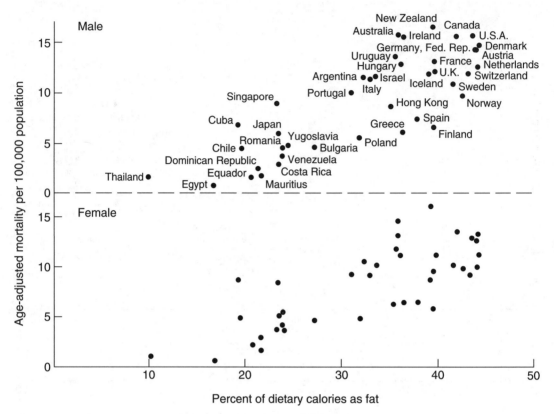

Figure 1b. Positive correlation between percentage of dietary calories as fat and age-adjusted mortality from colon cancer (Carroll, 1991). (Used with permission.)

cancer changes more quickly than breast cancer) and may require more than a generation to approximate the pattern in the host country. This suggests that factors operating early in life may be more important in determining future breast cancer risk (Adami et al., 1990).

In studies to date, the migrants have invariably moved from countries with lower to those with higher fat intake. Since the cancer pattern changes from that of the country of origin to that of the host country, this necessarily means an increase in those cancers that are positively correlated with dietary fat. It does not, however, prove that this is a causative relationship, since many other environmental changes are associated with the move.

The idea that dietary fat is one of the most important environmental variables comes primarily from the results of experimental studies which have shown consistently that animals on high-fat diets develop cancer at sites such as the breast and colon more readily than animals on low-fat diets (National Research Council, 1982; 1989). It should be noted, however, that the differences in cancer incidence and mortality associated with differences in dietary fat in the intercountry data are often substantially greater than the differences in cancer incidence observed in animals over a similar range of fat intake. In changing from low- to high-fat diets, there may thus be alterations in other components of the diet that influence the carcinogenic process. In this connection, it is interesting to

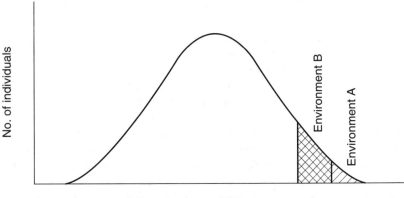

Figure 2. Diagram illustrating the possible relationship between genetic and environmental influences on carcinogenesis. In comparing data from two different countries, it is assumed that the population of each country has a similar range of genetic susceptibility to cancer, but a greater proportion of the more susceptible individuals may develop cancer under the environmental conditions of one country compared to the other (Carroll, 1986b). (Used with permission.)

note that rats on chow diet have been observed to develop fewer mammary tumors than those on semipurified diet, even when the level of fat is similar in the two diets (Carroll, 1975; Ip, 1987).

C. Time-Trend Studies

Environmental conditions are continually changing in any given country thereby providing additional opportunities to study the effects of the changing environments on cancer incidence and mortality (Lands et al., 1990). Time-trend studies have shown an increase in breast and colon cancer in Japan since World War II that has been accompanied by a marked increase in the level of dietary fat (Willett, 1989). As in the migrant studies, this cannot necessarily be assumed to be a causative relationship. The frequency of breast and colon cancer has also increased in a number of other countries in recent years (Kurihara et al., 1984), but the causes have not been investigated in any detail. Incidence of cancers of the breast, prostate, and to a lesser extent colorectal cancer, are also increasing in the United States (Newman, 1990). This may be due in part to increased detection of existing tumors, but may also reflect changes in actual risk (Liff et al., 1991; Potosky et al., 1990).

As in the migrant studies, time-trend studies have generally shown an increase in dietary fat intake and this has been associated with increases in types of cancer that are positively correlated with dietary fat in the intercountry studies. There is as yet little direct evidence that a decrease in dietary fat intake would result in reduced incidence of cancer at those sites.

D. Cohort Studies

In cohort studies, groups of individuals who were originally free of disease are followed prospectively with time, and attempts are made to relate environmental factors such as diet to development of the disease in particular individuals. Data on dietary fat and breast cancer have been reported for a number of such studies in recent years (Howe et al.,

1991; Jones et al., 1987; Knekt et al., 1990; Mills et al., 1989a; Willett et al., 1987). None has provided strong evidence for a positive association and in some cases a negative correlation was observed (Willett et al., 1987).

In a cohort study of diet and pancreatic cancer among 34,000 Seventh-Day Adventists, Mills et al. (1988b) observed that the protective effect of frequent consumption of vegetables and fruit was more important than any increased risk from frequent consumption of meat or other animal products. Bosland (1988) reviewed the etiopathogenesis of prostate cancer and concluded that a high intake of dietary fat was associated with elevated risk. However, a prospective study of prostate cancer in approximately 8000 men of Japanese ancestry in Hawaii showed no association with total fat intake during a follow-up period of about 20 years (Severson et al., 1989). Another cohort study of diet and prostate cancer in approximately 14,000 Seventh-Day Adventist men followed for 6 years showed no relationship with body-mass index and no association with animal product consumption after allowing for the protective influence of increased fruit and vegetable consumption (Mills et al., 1989a). A prospective study of more than 17,000 policy holders of the Lutheran Brotherhood Insurance Society with a 20-year follow-up likewise showed no association of prostate cancer with dietary factors, including meats, dairy products, fruits, or vegetables (Hsing et al., 1990). Increased risk of urothelial cancer associated with high intake of beef and pork and with several fried foods was reported by Steineck et al. (1988, 1990).

Although cohort studies offer an attractive approach to studying the role of dietary fat in cancer, they have some serious limitations (Freudenheim and Marshall, 1988; Goodwin and Boyd, 1987; Hegsted, 1989; Prentice et al., 1988). It is difficult to obtain an accurate assessment of the diet of individuals over time, especially when the assessment is based on self-administered questionnaires. Another serious problem is that the range of fat intake in cohort studies is generally less than that for intercountry studies and may be insufficient to distinguish effects of dietary fat from the influence of other factors that might affect carcinogenesis (Hebert and Kabat, 1991).

In spite of these limitations, Willett et al. (1990) have recently reported a positive association between dietary animal fat and risk of colon cancer in the same cohort of women as those for the study on breast cancer referred to above (Willett et al., 1987). In the colon cancer study, positive associations were observed for both saturated and monounsaturated fat, the major constituents of animal fat, but not for vegetable fat or linoleic acid. Total energy intake was not significantly associated with risk of colon cancer. However, the positive associations with total, saturated, and monounsaturated fats were weak and non-significant until adjusted for total energy intake.

The dichotomy between breast and colon cancer in these reports obviously requires explanation and more data may be needed to resolve the issue. In studies on migrants and time-trend studies within countries, the incidence of breast cancer has generally changed more slowly than that of colon cancer (Willett, 1989). This may indicate a longer latent period for breast cancer, and changes in dietary intake may be greater over a longer period of time.

E. Case–Control Studies

These are retrospective rather than prospective studies in which individuals with cancer are matched with hospital, community or population controls of similar age and sex, and an effort is made to identify factors that may have led to development of cancer in some individuals and not in others.

Like the cohort studies, these have not generally provided strong evidence for an association between dietary fat and cancer (Hulka, 1989; Willett, 1989), although a combined analysis of 12 case–control studies on breast cancer by Howe et al. (1990a) showed a consistent, statistically significant, positive association with saturated fat intake in postmenopausal women (relative risk for highest vs lowest quartile 1.46, $p < 0.0001$). Some other recent case–control studies on breast cancer have also shown positive associations with dietary fat (Brisson et al., 1989; Ewertz and Gill, 1990; Gerber et al., 1989, 1990; Iscovich et al., 1989; Pryor et al., 1989; Richardson et al., 1991; Toniolo et al., 1989; Van't Veer et al., 1990, 1991; Yu et al., 1990), although they may not always be clearly dissociated from increased energy consumption (Willett, 1990b). Other studies have not shown an association with dietary fat or have not specifically addressed the question (Katsouyanni et al., 1988; Lee et al., 1991; Le Marchand et al., 1988; Mills et al., 1988b; Rohan et al., 1990; Zaridze et al., 1991). Results of these studies are summarized in the Appendix Table.

Willett (1989) reviewed epidemiological studies on both breast and colon cancer and concluded that the evidence relating diet to colon cancer, although not conclusive, was stronger than that for breast cancer. This conclusion was based mainly on the results of cohort and case–control studies. Other recent case–control studies have generally shown a positive correlation between colorectal cancer and dietary fat (Freudenheim et al., 1990; Gerhardsson de Verdier et al., 1990; Graham et al., 1988; Slattery et al., 1988; West et al., 1989; Whittemore et al., 1990) or animal products (Benito et al., 1990; La Vecchia et al., 1988). Some differences in fat metabolism between cases and controls were observed by Neoptolemos et al. (1988) (See also the Appendix Table).

A number of case–control studies have been concerned with the role of diet in pancreatic cancer (Appendix Table). Ghadirian et al. (1991) reported increased risk associated with intake of total energy, total and saturated fat, and cholesterol. Howe et al. (1990b) also reported an association with total energy but not with total fat. Farrow and Davis (1990) found no association with total fat and Zatonski et al. (1991) found an inverse association with fat, particularly unsaturated fat, although there was a strong positive correlation with dietary cholesterol. Falk et al. (1988) and Olsen et al. (1989) observed increased risk associated with consumption of meat products and La Vecchia et al. (1990) reported an insignificant trend for increased risk associated with intake of meat, eggs, and margarine.

The role of diet in prostate cancer has been investigated in several recent case–control studies (Appendix Table), and some have shown evidence of increased risk associated with dietary fat (Mettlin et al., 1989; Slattery et al., 1990; West et al., 1991). Ohno et al. (1988) reported an increased risk with low β-carotene and vitamin A intake but found no association with dietary fat. Rose and Connolly (1991) summarized the results of eight earlier case–control studies on prostate cancer, all but one of which showed a positive association with dietary fat.

A positive association between lung cancer and dietary fat and cholesterol was reported by Goodman et al. (1988) for men but not for women. Jain et al. (1990) also observed an increased risk of lung cancer associated with cholesterol intake. One study on ovarian cancer (Shu et al., 1989) showed that risk was significantly correlated with increased intake of animal fats, but another showed no relation to dietary fat (Slattery et al., 1989).

Other recent case–control studies have examined effects of diet on cancer of the oral cavity and pharynx (Franceschi et al., 1991), cancers of the bladder (La Vecchia et al., 1989), other parts of the urinary tract (Steineck et al., 1990), and non-Hodgkin's lymphoma (Franceschi et al., 1989). The latter two studies showed evidence of an association between dietary fat and increased risk. Mettlin et al. (1990) reported that consumption of whole milk was associated with increased risk for cancer at a number of different sites.

Some of the studies now being reported are part of a multicentric, case–control program of the International Agency for Research on Cancer (IARC) with the acronym SEARCH. Dietary investigation is a dominant theme in two of these studies, one on pancreatic cancer and one on breast and colon cancer in women (Saracci, 1990).

For investigating relationships between dietary fat and cancer, case–control studies have a number of disadvantages. As with cohort studies, the range of dietary fat intake in cases and controls is generally not as great as for intercountry studies, and determining dietary intake of individuals in the past poses even greater difficulties than obtaining such information for prospective cohort studies (Vogel and McPherson, 1989).

Jain et al. (1989) compared dietary intake in a group of 94 control subjects from a case–control study of diet and colorectal cancer after an interval of 7 years and found that dietary habits had changed in a substantial number of people. Comparison of the current with the earlier intake showed good reliability for macrocomponents when no dietary change had occurred but poorer reliability for microcomponents and for subjects reporting a dietary change.

The choice of controls also presents potential difficulties. There is a possibility that the diets of hospital controls, as well as those of the cases themselves, may be influenced by the illnesses diagnosed and that the diets of population controls may be influenced by a particular interest in nutrition (Willett, 1990a).

A major problem with case–control studies is that the cases by definition are all genetically prone or have been sufficiently initiated for cancer to develop under particular environmental conditions. This cannot be assumed for the controls. As noted earlier, even in countries with high incidence of breast cancer such as the United States, only about one in nine women develop the disease. This suggests that in a group of control women, only a relatively small proportion will develop breast cancer, regardless of environmental factors such as the level of dietary fat. This argument also applies to cancer at other sites. Case–control studies are thus not well-suited for investigating effects of diet in cancer promotion in the absence of evidence that the cases and controls are at comparable risk in terms of initiation.

F. Intervention Studies

The aim of these studies is to provide direct evidence in humans that a particular change in diet, such as a reduction in dietary fat, will alter the risk of developing particular kinds of cancer. The advantages of this approach are that diets can be designed to compare relatively large differences in dietary fat intake and that study groups can be followed prospectively. Preliminary studies have already demonstrated the feasibility of this approach in women at risk of breast cancer (Boyd et al., 1988, 1990; Henderson et al., 1990, 1991; Holm, 1990; Holm et al., 1990) and in breast cancer patients (Boyar et al., 1988; Nordevang et al., 1990), although it would be desirable to have further documentation over a wider socioeconomic and ethnic range.

The reduction in fat intake is largely replaced by carbohydrate, although some increase in dietary protein has also been reported (Nordevang et al., 1990). In general, there is a tendency for overall caloric intake to decrease and this is accompanied by some reduction in weight and a decrease in serum cholesterol levels (Boyd et al., 1988; Henderson et al., 1990). These changes tend to be greater during the early intervention period but have persisted in longer term studies. Dougherty et al. (1988) have pointed out that a low-fat diet is richer in essential nutrients than a high-fat diet.

A major disadvantage of intervention trials is the high cost and labor intensive nature of such studies, which may need to be continued for a relatively long period of time with large numbers of individuals in order to obtain a clear-cut answer. One way of reducing the number of individuals that need to be studied is by recruiting those at higher risk, as in the study of Boyd et al. (1988). Another way to make such studies more cost effective is to broaden the scope of the investigation to study effects of reducing dietary fat on risk of other diseases, such as cardiovascular disease, as proposed in a modified version of the Women's Health Trial (Smigel, 1990).

Another approach in intervention studies is to investigate effects of reducing dietary fat on recurrence of cancer rather than on primary development (Wynder et al., 1990). There is some rationale for this in the case of breast cancer, which has been found to recur less frequently in Japan, where fat intake is substantially lower than in the United States. Verrault et al. (1988) and Holm et al. (1989) have reported that high-fat diets are associated with prognostic indicators of a less favorable outcome for women with breast cancer. These include larger tumors and more axillary node involvement, the latter being associated with higher saturated fat intake.

III. Discussion

A. Limitations of Study Design

Early enthusiasm for the proposal that high-fat diets increase the risk of cancers of the breast, colon, and other sites was based mainly on intercountry correlations, studies on migrants, and the results of experiments on animal cancer models. This enthusiasm was subsequently tempered by the results of cohort and case–control studies which often provided only weak or equivocal evidence for a positive association between dietary fat and cancer. There have also been suggestions that cancer is influenced more by energy balance than by any specific effect of dietary fat (Kritchevsky, 1990; Pariza, 1987, 1988).

The results of recently reported studies have not provided much further clarification of the role of dietary fat in cancer. Those who find the data from intercountry comparisons and animal experiments more convincing continue to believe that dietary fat is an important factor in observed geographical differences in cancer incidence and mortality at sites such as breast and colon. Those who place more credence in cohort and case–control studies continue to be skeptical and suggest that, if there is a relationship, the evidence for colon cancer is more convincing than that for cancer at other sites.

In the report, an attempt has been made to discuss the strengths and weaknesses of the different approaches to investigating the role of dietary lipids in cancer. (See also Colditz and Willett, 1991; Higginson and Sheridan, 1991). At this point in time, ecologic studies, supported by results of animal experimentation, provide a valid basis for thinking that dietary lipids have a significant effect on cancer incidence and mortality. Furthermore, the evidence from experimental studies indicates that any such effects of dietary lipids are exerted primarily at the promotional stage of carcinogenesis.

It is important, however, to consider why the results of case–control and cohort studies have not provided strong support for these conclusions. As discussed earlier, case–control studies do not appear to be well-suited for studying factors affecting cancer promotion, because the cases and controls are not comparable in terms of initiation. Cohort studies have an advantage over case–control studies in that the cases are not preselected and diets can be followed prospectively rather than retrospectively, which depends on dietary recall. The diagnosis of cancer is also likely to be more reliable in cohort studies than in intercountry studies, where the reliability may vary considerably from one country to another.

For cohort studies, the dietary intake is assessed on an individual basis, usually from completed questionnaires. The variations in dietary fat intake within the cohort are generally less than those covered by the intercountry studies. Thus, there is greater potential for overlap within different segments of the cohort. In such circumstances, variations in the dietary intake of individuals with time can also assume greater significance since a particular individual may not consistently remain within a specific sub-group of the cohort. Although some cohorts, such as those of Willett et al. (1987), have been followed for a considerable period of time, the numbers of individuals and the time span are still considerably less than those of intercountry studies.

For intercountry studies, dietary assessment is usually based on food disappearance data. It thus provides no information on individual intakes of dietary lipids and greatly overestimates intake when expressed as g/person/d. However, when fat intake is expressed as percent of total caloric intake, disappearance data give a reasonable approximation to values obtained by more rigorous methods. In any population there will be considerable individual variation in dietary fat intake, but, in comparing two countries with large differences, based on disappearance data, it seems reasonable to conclude that there will be relatively little overlap between the intakes of individuals within those countries. Since disappearance data for many countries have now been collected for 40 or more years, it is also possible to have an idea of intercountry differences over an extended period of time.

The above considerations provide some possible reasons for the relative lack of support of the dietary lipid hypothesis by case–control and cohort studies. (See also Byar and Freedman, 1989; Goodwin and Boyd, 1987; Hebert and Miller, 1988; Hulka, 1989; Prentice and Sheppard, 1989; and Schatzkin et al., 1989). In referring to case–control and cohort studies, Greenwald (1989) has expressed the view that when so many epidemiological studies give such varied results, it is questionable whether much more can be gained by further studies of this type.

B. Theoretical Explanations for Conflicting Results

It is pertinent to speculate, however, why case–control and prospective studies have generally provided more consistent evidence for a positive association of dietary fat with colon cancer than with breast cancer. One possibility is that the average latent period may be longer for breast cancer than for colon cancer. Dividing cells are more susceptible to mutagenic agents than differentiated non-dividing cells, and it therefore seems probable that initiation of breast cancer occurs more frequently at an early age when the breast is developing, whereas this may not be true for cancer of the colon where epithelial cells continue to divide during adult life.

The idea of early initiation of breast cancer is reinforced by evidence that incidence is influenced by factors such as age of menarche, age at first pregnancy, and parity (de Waard and Trichopoulos, 1988; Kelsey and Gammon, 1990). The initiation process may be influenced by the latter two factors because pregnancy tends to hasten differentiation of the glandular epithelial cells (Russo et al., 1990). The slower rate of change in incidence of breast cancer relative to colon cancer in migrants and in time-trend studies is also compatible with the idea that initiation of breast cancer occurs at an early age and that effects of a promoting agent such as dietary fat may be exerted at an early age to a greater extent than for colon cancer.

As discussed earlier, the pre-selection of individuals with cancer in case–control studies makes such studies unsuitable for investigating effects of dietary lipids on cancer promotion. In other kinds of epidemiological studies, including intercountry studies, migrant studies, time-trend studies, and cohort studies, it is also difficult to distinguish clearly between effects of initiation and promotion in carcinogenesis. This remains a problem, even in the case of intervention trials. In such trials, any differences in cancer incidence associated with changes in the diet would presumably be independent of effects of initiation by non-dietary carcinogens, but changes in diet might still lead to greater or lesser exposure to dietary carcinogens as well as to promoting agents.

In human studies on diet and carcinogenesis, it is also difficult to resolve the question of the relative importance of energy intake and dietary fat, because they are so strongly correlated with one another (Carroll and Khor, 1975). It is well known that caloric restriction inhibits carcinogenesis in experimental animals (Kritchevsky, 1990; Ruggeri, 1991). Welsch et al. (1990) expressed the opinion that enhancement of mammary carcinogenesis by dietary fat is dependent on ad libitum feeding. However, Freedman et al. (1990) concluded from their survey of experimental studies that dietary fat had an effect on mammary carcinogenesis which was independent of caloric intake. Other recent reviews of the influence of dietary fat on carcinogenesis in experimental animal models include those of Angres and Beth (1991), Birt (1990), Erickson and Hubbard (1990), Kritchevsky and Klurfeld (1991), Rogers and Longnecker (1988), Weisburger and Wynder (1991), and Zhao et al. (1991). The latter group concluded from an analysis of 14 studies that dietary fat has an important and specific role in the promotion of rat colon carcinoma.

The correlation analysis of international data by Hursting et al. (1990) led to the conclusion that total fat intake was strongly associated with cancers of the breast, colon, and prostate, even when adjusted for total caloric intake. Saturated fat was also associated with incidence of cancers of the breast, colon and prostate. Polyunsaturated fat was associated with incidence of breast and prostate but not with colon cancer.

Decreased caloric intake as a result of inadequate food supplies may have an inhibitory effect on carcinogenesis in some parts of the world, but it does not seem practical to encourage voluntary reduction of dietary intake as a means of reducing cancer risk when food is readily available. It has been observed, however, in feasibility studies with low-fat diets (Boyd et al., 1988; Henderson et al., 1990) that caloric intake tends to decrease when the level of fat in the diet is reduced. This may occur because of the more bulky nature and lower energy density of low-fat diets. If such diets are able to reduce the risk of cancer, it may not matter whether the effect is related specifically to dietary fat or caloric intake.

Any approach to risk reduction is nevertheless more appealing if a scientifically-based rationale can be provided. For colon cancer, it has been suggested that high-fat diets increase the concentration in the colon of bile acids and possibly of fatty acids as well, which in turn can act as promoters of carcinogenesis (Newmark et al., 1984; Reddy, 1986). These effects may be modified by other dietary components, such as calcium, which could bind the acids and prevent their promoting action (Lipkin, 1991; Lipkin et al., 1991).

Effects of dietary fat on sex hormones was one of the first mechanisms proposed to explain its effects on mammary cancer (Chan and Cohen, 1975). This has been a continuing theme of research (Adlercreutz, 1990a,b; Cohen, 1986; Key and Pike, 1988; Pike, 1990; Welsch, 1986), but the role of hormones has been surprisingly elusive, and there is still no consensus on the relationship of diet to hormonal changes associated with breast cancer (Adlercreutz, 1990a; Kelsey and Gammon, 1990). Attempts to relate hormonal changes to diet and prostatic cancer have likewise had little success (Rose and Connelly, 1991). Additional suggested mechanisms for effects of diet on mammary cancer include effects on the immune system, on prostaglandin synthesis, on lipid peroxidation, on membrane fluidity, on intercellular communication, and on response to growth factors (Cohen, 1986; Welsch, 1987).

Another recently proposed mechanism is based on evidence that the adipose tissue of the mammary gland has an important influence on development and proliferation of the mammary parenchyma (Carroll and Parenteau, 1991). Since adipose tissue represents the major site of energy storage in the body, it is likely to reflect changes in energy balance to a greater extent than body weight as a whole. The intimate association between adipose tissue and glandular tissue in the mammary gland should facilitate transfer of substances such as eicosanoids, estrogens, or other growth-promoting factors that might be present in larger or smaller amounts as the volume of adipose tissue increases or decreases under the influence of diet. This could perhaps mediate effects of high-fat versus low-fat diets and might also help to explain other dietary effects as well as effects of caloric restriction or exercise (Cohen et al., 1988; Simopoulos, 1990; Weindruch et al., 1991).

This proposed mechanism is also compatible with evidence that obesity is a risk factor for breast cancer (de Waard and Trichopoulos, 1988; Kelsey and Gammon, 1990; Rose and Connolly, 1990; Swanson et al., 1989), although this has not been observed consistently (London et al., 1989; Schapira et al., 1991). Le Marchand et al. (1988) obtained evidence for a protective role of adolescent obesity against premenopausal breast cancer but found that adult weight and a positive energy balance in adult life were positively associated with postmenopausal risk of breast cancer. Ballard-Barbash et al. (1990a) in a 10-year follow-up study of 5599 women from the National Health and Nutrition Examination Survey also observed a positive correlation between breast cancer and adult body weight gain, this after correction for various possible confounders. There was no association between body mass at baseline examination and subsequent breast cancer. There is also evidence from other studies that increased central to peripheral body fat distribution predicts breast cancer risk independently of the degree of adiposity (Ballard-Barbash et al., 1990b).

Goodwin and Boyd (1990) reviewed the literature on body size in relation to breast cancer prognosis and concluded that increased body size had a modest inverse effect that was independent of other prognostic factors. It was most apparent in postmenopausal women and may be greater in those with uninvolved axillary lymph nodes.

Reducing the fat content of the diet tends to decrease serum cholesterol levels, and there has been some concern over evidence that low serum cholesterols are actually associated with increased cancer rates, particularly cancer of the colon (McMichael, 1991). However, the low serum cholesterols may sometimes be a consequence of undetected cancer (Kritchevsky et al., 1991; Winawer et al., 1990), and the fact that colon cancer is relatively rare in many parts of the world where most people have low serum cholesterol levels indicates that there is no consistent relationship. It thus appears improbable that reducing the fat content of the diet is likely to increase the risk of cancer. Boyd and McGuire (1990) have reviewed evidence for an association between plasma high density lipoprotein (HDL) levels and risk of breast cancer. This association can be observed in demographic patterns, and preliminary studies have also shown that high-risk women with mammary dysplasia tend to have higher levels of HDL cholesterol (Boyd et al., 1989).

In another study, mammary dysplasia was associated with evidence of increased lipid peroxidation, as indicated by higher urinary levels of malonaldehyde (Boyd and McGuire, 1990). The role of lipid peroxidation and of antioxidants in carcinogenesis is of considerable interest and warrants further investigation. Experimental studies in animals have shown that dietary polyunsaturated fats promote mammary cancer more effectively than saturated fats (Carroll and Khor, 1975; Ip, 1987), but epidemiological data have not provided clear evidence regarding the effects of different types of dietary fat (Carroll et al., 1986; Hursting et al., 1990).

Eid and Berry (1988) analyzed the fatty acid composition of subcutaneous adipose tissue as a measure of the type of fat ingested and reported that the quality of fat did not appear to be a major factor in the development of breast carcinoma. Gonzales et al. (1991) have recently reported that the inhibitory effect of dietary fish oil on mammary carcinogenesis is associated with increased levels of tumor lipid peroxidation products. This contrasts with results of the studies of Boyd and McGuire (1990) referred to above. Although the evidence regarding lipid peroxidation is somewhat inconsistent, it is important to try to identify markers that are associated with increased cancer risk and that might be modified by dietary means.

IV. Conclusions

There is substantial but not conclusive evidence that high-fat diets increase the risk of developing cancers of the breast, colon, prostate and possibly other sites, compared to low-fat diets. It is difficult to dissociate effects of dietary fat from those of energy intake in human studies because they are so closely correlated with one another. However, decreasing the fat content of the diet appears to be a more practical approach to reducing the risk of cancer than voluntary restriction of energy intake in the presence of an abundant food supply.

Intercountry comparisons suggest that a reduction of dietary fat to less than 30 percent of total calories is required to have a measurable effect on cancer incidence and mortality. This is compatible with results of cohort and case–control studies that have failed to show strong associations between breast cancer and dietary fat over ranges above 30 percent of calories but does not explain the better correlation between colon cancer and dietary fat in some of these studies. It is not clear from the intercountry data whether there is a linear correlation between cancer incidence and mortality and dietary fat at levels below 30 percent of energy. A level of about 20 percent of energy appears to be the minimum that can be readily achieved without drastic alteration of the typical North American diet.

Individuals differ in their susceptibility to cancer and in some cases groups with increased susceptibility can be recognized. For example, certain types of benign breast disease are associated with increased risk of breast cancer, and individuals with intestinal polyposis have an increased risk of developing colon cancer. However, any attempt to achieve a significant reduction in cancer incidence by decreasing the fat content of the diet would probably need to be applied to populations as a whole.

The main sources of fat in the diet are the visible fats and oils used as spreads, cooking fats and salad oils, and the fats in meats and dairy products. The visible fats and oils provide relatively little in terms of essential nutrients but add flavor and variety to the diet. The amounts used can be reduced, however, without basic changes in the diet as a whole. Meats and dairy products are both good sources of essential nutrients, and the approach in this case could be to use lower fat products, which are now becoming more widely available. Most other components of the diet contribute relatively little to the overall fat content.

Given the totality of data available, the most critical gap in knowledge at the present time is the lack of direct evidence that risk of cancer can be reduced by decreasing the fat content of the diet. It appears that this gap can only be filled by intervention trials, which are expensive and time consuming. By studying individuals with increased risk of cancer, it may be possible to obtain answers with lesser numbers of subjects, but such answers will not necessarily be applicable to whole populations. Thus, there seems little alternative to population-based intervention studies if one wishes to obtain a definitive answer.

V. Bibliography*

Adami, H.-O.; Adams, G.; Boyle, P.; Ewartz, M.; Lee, N.C.; Lund, E.; Miller, A.B.; Olsson, H.; Steel, M.; Trichopoulos, D.; Tulinius, H. 1990. Breast-cancer etiology. *Int. J. Cancer* 5(Suppl.):22–39.

Adlercreutz, H. 1990a. Diet, breast cancer, and sex hormone metabolism. *Ann. N. Y. Acad. Sci.* 595:281–290.

Adlercreutz, H. 1990b. Western diet and Western diseases: some hormonal and biochemical mechanisms and associations. *Scand. J. Clin. Invest.* 50(Suppl.):3–23.

Angres, G.; Beth, M. 1991. Effects of dietary constituents on carcinogenesis in different tumor models: an overview from 1975 to 1988. In: Alfin-Slater, R.B.; Kritchevsky, D.; eds. *Human nutrition: a comprehensive treatise.* Vol. 7. Cancer and nutrition. New York: Plenum Press. p. 337–485.

Armstrong, B.; Doll, R. 1975. Environmental factors and cancer incidence and mortality in different countries, with special reference to dietary practices. *Int. J. Cancer* 15:617–631.

Ballard-Barbash, R.; Schatzkin, A.; Taylor, P.R.; Kahle, L.L. 1990a. Association of change in body mass with breast cancer. *Cancer Res.* 50:2152–2155.

Ballard-Barbash, R.; Schatzkin, A.; Carter, C.L.; Kannel, W.B.; Kreger, B.E.; D'Agostino, R.B.; Splansky, G.L.; Anderson, K.M.; Helsel, W.E. 1990b. Body fat distribution and breast cancer in the Framingham Study. *J. Natl. Cancer Inst.* 82:286–290.

Benito, E.; Obrador, A.; Stiggelbout, A.; Bosch, F.X.; Mulet, M.; Munoz, N.; Kaldor, J. 1990. A population-based case–control study of colorectal cancer in Majorca. I. Dietary factors. *Int. J. Cancer* 45:69–76.

Birt, D.F. 1990. The influences of dietary fat on carcinogenesis: lessons from animal models. *Nutr. Rev.* 48:1–5.

Bosland, M.C. 1988. The etiopathogenesis of prostatic cancer with special reference to environmental factors. *Adv. Cancer Res.* 51:1–106.

Boyar, A.P.; Rose, D.P.; Loughridge, J.R.; Engel, A.; Palgi, A.; Laakso, K.; Kimo, D.; Wynder, E.L. 1988. Responses to a diet low in total fat in women with postmenopausal breast cancer. *Nutr. Cancer* 11:93–99.

Boyd, N.F.; Cousins, M.; Beaton, M.; Fishell, E.; Wright, B.; Fish, E.; Kriukov, V.; Lockwood, G.; Tritchler, D.; Hanna, W.; Page, D.L. 1988. Clinical trial of low-fat, high-carbohydrate diet in subjects with mammographic dysplasia: report of early outcomes. *J. Natl. Cancer Inst.* 80:1244–1248.

Boyd, N.F.; Cousins, M.; Lockwood, G.; Tritchler, D. 1990. The feasibility of testing experimentally the dietary fat–breast cancer hypothesis. *Br. J. Cancer* 62:878–881.

Boyd, N.F.; McGuire, V. 1990. Evidence of association between plasma high-density lipoprotein cholesterol and risk factors in breast cancer. *J. Natl. Cancer Inst.* 82:460–468.

Boyd, N.F.; McGuire, V.; Fishell, E.; Kuriov, V.; Lockwood, G.; Tritchler, D. 1989. Plasma lipids in premenopausal women with mammographic dysplasia. *Br. J. Cancer* 59:766–771.

Brisson, J.; Verreault, R.; Morrison, A.S.; Tennina, S.; Meyer, F. 1989. Diet, mammographic features of breast tissue, and breast cancer risk. *Am. J. Epidemiol.* 130:14–24.

Byar, D.P.; Freedman, L.S. 1989. Clinical trials in diet and cancer. *Prev. Med.* 18:203–219.

Carroll, K.K. 1975. Experimental evidence of dietary factors and hormone-dependent cancers. *Cancer Res.* 35:3374–3383.

Carroll, K.K. 1986a. Experimental studies on dietary fat and cancer in relation to epidemiological data. *Prog. Clin. Biol. Res.* 222:231–248.

*This bibliography contains all reference citations that are either in the text or the tables or both.

Carroll, K.K. 1986b. Diet and mammary carcinogenesis. In: Vahouny, G.V.; Kritchevsky, D.; eds. *Dietary fiber: basic and clinical aspects.* New York: Plenum Press. p. 433–439.

Carroll, K.K. 1991. Nutrition and cancer: fat. In: Rowland, I.R., ed. *Nutrition, toxicity, and cancer.* Boca Raton, FL: CRC Press. p. 439–453.

Carroll, K.K.; Braden, L.M.; Bell, J.A.; Kalamegham, R. 1986. Fat and cancer. *Cancer* 58(Suppl.):1818–1825.

Carroll, K.K.; Khor, H.T. 1975. Dietary fat in relation to tumorigenesis. *Prog. Biochem. Pharmacol.* 10:308–353.

Carroll, K.K.; Parenteau, H.I. 1991. A proposed mechanism for effects of diet on mammary cancer. *Nutr. Cancer* 16:79–83.

Chan, P.-C.; Cohen, L.A. 1975. Dietary fat and growth promotion of rat mammary tumors. *Cancer Res.* 35:3384–3386.

Cohen, L.A. 1986. Dietary fat and mammary cancer. In: Reddy, B.S.; Cohen, L.A.; eds. *Diet, nutrition and cancer: a critical evaluation.* Vol. I. Macronutrients and cancer. Boca Raton, FL: CRC Press. p. 77–100.

Cohen, L.A.; Choi, K.; Wang, C.-X. 1988. Influence of dietary fat, caloric restriction, and voluntary exercise on *N*-nitrosomethyl urea-induced mammary tumorigenesis in rats. *Cancer Res.* 48:4276–4283.

Colditz, G.A.; Willett, W.C. 1991. Epidemiologic approaches to the study of diet and cancer. In: Alfin-Slater, R.B.; Kritchevsky, D.; eds. *Human nutrition: a comprehensive treatise.* Vol. 7. Cancer and nutrition. New York: Plenum Press. p. 51–57.

De Waard, F.; Trichopoulos, D. 1988. A unifying concept of the aetiology of breast cancer. *Int. J. Cancer* 41:666–669.

Dougherty, R.W.; Fong, A.K.H.; Iacono, J.M. 1988. Nutrient content of the diet when fat is reduced. *Am. J. Clin. Nutr.* 48:970–979.

Eid, A.; Berry, E.M. 1988. The relationship between dietary fat, adipose tissue composition, and neoplasms of the breast. *Nutr. Cancer* 11:173–177.

Erickson, K.L.; Hubbard, N.E. 1990. Dietary fat and tumor metastasis. *Nutr. Rev.* 48:6–14.

Ewertz, M.; Gill, C. 1990. Dietary factors and breast-cancer risk in Denmark. *Int. J. Cancer* 46:779–784.

Falk, R.T.; Pickle, L.W.; Fontham, E.T.; Correa, P.; Fraumeni, J.F. 1988. Life-style risk factors for pancreatic cancer in Louisiana: a case–control study. *Am. J. Epidemiol.* 128:324–336.

Farrow, D.C.; Davis, S. 1990. Diet and the risk of pancreatic cancer in men. *Am. J. Epidemiol.* 132:423–431.

Food and Agriculture Organization of the United Nations. 1980. *Food balance sheets 1975–77. Average and per caput food supplies, 1961–65; Average, 1967 to 1977.* Available from: FAO, Rome.

Franceschi, S.; Bidoli, E.; Barón, A.E.; Barra, S.; Talamini, R.; Serraino, D.; La Vecchia, C. 1991. Nutrition and cancer of the oral cavity and pharynx in north-east Italy. *Int. J. Cancer* 47:20–25.

Franceschi, S.; Serraino, D.; Carbone, A.; Talamini, R.; La Vecchia, C. 1989. Dietary factors and non-Hodgkin's lymphoma: a case–control study in the northeastern part of Italy. *Nutr. Cancer* 12:333–341.

Freedman, L.S.; Clifford, C.; Messina, M. 1990. Analysis of dietary fat, calories, body weight, and the development of mammary tumors in rats and mice: a review. *Cancer Res.* 50:5710–5719.

Freudenheim, J.L.; Graham, S.; Marshall, J.R.; Haughey, B.P.; Wilkinson G. 1990. A case–control study of diet and rectal cancer in western New York. *Am. J. Epidemiol.* 131:612–624.

Freudenheim, J.L.; Marshall, J.R. 1988. The problem of profound mismeasurement and the power of epidemiological studies of diet and cancer. *Nutr. Cancer* 11:243–250.

Gerber, M.; Richardson, S.; Cavallo, F.; Marubini, E.; de Paulet, P.C.; de Paulet, A.C.; Pujol, H. 1990. The role of diet history and biologic assays in the study of diet and breast cancer. *Tumori* 76:321–330.

Gerber, M.; Richardson, S.; De Paulet, P.C.; Pujol, H.; De Paulet, A.C. 1989. Relationship between vitamin E and polyunsaturated fatty acids in breast cancer: nutritional and metabolic aspects. *Cancer* 64:2347–2353.

Gerhardsson de Verdier, M.; Hagman, U.; Steineck, G.; Rieger, A.; Norell, S.E. 1990. Diet, body mass and colorectal cancer: a case–referent study in Stockholm. *Int. J. Cancer* 46:832–838.

Ghadirian, P.; Simard, A.; Baillargeon, J.; Maisonneuve, P.; Boyle, P. 1991. Nutritional factors and pancreatic cancer in the francophone community in Montreal, Canada. *Int. J. Cancer* 47:1–6.

Gonzales, M.J.; Schemmel, R.A.; Gray, J.I.; Dugan, J.; Sheffield, L.G.; Welsch, C.W. 1991. Effect of dietary fat on growth of MCF-7 and MDA-MB231 human breast carcinomas in athymic nude mice; relationship between carcinoma growth and lipid peroxidation product levels. *Carcinogenesis* 12:1231–1235.

Goodman, M.T.; Kolonel, L.N.; Yoshizawa, C.N.; Hankin, J.H. 1988. The effect of dietary cholesterol and fat on the risk of lung cancer in Hawaii. *Am. J. Epidemiol.* 128:1241–1255.

Goodwin, P.J.; Boyd, N.F. 1987. Critical appraisal of the evidence that dietary fat intake is related to breast cancer risk in humans. *J. Natl. Cancer Inst.* 79:473–485.

Goodwin, P.J.; Boyd, N.F. 1990. Body size and breast cancer prognosis: a critical review of the evidence. *Breast Cancer Res. Treat.* 16:205–214.

Graham, S.; Marshall, J.; Haughey, B.; Mittelman, A.; Swanson, M.; Zielezny, M.; Byers, T.; Wilkinson, G.; West, D. 1988. Dietary epidemiology of cancer of the colon in western New York. *Am. J. Epidemiol.* 128:490–503.

Greenwald, P. 1989. Strengths and limitations of methodologic approaches to the study of diet and cancer: summary and future perspectives with emphasis on dietary fat and breast cancer. *Prev. Med.* 18:163–166.

Hebert, J.R.; Kabat, C.C. 1991. Distribution of smoking and its association with lung cancer: implications for studies in the association of fat with cancer. *J. Natl. Cancer Inst.* 83:872–874.

Hebert, J.R.; Miller, D.R. 1988. Methodologic considerations for investigating the diet–cancer link. *Am. J. Clin. Nutr.* 47:1068–1077.

Hegsted, D.M. 1989. Errors of measurement. *Nutr. Cancer* 12:105–107.

Henderson, M.M.; Kushi, L.H.; Thompson, D.J.; Gorbach, S.L.; Clifford, C.K.; Insull, W.; Moskowitz, M.; Thompson, R.S. 1990. Feasibility of a randomized trial of a low-fat diet for the prevention of breast cancer: dietary compliance in the Women's Health Trial Vanguard Study. *Prev. Med.* 19:115–133.

Henderson, M.M.; White, E.; Thompson, R.S. 1991. Cancer incidence in Seattle Women's Health Trial participants by group and time since randomization. *J. Natl. Cancer Inst.* 83:1260–1261.

Higginson, J.; Sheridan, M.J. 1991. Nutrition and human cancer. In: Alfin-Slater, R.B.; Kritchevsky, D.; eds. *Human nutrition: a comprehensive treatise*. Vol. 7. Cancer and nutrition. New York: Plenum Press. p. 1–50.

Holm, L.-E. 1990. Nutritional intervention studies in cancer prevention. *Med. Oncol. Tumor Pharmacotherap.* 7:209–215.

Holm, L.-E.; Callmer, E.; Hjalmar, M.-L.; Lidbrink, E.; Nilsson, B.; Skoog, L. 1989. Dietary habits and prognostic factors in breast cancer. *J. Natl. Cancer Inst.* 81:1218–1223.

Holm, L.-E.; Nordevang, E.; Ikkala, E.; Hallstrom, L.; Callmer, E. 1990. Dietary intervention as adjuvant therapy in breast cancer patients—a feasibility study. *Breast Cancer Res. Treat.* 16:103–109.

Howe, G.R.; Friedenreich, C.M.; Jain, M.; Miller, A.B. 1991. A cohort study of fat intake and risk of breast cancer. *J. Natl. Cancer Inst.* 83:336–340.

Howe, G.R.; Hirohata, T.; Hislop, T.G.; Iscovich, J.M.; Yuan, J.-M.; Katsouyanni, K.; Lubin, F.; Marubini, E.; Modan, B.; Rohan, T.; Toniolo, P.; Shunzhang, Y. 1990a. Dietary factors and risk of breast cancer: combined analysis of 12 case–control studies. *J. Natl. Cancer Inst.* 82:561–569.

Howe, G.R.; Jain, M.; Miller, A.B. 1990b. Dietary factors and risk of pancreatic cancer: results of a Canadian population-based case–control study. *Int. J. Cancer* 45:604–608.

Hsing, A.W.; McLaughlin, J.K.; Schuman, L.M.; Bjelke, E.; Gridley, G.; Wacholder, S. 1990. Diet, tobacco use, and fatal prostate cancer: results from the Lutheran Brotherhood Cohort Study. *Cancer Res.* 50:6836–6840.

Hulka, B.S. 1989. Dietary fat and breast cancer: case–control and cohort studies. *Prev. Med.* 18:180–193.

Hursting, S.D.; Thornquist, M.; Henderson, M.M. 1990. Types of dietary fat and the incidence of cancer at five sites. *Prev. Med.* 19:242–253.

Ip, C. 1987. Fat and essential fatty acid in mammary carcinogenesis. *Am. J. Clin. Nutr.* 45:218–224.

Iscovich, J.M.; Iscovich, R.B.; Howe, G.; Shiboski, S.; Kaldor, J.M. 1989. A case–control study of diet and breast cancer in Argentina. *Int. J. Cancer* 44:770–776.

Jain, M.; Burch, J.D.; Howe, G.R.; Risch, H.A.; Miller, A.B. 1990. Dietary factors and risk of lung cancer: results from a case–control study, Toronto, 1981–1985. *Int. J. Cancer* 45:287–293.

Jain, M.; Howe, G.R.; Harrison, L.; Miller, A.B. 1989. A study of repeatability of dietary data over a seven-year period. *Am. J. Epidemiol.* 129:422–429.

Jones, D.Y.; Schatzkin, A.; Green, S.B.; Block, G.; Brinton, L.A.; Ziegler, R.G.; Hoover, R.; Taylor, P.R. 1987. Dietary fat and breast cancer in the National Health and Nutrition Examination Survey I Epidemiologic Follow-up Study. *J. Natl. Cancer Inst.* 79:465–471.

Katsouyanni, K.; Willett, W.; Trichopoulos, D.; Boyle, P.; Trichopoulou, A.; Vasilaros, S.; Papadiamantis, J.; MacMahon, B. 1988. Risk of breast cancer among Greek women in relation to nutrient intake. *Cancer* 61:181–185.

Kelsey, J.L.; Gammon, M.D. 1990. Epidemiology of breast cancer. *Epidemiol. Rev.* 12:228–240.

Key, T.J.A.; Pike, M.C. 1988. The role of estrogens and progestins in the epidemiology and prevention of breast cancer. *Eur. J. Cancer Clin. Oncol.* 24:29–43.

Knekt, P.; Albanes, D.; Seppänen, R.; Aromaa, A.; Järvinem, R.; Hyvonen, L.; Teppo, L.; Pukkala, E. 1990. Dietary fat and risk of breast cancer. *Am. J. Clin. Nutr.* 52:903–908.

Kolonel, L.N.; Yoshizawa, C.N.; Hankin, J.H. 1988. Diet and prostatic cancer: a case–control study in Hawaii. *Am. J. Epidemiol.* 127:999–1012.

Kritchevsky, D. 1990. Nutrition and breast cancer. *Cancer* 66:1321–1325.

Kritchevsky, D.; Klurfeld, D.M. 1991. Fat and cancer. In: Alfin-Slater, R.B.; Kritchevsky, D.; eds. *Human nutrition: a comprehensive treatise.* Vol. 7. Cancer and nutrition. New York: Plenum Press. p. 127–140.

Kritchevsky, S.B.; Wilcosky, T.C.; Morris, D.L.; Truong, K.N.; Tyroler, H.A. 1991. Changes in plasma lipid and lipoprotein cholesterol and weight prior to the diagnosis of cancer. *Cancer Res.* 51:3198–3203.

Kune, S.; Kune, G.A.; Watson, L.F. 1987. Case–control study of dietary etiological factors: the Melbourne colorectal cancer study. *Nutr. Cancer* 9:21–42.

Kurihara, M., Aoki, K., Tominaga, S. 1984. *Cancer mortality statistics of the World.* Nayoga, Japan: University of Nagoya Press.

Lands, W.E.M.; Hamazaki, T.; Yanasaki, K.; Okuyama, H.; Sakai, K.; Goto, Y.; Hubbard, V.S. 1990. Changing dietary patterns. *Am. J. Clin. Nutr.* 51:991–993.

La Vecchia, C.; Negri, E.; D'Avanzo, B.; Ferraroni, M.; Gramenzi, A.; Savoldelli, R.; Boyle, P.; Franceschi, S. 1990. Medical history, diet, and pancreatic cancer. *Oncology* 47:463–466.

La Vecchia, C.; Negri, E.; Decarli, A.; D'Avanzo, B.; Francechi, S. 1989. Dietary factors in the risk of bladder cancer. *Nutr. Cancer* 12:93–101.

La Vecchia, C.; Negri, E.; Decarli, A.; D'Avanzo, B.; Gallotti, L.; Gentile, A.; Franceschi, S. 1988. A case–control study of diet and colo-rectal cancer in northern Italy. *Int. J. Cancer* 41:492–498.

Lee, H.P.; Gourley, L.; Duffy, S.W.; Estève, J.; Lee, J.; Day, N.E. 1991. Dietary effects on breast-cancer risk in Singapore. *Lancet* 337:1197–1200.

Le Marchand, L.; Kolonel, L.N.; Earle, M.E.; Mi, M.-P. 1988. Body size at different periods of life and breast cancer risk. *Am. J. Epidemiol.* 128:137–152.

Liff, J.M.; Sung, J.F.C.; Chow, W.-H.; Greenberg, R.S.; Flanders, W.D. 1991. Does increased detection account for the rising incidence of breast cancer? *Am. J. Publ. Health* 81:462–465.

Lipkin, M. 1991. Application of intermediate biomarkers to studies of cancer prevention in the gastrointestinal tract: introduction and perspective. *Am. J. Clin. Nutr.* 54:1885–1925.

Lipkin, M.; Newmark, H.L.; Kelloff, G.; editors. 1991. *Calcium, vitamin D, and prevention of colon cancer.* Boca Raton, FL: CRC Press.

London, S.J.; Colditz, G.A.; Stampfer, M.J.; Willett, W.C.; Rosner, B.; Speizer, F.E. 1989. Prospective study of relative weight, height, and risk of breast cancer. *J. Am. Med. Assoc.* 262:2853–2858.

McMichael, A.J. 1991. Serum cholesterol and human cancer. In: Alfin-Slater, R.B.; Kritchevsky, D.; eds. *Human nutrition: a comprehensive treatise.* Vol. 7. Cancer and nutrition. New York: Plenum Press. p. 141–158.

McMichael, A.J.; Giles, G.C. 1988. Cancer in migrants to Australia: extending the descriptive epidemiological data. *Cancer Res.* 48:751–756.

Mettlin, C.; Schoenfeld, E.R.; Natarajan, N. 1990. Patterns of milk consumption and risk of cancer. *Nutr. Cancer* 13:89–99.

Mettlin, C.; Selenskas, S.; Natarajan, N.; Huben, R. 1989. Beta-carotene and animal fats and their relationship to prostate cancer risk: a case–control study. *Cancer* 64:605–612.

Mills, P.K.; Annegers, J.F.; Phillips, R.L. 1988. Animal product consumption and subsequent fatal breast cancer risk among Seventh-Day Adventists. *Am. J. Epidemiol.* 127:440–453.

Mills, P.K.; Beeson, W.L.; Abbey, D.E.; Fraser, G.E.; Phillips, R.L. 1988. Dietary habits and past medical history as related to fatal pancreas cancer among adventists. *Cancer* 61:2578–2585.

Mills, P.K.; Beeson, W.L.; Phillips, R.L.; Fraser, G.E. 1989a. Dietary habits and breast cancer incidence among Seventh-Day Adventists. *Cancer* 64:582–590.

Mills, P.K.; Beeson, W.L.; Phillips, R.L.; Fraser, G.E. 1989b. Cohort study of diet, lifestyle, and prostatic cancer in Adventist men. *Cancer* 64:598–604.

National Research Council, Committee on Diet and Health. 1989. *Diet and health: implications for reducing chronic disease risk.* Washington, DC: National Academy Press. p. 14.

National Research Council, Committee on Diet, Nutrition and Cancer. 1982. *Diet, nutrition and cancer.* Washington, DC: National Academy Press.

Neoptolemos, J.P.; Clayton, H.; Heagerty, A.M.; Nicholson, M.J.; Johnson, B.; Mason, J.; Manson, K.; James, R.F.; Bell, P.R. 1988. Dietary fat in relation to fatty acid composition of red cells and adipose tissue in colorectal cancer. *Br. J. Cancer* 58:575–579.

Newman, M.E. 1990. New cancer statistics show losses, gains. *J. Natl. Cancer Inst.* 82:1238–1239.

Newmark, H.L.; Wargovich, M.J.; Bruce, W.R. 1984. Colon cancer and dietary fat, phosphate, and calcium: a hypothesis. *J. Natl. Cancer Inst.* 72:1323–1325.

Nordevang, E.; Ikkala, E.; Callmer, E.; Hallstrom, L.; Holm, L.-E. 1990. Dietary intervention in breast cancer patients: effects on dietary habits and nutrient intake. *Eur. J. Clin. Nutr.* 44:681–687.

Ohno, Y.; Yoshida, O.; Oishi, K.; Okada, K.; Yamabe, H.; Schroeder, F.H. 1988. Dietary β-carotene and cancer of the prostate: a case–control study in Kyoto, Japan. *Cancer Res.* 48:1331–1336.

Oishi, Y.; Okada, K.; Yoshida, O.; Yamabe, H.; Ohno, Y.; Hayes, R.B.; Schroeder, F.H. 1988. A case–control study of prostatic cancer with reference to dietary habits. *Prostate* 12:179–190.

Olsen, G.W.; Mandel, J.S.; Gibson, R.W.; Wattenberg, L.W.; Schuman, L.M. 1989. A case–control study of pancreatic cancer and cigarettes, alcohol, coffee and diet. *Am. J. Public Health* 79:1016–1019.

Pariza, M.W. 1987. Fat, calories, and mammary carcinogenesis: net energy effects. *Am. J. Clin. Nutr.* 45:261–263.

Pariza, M.W. 1988. Dietary fat and cancer risk: evidence and research needs. *Cancer Res.* 8:167–183.

Phillips, R.L.; Garfinkel, L.; Kuzma, J.W.; Beeson, W.L.; Lotz, T.; Brin, B. 1980. Mortality among California Seventh-Day Adventists for selected cancer sites. *J. Natl. Cancer Inst.* 65:1097–1107.

Pike, M.C. 1990. Reducing cancer risk in women through lifstyle-mediated changes in hormone levels. *Cancer Detect. Prevent.* 14:595–607.

Potosky, A.L.; Kessler, L.; Gridley, G.; Brown, C.C.; Horm, J.W. 1990. Rise in prostatic cancer incidence associated with increased use of transurethral resection. *J. Natl. Cancer Inst.* 82:1624–1628.

Prentice, R.L.; Kakar, F.; Hursting, S.; Sheppard, L.; Klein, R.; Kushi, H. 1988. Aspects of the rationale for the Women's Health Trial. *J. Natl. Cancer Inst.* 80:802–814.

Prentice, R.L.; Sheppard, L. 1989. Validity of international, time-trend, and migrant studies of dietary factors and disease risk. *Prev. Med.* 18:167–179.

Pryor, M.; Slattery, M.L.; Robison, L.M.; Egger, M. 1989. Adolescent diet and breast cancer in Utah. *Cancer Res.* 49:2161–2167.

Reddy, B.S. 1986. Diet and colon cancer: evidence from human and animal model studies. In: Reddy, B.S.; Cohen, L.A.; eds. *Diet, nutrition and cancer: a critical evaluation.* Vol. 1. Macronutrients and cancer. Boca Raton, FL: CRC Press. p. 47–65.

Richardson, S.; Gerber, M.; Cenée, S. 1991. The role of fat, animal protein and some vitamin consumption in breast cancer: a case–control study in southern France. *Int. J. Cancer* 48:1–9.

Rogers, A.E.; Longnecker, M.P. 1988. Biology of disease—dietary and nutritional influences on cancer: a review of epidemiologic and experimental data. *Lab. Invest.* 59:729–759.

Rohan, T.E.; Cook, M.G.; Potter, J.D.; McMichael, A.J. 1990. A case–control study of diet and benign proliferative epithelial disorders of the breast. *Cancer Res.* 50:3176–3181.

Rose, D.P.; Connolly, J.M. 1990. Dietary prevention of breast cancer. *Med. Oncol. Tumor Pharmacother.* 7:121–130.

Rose, D.P.; Connolly, J.M. 1991. Dietary fat, fatty acids and prostate cancer. *Lipids* (In press).

Ross, R.K.; Shimizu, H.; Paganini-Hill, A.; Honda, G.; Henderson, B.E. 1987. Case–control studies of prostate cancer in blacks and whites in southern California. *J. Natl. Cancer Inst.* 78:869–874.

Ruggeri, B. 1991. The effects of caloric restriction on neoplasia and age-related degenerative processes. In: Alfin-Slater, R.B.; Kritchevsky, D.; eds. *Human nutrition: a comprehensive treatise.* Vol. 7. Cancer and nutrition. New York: Plenum Press. p. 187–210.

Russo, J.; Gusterson, B.A.; Rogers, A.E.; Russo, I.H.; Wellings, S.R.; Van Zwieten, M.J. 1990. Biology of disease: comparative study of human and rat mammary tumorigenesis. *Lab. Invest.* 62:244–278.

Saracci, R. 1990. The diet and cancer hypothesis: current trends. *Med. Oncol. Tumor Pharmacother.* 7:99–107.

Schapira, D.V.; Kumar, N.B.; Lyman, G.H.; Cox, C.E. 1991. Obesity and body fat distribution and breast cancer prognosis. *Cancer* 67:523–528.

Schatzkin, A.; Greenwald, P.; Byar, D.P.; Clifford, C.K. 1989. The dietary fat–breast cancer hypothesis is alive. *J. Am. Med. Assoc.* 261:3284–3287.

Severson, R.K.; Nomura, A.M.Y.; Grove, J.S.; Stemmerman, G.N. 1989. A prospective study of demographics, diet, and prostate cancer among men of Japanese ancestry in Hawaii. *Cancer Res.* 49:1857–1860.

Shu, O.X.; Gao, Y.T.; Yuan, J.M.; Ziegler, R.G.; Brinton, L.A. 1989. Dietary factors and epithelial ovarian cancer. *Br. J. Cancer* 59:92–96.

Simard, A.; Vobecky, J.; Vobecky, J.S. 1990. Nutrition and lifestyle factors in fibrocystic disease and cancer of the breast. *Cancer Detect. Prev.* 14:567–572.

Simopoulos, A.P. 1990. Energy imbalance and cancer of the breast, colon, and prostate. *Med. Oncol. Tumor Pharmacother.* 7:109–120.

Slattery, M.L.; Schumacher, M.C.; Smith, K.R.; West, D.W.; Abd-Elghany, N. 1988. Physical activity, diet, and risk of colon cancer in Utah. *Am. J. Epidemiol.* 128:989–999.

Slattery, M.L.; Schumacher, M.C.; West, D.W.; Robison, L.M.; French, T.K. 1990. Food-consumption trends between adolescent and adult years and subsequent risk of prostate cancer. *Am. J. Clin. Nutr.* 52:752–757.

Slattery, M.L.; Schuman, K.L.; West, D.W.; French, T.K.; Robison, L.M. 1989. Nutrient intake and ovarian cancer. *Am. J. Epidemiol.* 130:497–502.

Smigel, K. 1990. Low-fat diet trial set to take off. *J. Natl. Cancer Inst.* 82:1736–1737.

Steineck, G.; Hagman, U.; Gerhardsson de Verdier, M.; Norell, S.E. 1990. Vitamin A supplements, fried foods, fat and urothelial cancer: a case–referrant study in Stockholm in 1985–87. *Int. J. Cancer* 45:1006–1011.

Steineck, G.; Norell, S.E.; Feyething, M. 1988. Diet, tobacco, and urothelial cancer: a 14-year follow-up of 16,477 subjects. *Acta Oncol.* 77:323–327.

Swanson, C.A.; Brinton, L.A.; Taylor, P.R.; Licitra, L.M.; Ziegler, R.G.; Schairer, C. 1989. Body size and breast cancer risk assessed in women participating in the breast cancer detection demonstration project. *Am. J. Epidemiol.* 130:1133–1141.

Toniolo, P.; Riboli, E.; Protta, F.; Charrel, M.; Cappa, A.P. 1989. Calorie-providing nutrients and risk of breast cancer. *J. Natl. Cancer Inst.* 81:278–286.

Tuyns, A.J.; Kaaks, R.; Haelterman, M. 1988. Colorectal cancer and the consumption of foods: a case–control study in Belgium. *Nutr. Cancer* 11:189–204.

U.S. Department of Health and Human Services. 1988. *The Surgeon General's report on nutrition and health.* DHHS (PHS) Publication No. 88-50210. p. 194. Available from: U.S. Government Printing Office, Washington, DC.

Van't Veer, P.; Kok, F.J.; Brants, H.A.; Ockhuizen, T.; Sturmans, F.; Hermus, R.J. 1990. Dietary fat and the risk of breast cancer. *Int. J. Epidemiol.* 19:12–18.

Van't Veer, P.; van Leer, E.M.; Rietdij, A.; Kok, F.J.; Schouten, E.G.; Hermus, R.J.; Sturmans, F. 1991. Combination of dietary factors in relation to breast-cancer occurrence. *Int. J. Cancer* 47:649–653.

Verreault, R.; Brisson, J.; Deschenes, L.; Naud, F.; Meyer, F.; Belanger, L. 1988. Dietary fat in relation to prognostic indicators in breast cancer. *J. Natl. Cancer Inst.* 80:819–825.

Vogel, V.G.; McPherson, R.S. 1989. Dietary epidemiology of colon cancer. *Hematol. Oncol. Clin. North Am.* 3:35–63.

Weindruch, R.; Albanes, D.; Kritchevsky, D. 1991. The role of calories and caloric restriction in carcinogenesis. *Hematol. Pathol. Clin. North. Am.* 5:79–89.

Weisburger, J.H.; Wynder, E.L. 1991. Dietary fat intake and cancer. *Hematol. Oncol. Clin. North Am.* 5:7–23.

Welsch, C.W. 1986. Interrelationship between dietary fat and endocrine processes in mammary gland tumorigenisis. *Prog. Clin. Biol. Res.* 222:623–654.

Welsch, C.W. 1987. Enhancement of mammary tumorigenesis by dietary fat: review of potential mechanisms. *Am. J. Clin. Nutr.* 45:192–202.

Welsch, C.W.; House, J.L.; Herr, B.L.; Eliasberg, S.J.; Welsch, M.A. 1990. Enhancement of mammary carcinogenesis by high levels of dietary fat: a phenomenon dependent on ad libitum feeding. *J. Natl. Cancer Inst.* 82:1615–1620.

West, D.W.; Slattery, M.L.; Robison, L.M.; French, T.K.; Mahoney, A.W. 1991. Adult dietary intake and prostate cancer rate in Utah: a case–control study with special emphasis on aggressive tumors. *Cancer Causes Control* 2:85–94.

West, D.W.; Slattery, M.L.; Robison, L.M.; Schuman, K.L.; Ford, M.H.; Mahoney, A.W.; Lyon, J.L.; Sorensen, A.W. 1989. Dietary intake and colon cancer: sex- and anatomic site-specific associations. *Am. J. Epidemiol.* 130:883–894.

Whelan, L.; Parkin, D.M.; Masuyer, E., editors. 1990. *Patterns of cancer in five continents.* Lyon, France: International Agency for Research in Cancer.

Whittemore, A.S.; Wu-Williams, A.H.; Lee, M.; Shu, Z.; Gallagher, R.P.; Deng-ao, J.; Lun, Z.; Xianghui, W.; Kun, C.; Jung, D.; Teh, C.-Z.; Chengde, L.; Yao, X.J.; Paffenbarger, R.S., Jr.; Henderson, B.E. 1990. Diet, physical activity, and colorectal cancer among Chinese in North America and China. *J. Natl. Cancer Inst.* 82:915–926.

Willett, W. 1989. The search for the causes of breast and colon cancer. *Nature* 338:389–393.

Willett, W.C. 1990a. Epidemiologic studies of diet and cancer. *Med. Oncol. Tumor Pharmacother.* 7:93–97.

Willett, W.C. 1990b. Total energy intake and nutrient composition: dietary recommendations for epidemiologists. *Int. J. Cancer* 46:770–771.

Willett, W.C.; Stampfer, M.J.; Colditz, G.A.; Rosner, B.A.; Hennekens, C.H.; Speizer, F.E. 1987. Dietary fat and the risk of breast cancer. *N. Engl. J. Med.* 316:22–28.

Willett, W.C.; Stampfer, M.J.; Colditz, G.A.; Rosner, B.A.; Speizer, F.E. 1990. Relation of meat, fat, and fiber intake to the risk of colon cancer in a prospective study among women. *N. Engl. J. Med.* 323:1664–1672.

Winawer, S.J.; Flehinger, B.J.; Buchalter, J.; Herbert, E.; Shike, M. 1990. Declining serum cholesterol levels prior to diagnosis of colon cancer: a time-trend, case–control study. *J. Am. Med. Assoc.* 263:2083–2085.

World Health Organization. 1990. Causes of death. *World health statistics annual.* Geneva: World Health Organization.

Wynder, E.L.; Morabia, A.; Rose, D.P.; Cohen, L.A. 1990. Clinical trials of dietary intervention to enhance cancer survival. *Prog. Clin. Biol. Res.* 346:217–229.

Yu, S.-Z.; Lu, R.-F.; Xu, D.D.; Howe, G.B. 1990. A case–control study of dietary and nondietary risk factors for breast cancer in Shanghai. *Cancer Res.* 50:5017–5021.

Zaridze, D.; Lifanova, Y.; Maximovitch, D.; Day, N.E.; Duffy, S.W. 1991. Diet, alcohol consumption and reproductive factors in a case–control study of breast cancer in Moscow. *Int. J. Cancer* 48:493–501.

Zatonski, W.; Przewozniak, K.; Howe, G.R.; Maisonneuve, P.; Walker, A.M.; Boyle, P. 1991. Nutritional factors and pancreatic cancer: a case–control study from south-west Poland. *Int. J. Cancer* 48:390–394.

Zhao, L.P.; Kushi, L.H.; Klein, R.D.; Prentice, R.L. 1991. Quantitative review of studies of dietary fat and rat colon carcinoma. *Nutr. Cancer* 15:169–177.

Appendix

Criteria for Inclusion of Articles in Appendix Tables

Articles in peer-reviewed journals related to the topic of this review were selected primarily on the basis of date and content. In general, papers appearing in 1987 or thereafter were included, provided that they presented original data from studies in humans. Certain items tabulated for the sake of completeness may not have been cited in the body of the text if their weight or relevance did not add significantly to development of the author's argument. Reviews have not been listed except as they included new data or useful meta-analyses.

APPENDIX TABLE   Lipids and Cancer (By Site)

		I. Breast Cancer	
Study	Type/Location	Subject Number and Description	Methods
Boyd et al., 1988	Intervention Toronto, Canada	295 ♀ ≥ 30 yr with dysplasia in ≥50% of breast volume diagnosed within 3 mo of study. 227 out of 295 subjects (77%) completed the full year. 32% of the intervention group dropped out before 1 yr.	Subjects were randomly assigned to either: "Control diet" containing ≈36% calories as fat or "Intervention diet" containing ≈15% calories from fat. Diets were balanced isocalorically with the addition of carbohydrate to the intervention diet. Compliance measured by random diet records and 24-hr recalls throughout the 1 yr trial. Dependent variables were differences between baseline and end-of-trial mammographies and histology when available.
Boyd et al., 1989	Cross-sectional Toronto, Canada	2 groups of premenopausal ♀: I. No dysplasia (ND): (n = 16) <25% of the breast with mammographic evidence of dysplasia. II. Dysplasia (D): (n = 30) >75% of the breast having mammographic evidence of dysplasia. 50% of eligible subjects participated.	Subjects recruited by mail then by phone. Interviewed at home. Measurements included: demographics, 7-d diet recall and a 4-d (including 1 weekend d) diet diary kept by subjects. Subjects trained in portion size estimation and supplied with digital scales, measuring cups, and spoons. Fasted blood samples were collected during the follicular and luteal phases of menstruation. Luteal blood was used for assessment of lipid chemistry (triglycerides, total cholesterol, HDL, LDL).
Brisson et al., 1989	Case–control Quebec, Canada	290 cases of newly diagnosed *breast cancer*. 645 age-matched control ♀ without BC enrolled in a longitudinal BC-screening program/study.	All subjects were interviewed about demographics, menstrual history, height and weight, smoking history, physical activity, drug use history, and diet history. 114-item food-frequency questionnaire. Reference period: the previous yr. Food models were used to estimate portions sizes. All subjects had mammograms; for cases the unaffected breast was evaluated, for controls random selection. All evaluations were done blindly.
Eid and Berry, 1988	Cross-sectional Jerusalem, Israel	85 consecutive patients undergoing needle biopsies were divided (post-biopsy) into 3 groups: Carcinoma (C; n = 37), Fibroadenoma (F; n = 27) Other types (O; n = 21)	Adipose tissue samples were collected from breast and buttocks of all subjects and used as a surrogate measure of the quality of habitual dietary fat intake.
Ewertz and Gill, 1990	Case–control Denmark	1474 cases of *breast cancer* diagnosed over period 1983–1984. 1322 age-stratified randomly-selected controls.	Cases mailed questionnaire 1 yr after diagnosis. Controls matched to cases for date of diagnosis. 21-item food-frequency questionnaire designed to "include 80% of the consumption of fat and β-carotene in the study population." Food models were used to estimate portion sizes. Subjects also asked about supplement use, caffeinated beverages, sugar, and artificial sweeteners.

I. Breast Cancer

Results	Comments
The mean fat intake of the intervention group was reduced from 37% at baseline to 23% by 4 mo and continued at that level throughout the trial. Carbohydrate intake increased from 43% to 56% of calories and remained there for the duration of the trial. At 1 yr there were 172 sets of mammographs for comparison. 45% of the control group had reduction of dysplasia, 15% had evidence of increase. 29% of intervention group showed improvement with 10% showing a deterioration. There were no significant differences between groups.	Potential self-selection bias: subjects were examined under their volition, all subjects were highly educated, all subjects had been diagnosed with mammary dysplasia. No real control group. Length of trial may have been too short to demonstrate a discernible effect. No indication of diet during exposure period prior to diagnosis. Diets were not isocaloric as intervention did not completely compensate for calories lost from fat reduction.
Groups differed in family history (D > ND for family history of breast cancer) and anthropometrics (D < ND for weight and skinfold thickness). Based on 4-d diaries, the only difference was alcohol consumption (D > ND). There were significant differences in blood lipids (triglycerides, HDL and LDL) between groups (D < ND for Trig. and LDL, D > ND for HDL). There were significant independent associations between mammographic patterns, family history and HDL cholesterol. Triglyceride levels were independently associated with family history.	Small sample from limited geographical area. High refusal rates (50% of eligible subjects). Potential self-selection bias as all subjects were participating in a preventative screening program. No socio-economic (SES) data presented.
In controls, ↑ in energy-adjusted saturated fat intake was associated with ↑ high-risk mammographic features; however, there was no effect from energy-adjusted dietary polyunsaturated fat or cholesterol. ↑ carotenoid and fiber intakes were associated with a ↓ in high risk features on mammograms. Retinol had no effect on mammogram features.	No comparisons in terms of risk of BC related to intake. Analysis limited to associations between mammogram features and diet. Supplement use not reported. Dependent variables, mammogram features were derived from subjective evaluation of the observer. The relationship of mammographic features to dietary components and breast cancer risk factors was assessed in controls only. The dietary design of this study was cross-sectional not case–control. Potential for self-selection bias as all controls were from a pool of volunteers involved in an ongoing BC screening program.
No differences except for stearic and linolenic acids which were lower in group F than either of the other 2 groups. F was significantly thinner and younger than either of the other groups.	No diet data, no matching for any variables, no controls.
There was a significant trend for increased risk with increased intake of total fat. There were no changes in these findings after adjustment for socioeconomic status (SES), age at first menarche, natural menopause, parity, and age at first birth. There was no association between β-carotene intake and risk of breast cancer. Nonsignificant elevation in risk with the use of all common vitamin supplements. More cases (72%) than controls (67%) used supplements.	Reference period not clearly defined. The rationale stated for delay of a yr after diagnosis was "to avoid asking questions on diet during a period where adjuvant chemotherapy was administered ..." This implies that the diet data referred to intake patterns after diagnosis which would not reflect risk, rather response to the disease.

(continued)

APPENDIX TABLE   (*continued*)

Study	Type/Location	Subject Number and Description	Methods
Gerber et al., 1990	Case–control Milan, Italy Montpelier, France	317 cases of primary nonmetastasizing breast cancer (214 Italy, 103 France). 318 hospital-based controls (215 Italy, 103 France).	Fasting blood drawn the d after admission and frozen at −18°C analyzed for levels of retinol, β-carotene, vitamin E, vitamin C, and riboflavin. Subjects interviewed about demographics and medical history. Food-frequency questionnaire was used to assess dietary habits. The Italians were asked about all foods eaten; whereas the French were only asked about key lipid and vitamin-rich foods. Reference period was the previous yr unless diet had changed in which case subjects were asked about the previous 12 mo. Subjects estimated portion sizes.
Gerber et al., 1989	Case–control France	120 cases of *breast cancer*. 109 controls hospitalized for nonmalignant and non-CVD-related neurological disorders. Recruitment over a 4-yr period (1982–1986).	Subjects given a structured interview containing: SES data, menopausal status, reproductive and health history, and 55-item food-frequency questionnaire. Subjects were asked about duration of nutritional habits and if there had been a change within previous yr to refer to diet prior to changes. Subjects' estimation of portion sizes was based on specified units of measure (e.g., weight, spoon). Fasting blood samples were drawn the day after admission to hospital and stored at −18°C for unknown duration. Lipid measures included triglycerides (TG), total cholesterol (TC), monounsaturated (MUFA), poly-unsaturated (PUFA), and saturated (SFA) fatty acids. Vitamin E measured by HPLC.
Holm et al., 1989	Cohort Stockholm, Sweden	240 ♀ who had surgery for breast cancer between 1983–1986. 12% premenopausal, 86% postmenopausal, 2% unknown. Mean age at diagnosis was 58 yr.	All subjects were interviewed at home within 4 mo of surgery. Diet reference period was the yr prior to diagnosis. Subjects estimated portion sizes. Data also collected about demographics, reproductive history, anthropometrics (self-reported), smoking, physical activity history, and alcohol intake. Tumor size, presence of local lymphatic metastases, and estrogen receptor status were correlated with dietary factors.
Howe et al., 1991	Cohort Toronto, Canada	519 cases of newly-diagnosed, histologically-confirmed breast cancer. The study sample was selected from a larger cohort of 56,837 ♀ enrolled in the diet-history collection phase of a larger breast screening intervention trial.	Beginning in 1982, all new subjects and all those returning for screening filled out a diet-history questionnaire containing an 86-item food-frequency questionnaire. Subjects estimated portion sizes with the aid of photographs and standard serving sizes. Subjects were matched for age (± 1 yr), screening center, and date of enrollment (± 2 mo).

Results	Comments
A significant difference was found in total fat and cholesterol between cases and controls of both groups; in the French groups there was a difference in saturated and monounsaturated fat intake. No difference in lipid-soluble vitamin intake between groups. There was a higher serum level of cholesterol and plasma vitamin E in cases compared to controls of both groups. Increased risk associated with dietary cholesterol, total dietary lipids, plasma vitamin E, and serum zinc (only measured in Italian sample).	No community-based controls. No comparison of controls to each other or to community standards. Blood levels were correlated with past intake (data based on long retrospective period). Differences in quantification of diet records between 2 study sites. Blood assays were blinded and all vitamin assays were performed at the same lab. Storage time was not given.
Postmenopausal cases consumed more total fat ($p < 0.07$) and significantly more saturated and monounsaturated fats ($p < 0.05$) than postmenopausal controls. Plasma total cholesterol (TC) and vitamin E were higher in cases than controls. Differences in vitamin E were greater in premenopausal women as was the ratio vitamin E/TC (which was not significant in postmenopausal patients). Plasma vitamin E was significantly correlated with safflower oil intake in all subjects. Dietary vitamin E (adjusted for age and TC) was significantly associated with plasma vitamin E in both groups. Other significant findings relate to evidence of lower lipid peroxidation in cases than controls.	Possibly inappropriate control group (all were suffering neurological or spinal problems; no medication history was reported). No community-based control group. Although stage of disease was known, there was no analysis using this variable. Duration of sample storage not given. Relevant time frame for retrospective dietary information was not clear.
A bivariate analysis (by tumor size) showed that cases with tumors $\geq 20mm$ had fewer children and lower actual intakes of carbohydrate and fiber as a % of total calories and per 10MJ respectively than cases with tumors $\leq 20mm$. Those with larger tumors also consumed a higher % of total calories as total fat and monounsaturated fat. Cases with estrogen receptor-rich tumors consumed a greater % of total calories as carbohydrate and more retinol than those with low estrogen.	No control group. No documentation of time between diagnosis or onset of symptoms and surgery. No follow-up analysis was performed due to insufficient numbers of recurrent tumors.
There was a trend ($p = 0.052$) towards increased risk associated with increasing levels of total fat intake. The positive association between fat and risk was independent of other sources of calories. Similarly, there was an inverse association between carbohydrate consumption and risk that was also independent of other sources of calories.	All subjects were volunteers in a breast cancer prevention program. No comparison group outside this cohort. Menopausal status was not available for analysis. There was no adjustment or assessment of SES, or smoking status, no biochemistry, no evaluation of potential impact of other nutrients, nutritional supplements, or no analysis by food types.

(*continued*)

APPENDIX TABLE   (*continued*)

Study	Type/Location	Subject Number and Description	Methods
Iscovich et al., 1989	Case–control La Plata, Argentina	150 cases of histologically-confirmed breast cancer. 300 controls: 1 hospital-based and 1 community-based for each case, matched for age (± 5 yr). All subjects had to have resided in La Plata for at least 5 yr. Cases were drawn from 8 area hospitals over a 1-yr period. Hospital controls had to have been admitted within 3 mo of their matched case's diagnosis.	All subjects interviewed by non-blinded interviewers either in hospital or at home. Each case–control triplet was interviewed by the same interviewer. Data collected included demographic and SES factors, menstrual and reproductive history, family health history, smoking habits, and pharmaceutical drug use. 147-item food-frequency questionnaire was used; reference period was the 5-yr period up to 6 mo prior to the interview. Portion sizes were estimated from standard serving sizes derived from a previous pilot study.
Jones et al., 1987	Cohort USA	99 cases of confirmed breast cancer: 34 premenopausal, 65 post-menopausal. 5386 controls. All subjects were obtained from the cohort of 5485 ♀ who participated in the National Health and Nutrition Examination Survey I Epidemiologic Follow-up Study. All subjects were identified after the 10-yr period following NHANES I.	Diet data used in this report were obtained at the baseline period during NHANES I. All subjects supplied a 24-hr recall. Portion sizes were estimated by the subjects with the use of food models.
Katsouyanni et al., 1988	Case–control Athens, Greece	120 breast cancer cases. 120 hospital controls (patients in orthopedic ward in a different hospital than BC cases).	All subjects interviewed before discharge on first hospital admission. Data collected included demographics, socioeconomic, reproductive, and medical histories. 120-item food-frequency questionnaire. To assess the impact of individual nutrients on BC, nutrient intakes were calorie adjusted. Reference period was "the period preceding the onset of disease." Standard portions sizes were used to estimate intake.
Knekt et al., 1990	Cohort Finland	54 cases of histologically-confirmed breast cancer. 3934 controls. All subjects were selected from a larger cohort involved in a dietary survey of 10,054 during 1966–1972. 3988 ♀ aged 20–69 yr. Cases identified over a 20-yr period (1967–1986).	All subjects completed a self-administered questionnaire with information about residence, occupation, parity, and smoking. ♀ ≥ 50 yr were classified as postmenopausal. An unspecified diet history questionnaire was used to assess intake. Reference period was the usual food consumed during the previous yr.

Results	Comments
Because of risk differences, dietary analyses were all adjusted for age, age at birth of first child, husband's occupation, and body-mass index. Cases consumed significantly more total calories, fat, protein, carbohydrate, and total vitamin A than either control group.	The time frame between onset of symptoms, diagnosis, stage of disease, and the interview was not explained or controlled.
There was significantly increased risk associated with increased caloric consumption. Consumption of eggs was a significant risk factor for breast cancer, while whole milk and green leafy vegetables were protective.	The increased caloric intake of cases was not reflected in a greater degree of adiposity. The authors discuss possible reasons for this discrepancy and the association with breast cancer. The diet assessment was not sensitive enough to examine individual nutrient intakes. There was no biochemistry or any other assessment of nutritional status.
	There was no analysis presented for pre- vs. postmenopausal effects
There were a number of factors associated with increased risk including: SES, adiposity, age at menopause, family history, and age at menarche. After adjustment for risk factors, there were no significant differences between groups for nutrient intake.	Reliability of a single data point (24-hr recall) is questionable.
There was a significant inverse association found between both total fat and saturated fat intake and risk of breast cancer.	
Cases consumed significantly less total calories and macronutrients including total fat, protein and carbohydrates. Cases also ate less saturated, mono- and polyunsaturated fats than controls. There was a suggestion of a positive association between risk and monounsaturated fat intake ($p < 0.10$). Total vitamin A intake was inversely associated with BC risk. Cases consumed less total vitamin A and retinol than controls. There was no difference in adjusted β-carotene intake. There were no differences in actual or calorie-adjusted intakes of vitamin C between cases and controls. Similarly there was no association between vitamin C and risk of BC.	Inappropriate controls (about 25% had osteoarthritis which is known to affect antioxidant vitamin status). Potential mismatching due to different cachement area of controls.
	No demographics.
	No biochemistry.
	Diet data were related to the period preceding the onset of the disease which was not controlled nor was it documented.
	Supplement use not documented.
	Data collected over a 12-mo period; no control for seasonal variations in intakes.
	Portion sizes were estimated from averages in food tables.
Breast cancer risk was significantly inversely related to total energy and non-significantly inversely related to total fat, carbohydrate, and protein intakes. There was a positive association between energy-adjusted fat intake and risk. There was a trend for increased risk associated with intake of monounsaturated fat intake ($p < 0.05$) and cholesterol ($p < 0.09$). There were no interactions between risk factors, e.g., smoking, body-mass index, stature, geographic region, menopausal status, and parity, and the fat and risk relationship. There was an association between high milk intake ($p = 0.02$) and low meat intake ($p = 0.12$) and risk. Adjustment for energy strengthened the meat and risk relationship.	Variable time periods between reference period and diagnosis or onset of disease with a potential range of 2–20 yr.
	No biochemistry, no data on dietary supplements.
	Diet collection was not described.
	No descriptive data supplied.

(*continued*)

APPENDIX TABLE   (*continued*)

Study	Type/Location	Subject Number and Description	Methods
Lee et al., 1991	Case–control Singapore	200 cases of histologically-confirmed breast cancer consecutively admitted to 2 hospitals. 420 hospital-based controls age-matched (± 5 yr) and admitted to same hospitals as cases.	All subjects were interviewed in the hospital; cases within 1–3 wk of diagnosis. Data collected included menstrual and reproductive history, oral contraceptive use, breastfeeding, smoking history, family health history, occupation, education, language dialect used, and anthropometrics (weight and height). 90-item food-frequency questionnaire was used to assess intakes of animal and vegetable protein, fat, saturated fatty acids, mono- and polyunsaturated fatty acids, cholesterol, β-carotene, vitamin E, and caffeine and other methyl-xanthines. The reference period for cases was 1 yr prior to diagnosis. Photographs and portion models were used for subject estimation of portion sizes.
Le Marchand et al., 1988	Cohort- "nested case–control" Hawaii	580 cases of breast cancer identified from Hawaii Tumor Registry between 1972–1983. 2528 controls matched to cases for race of parent and mo and yr of birth. All subjects selected from a larger historical cohort of 38,084 ♀ born between 1918–1943. All subjects were living in Hawaii in 1943 and in 1972.	Weight and height was obtained from the 1942–1943 census. Adult height and weight was obtained from 1972 driver's licenses. Other body size measures included body surface area, Quetelet and Cole's body mass indices, and Benn's relative weight. Linkages were made with other data files to obtain age at birth of first child and parity. SES in 1942 was ascertained from occupation of head of the household. SES in 1972 was based on education for adults living in the same census tract in 1972 based on 1970 census data.
Mills et al., 1988a	"Nested" case–control California	142 cases of fatal breast cancer: 852 controls matched for age (age in 1960 ± 1 yr). All subjects were white ♀ selected from a larger cohort of 16,190 Seventh-Day Adventist ♀ who had completed a questionnaire in 1960. All subjects were self-reported to be without a previous history of cancer as of 1960.	All subjects completed a questionnaire in 1960 which contained data on: demographics, tobacco use, menstrual and reproductive characteristics, and disease history. There was a 21-item food-frequency questionnaire "which was not sufficiently detailed to allow analysis of specific nutrients." From 1960–1965 church members involved in data collection, identified deaths. From 1966–1980 deaths were identified from a central registry of all death certificates in California.
Pryor et al., 1989	Case–control Utah, USA	172 cases of ♀ with histologically-confirmed first primary breast cancer identified through the Utah state cancer registry. 190 control ♀ age-matched (± 5 yr). 70% of eligible cases and 80% of controls participated. All subjects were participants in a larger study: Cancer and Steroid Hormones (CASH).	All subjects were interviewed at home by telephone to ascertain the frequency of intake of certain foods during adolescence. Standard serving sizes were assigned to calculate individual nutrients. Total dietary calories were not assessed. Adjustment was made for age, SES, age at menarche, and age at first pregnancy in the analysis of diet and risk associations.

Results	Comments

All analyses were adjusted for age and other known risk factors.
In premenopausal ♀ there was a significant increase in risk associated
with intake of red meat and high proportion of total protein from animal
sources.
There were significantly decreased risks associated with intake of
polyunsaturated fatty acids, the ratio of PUFA:saturated fat, β-carotene,
soya protein, and total soya products.
There were no significant effects seen in postmenopausal ♀.

No community-based controls nor comparisons to
national intake standards.
Long retrospective period.
No dietary supplement use data.
Reference period for control group was not matched
to cases.
No correlations run between presumed non-nutritional
risk factors, e.g., smoking history, and dietary factors.
No distinction made with respect to type of red meat
or poultry.

Adjusted mean anthropometrics were lower for cases than controls in
1942. There was a negative association between premenopausal breast
cancer and adolescent body size.
This was a statistically significant effect for girls aged 10–14 in 1942
across all ethnic groups which was strongest for overweight ♀ who
remained overweight as adults.
Adult weight and gain in body-mass index since 1942 were associated
with increased postmenopausal risk.

No direct measure of diet.
Subjects did not have to be born in Hawaii. Subjects
were predominantly Oriental (50.5% Japanese,
25% Hawaiian/part Hawaiian, 9% Chinese, 4.7%
Philipino, 7.9% white, 2.9% of other ethnic origin).
Menopausal status defined by age at diagnosis.
Premenopausal were <50 yr at diagnosis, post-
menopausal >50 yr.
No family health history.

There were no significant relationships between meat (no distinction
between beef and poultry), milk, cheese, and egg consumption and risk.
There was a non-significant trend between meat and risk in ♀
experiencing early (≤ 48 yr) menopause.

Limited data from food-frequency questionnaire prevented examination of role of individual nutrients.
There was no distinction made on the questionnaire
between red meat and poultry and no data of fish intake.
Variable length of time between onset and death from
breast cancer could have resulted in some subjects being
in early stages of cancer at the time of the original
questionnaire.
It was not possible to ascertain the actual menopausal
status of all subjects.
Some cases may have become postmenopausal prior to
onset of disease.

There was a non-significant trend towards lowered risk associated with
the upper three quartiles of fat intake in pre- but not postmenopausal ♀.
↑ risk associated with ↑ body-mass index at age 12 in pre- but not postmenopausal subjects. Fat from milk, cheese, and yogurt was associated
with lowered risk in both pre- and postmenopausal ♀ (the trend was significant in the latter group, p = 0.01). There was a significant (p < 0.01)
trend towards a protective effect from fiber intake in premenopausal ♀.
The opposite was true for the postmenopausal group (the elevated odds
ratio could have been due to large variability in the data). Fiber from
grains significantly lowered risk in both pre- and postmenopausal groups.
In premenopausal group, fiber from other sources, i.e., fruits and vegetables, lowered risk whereas in postmenopausal group the risk ↑.

>50% of subjects had >12 yr of formal education,
77% of subjects were Mormons.
All subjects were identified from a larger study
cohort, CASH involved with health related issues.
Long and variable retrospective data collection
reference period for dietary data.
Neither total caloric intake nor other individual
nutrient intakes were assessed.

(*continued*)

APPENDIX TABLE   (*continued*)

Study	Type/Location	Subject Number and Description	Methods
Richardson et al., 1991	Case–control southern France	409 case of histologically-confirmed breast cancer. 515 age-matched hospital-based controls. Groups were similar for geographical area of residence.	All subjects interviewed in hospital about medical and reproductive history and SES factors. A 55-item food-frequency questionnaire was used to cover intake of food sources of lipid, animal protein, retinol, β-carotene, and vitamin E. Because the items represented sources of only these nutrients it was not possible to estimate total caloric intake or other nutrients. Subjects were asked to specify quantities of each item consumed. Reference period was recent 12 mo unless there had been a change, in which case previous diet was requested
Rohan et al., 1990	Case–control Australia	383 biopsy-confirmed cases of benign proliferative epithelial disorders (BPED). 192 controls without BPED (confirmed by biopsy). 383 community-based controls.	All subjects given a standardized questionnaire in their homes. Cases and biopsy controls interviewed just after diagnosis (intervals 2.8 and 2.9 mo, respectively). 179-item food-frequency questionnaire. Cases and biopsy controls were asked to record intake prior to diagnosis and disregard any changes made subsequent to diagnosis.
Simard et al., 1990	Cohort Montreal, Canada	68 cases of breast cancer. 340 cases of fibrocystic breast disease (FBD). 343 controls. All subjects selected from a larger cohort of 9089 ♀ participating in the National Breast Screening Study, an intervention trial of mammography and physical exams. Subjects were in the 4th and 5th yr of screening.	All subjects were given a questionnaire with items pertaining to religion, occupation, education, marital status, socioeconomic level, weight, and number of pregnancies. A food-frequency questionnaire containing 41 food categories was used. Controls and FBD patients completed a 24-hr dietary recall.
Toniolo et al., 1989	Case–control Italy	250 cases of breast cancer (free of metastases, except in regional lymph nodes. Controls were 499 ♀ from general population stratified by age (± 10 yr) and geographical area.	All subjects interviewed (unblinded) given modified food-frequency questionnaire structured by meals. Cases interviewed on average of 7.8 mo after diagnosis and after treatment or surgery. Indigenous foods and recipes were added to the database. General demographic data was obtained from electoral rolls. Standard portion sizes before cooking were estimated. Interview data included SES data, health and reproductive history.
Van't Veer et al., 1990, 1991	Case–control Netherlands	133 newly diagnosed cases of breast cancer. 238 community controls (for whom complete dietary data were available).	All subjects given a home interview about demographics, smoking history, health, and reproductive and hormone history. Cases within 6 mo of diagnosis. No interviews during chemotherapy. 236-item food-frequency questionnaire. Reference period 12 mo prior to diagnosis in cases and 12 mo preceding interview in controls. Portion sizes estimated by subjects using common households utensils. The focus of the 1990 report was fat intake; whereas the 1991 study assessed the potential impact of specific nutrients or diet patterns based on their hypothesized role in carcinogenesis, e.g., vitamins A and E as antioxidants.

Results	Comments
Total fat, saturated and monounsaturated fat were positively related to elevated risk.	Limited number of items on diet questionnaire, no supplement use data, no adjustment for total calories in analyses.
Saturated fat was significantly related to risk in postmenopausal ♀ as was increased Quetelet index (reflecting body mass). There was a significant increasing trend associated with intake of high-fat cheese, desserts, and chocolate and total food consumption. No change in risk associated with apparent intakes of vitamin E, retinol, or β-carotene.	No community-based controls. Reference period was variable and not necessarily related to onset or diagnosis of disease.
There was no change in risk associated with intake of total fat or any of the major subfractions, i.e., saturated, mono- or polyunsaturated fats. There was an increased risk associated with the highest levels of cholesterol intake, an effect that reached statistical significance in premenopausal ♀. Statistically significant trend towards decreased risk with ↑ intake of retinol and β-carotene when cases compared to community controls. There was a similar trend with biopsy controls but not statistically significant. Adjustment for energy intake eliminated the β-carotene trend but not the point estimate.	Portion sizes estimated. No analysis by food group. No data on supplement use. No matching of reference period for cases and all controls. Case group may have been self-selected as they differed from controls in self-examination practices.
Cases were significantly heavier and had a higher body-mass index than either of the other groups.	Possible selection bias as all subjects were in the latter stages of a breast cancer prevention program. Only controls and FBD patients completed 24-hr recall.
Cases had significantly less education. Cases consumed more poultry, fish, pastry, margarine, and alcohol and less milk, raw vegetables, pastas, sugar, butter, and coffee than the other groups.	No reference period given for the food-frequency data. Portion size estimation was not described. No pre- vs postmenopausal status analysis. No computation or adjustment for total calories.
Cases consumed more animal protein and fat. Reduced risk was associated with decreased intakes of fat especially saturated fat and animal protein.	Not blinded, no biochemistry, long period of time between diagnosis or treatment and study (on average 7.8 mo after diagnosis).
♀ who consumed <28% of total calories as fat had lower risk than those consuming >36% of calories as fat. Decreased risk was associated with intakes of <9.6% saturated fat and <5.9% of calories from animal protein. Intakes of retinol and β-carotene were slightly higher in cases. No difference in vitamin E or C intake between groups.	Retrospective diet data not necessarily indicative of diets prior to diagnosis. Smoking histories not reported.
The *1990 study* reported a significant ↑ risk associated with fat intake independent of total calories.	Small sample size.
The multivariate adjusted analysis for risk that compared the highest to lowest quintile of fat intake showed a 30% ↑ in risk per 10% of energy from fat.	Large nonresponse rate in selection of controls (238 out of a potential pool of 548) may have resulted in bias.
The *1991 study* reported that a diet with the combination of low fat and a high intake of fermented milk products and fiber conferred significant protective effects.	Cases and controls not matched on reference period, i.e., time between diagnosis and interview in cases. No supplement data, no analysis with other risk factors, e.g., smoking, hormones. No analyses by menopausal status.

(continued)

APPENDIX TABLE   (*continued*)

Study	Type/Location	Subject Number and Description	Methods
Verreault et al., 1988	Cross-sectional Quebec City, Canada	666 cases of newly diagnosed infiltrating breast cancer. Cases with distal metastases were excluded.	Subjects were interviewed at home 3–6 mo post-diagnosis. Data included demographics, menstrual and reproductive history, height and weight, smoking habits, physical activity, and medication history. 114-item food-frequency questionnaire, referenced to the yr prior to diagnosis. Food models were used to estimate portion sizes. The study compared prognostic indicators of breast cancer to dietary factors. The indicators included: axillary node involvement at diagnosis, estrogen receptor status, and histological features of the primary tumor.
Yu et al., 1990	Case–control Shanghai, China	186 cases of newly diagnosed histologically-confirmed breast cancer. 186 hospital control (HC) cancer patients (head and neck, stomach, and lung) from same hospitals as cases. 186 community controls (CC) matched for residential district to cases. All subjects were matched for age (± 5 yr).	All subjects interviewed at home to obtain data about: SES and menstrual and reproductive history. 68-item food-frequency questionnaire containing foods commonly found in Shanghai. Reference period was usual diet unless there had been a change within the last yr in which case usual diet before that time was determined. Quantification was determined with standard portion sizes.
Zaridze et al., 1991	Case–control Moscow, Russia	139 newly-diagnosed consecutive cases of breast cancer. None of the cases had previous treatments or distal metastases. 139 controls matched by age (± 2 yr) and neighborhood were recruited from same outpatient screening clinic as cases.	Cases were interviewed within 4 d of admission to the clinic. Diet assessed with 145-item food-frequency questionnaire. Reference period was the yr prior to diagnosis for cases and the yr prior to interview for controls. No portion size estimation method was reported.

II. Colorectal Cancer

Study	Type/Location	Subject Number and Description	Methods
Benito et al., 1990	Case–control Majorca, Spain	286 case of *colorectal cancer*: all residents for at least 10 yr and <80 yr old selected for 1984–1988. 295 community controls (CC) selected from 1982 census stratified by age and sex. 203 hospital controls (HC) selected from hospitals were 70% of cases diagnosed.	All subjects interviewed at home about demographics, SES, occupation, medical history, exposure to toxins, and pharmacological history. Cases interviewed within 3 mo of diagnosis. 99-item food-frequency questionnaire. Reference period was the previous year unless there had been a change within previous 6 mo, in which case they were asked about their diet prior to changes. Portion size estimation procedure not given.
Freudenheim et al., 1990	Case–control New York	422 cases of *rectal cancer* (277 ♂, 145 ♀). 422 sex-, race-, age- (± 5 yr), neighborhood-matched controls.	Subjects given a 2.5 hr interview consisting of 129-item food-frequency questionnaire. Reference period the previous yr for controls and for cases a yr prior to the onset of symptoms. Portion size estimated with the use of pictures. Additional information included smoking and alcohol use, and occupational and health histories, seasonality of intake, preparation, and food storage.

Results	Comments
After adjustment for total energy, age, body weight, and tumor size at diagnosis, ↑ in saturated fat intake was related to an ↑ frequency of node involvement at diagnosis in postmenopausal ♀. ↑ in polyunsaturated fat intake was associated with ↓ % of patients with positive nodes at diagnosis in both pre- and postmenopausal patients. Dietary fat was not related to estrogen-receptor status of tumors. There were no associations between dietary factors and histological features of the primary tumor.	No comparison group. No analysis for nutrients other than fat. No data on dietary supplement use.
Cases consumed significantly more calories, total fat (primarily from increased intake of monounsaturated fats) and protein than either controls. Total fat and monounsaturated fat intake was associated with increased risk after adjustment for other caloric sources. Cases were also more educated than either control group. ♀ with natural menopause ≥ 45 yr had significantly increased risk compared to ♀ who were younger at menopause.	Reference period unclear and potentially variable. No analysis by menopausal status in spite of differences in risk reported.
There were no significant effects of diet on risk in premenopausal ♀. In postmenopausal ♀ there was a significant ↑ in risk associated with protein intake and a marginally significant risk ($p < 0.06$) associated with saturated fat. There were significant protective effects associated with high intakes of polyunsaturated fats, mono- and disaccharides, cellulose, β-carotene, vitamin C, and potassium.	Possible bias associated with subjects involvement in screening clinic. No portion size estimation procedure given. Small sample size.

II. Colorectal Cancer

Significant trend for increased risk associated with education and weight. Increased risk for *colorectal* cancer associated with cereal (white bread and pasta). Risk for *colon* cancer was associated with fresh meats (lamb and game), and a protective effect for cruciferous vegetables. Increased risk for *rectal* cancer associated with dairy products and protection from cruciferous vegetables. There was no risk associated with type of oil, mode of consumption (crude or cooked), or quantity or frequency of consumption in common dishes. Significant increases in risk associated with cereals, potatoes, pastry, eggs, and number of meals/d. Combination of high consumption of fresh meat, dairy products, and cereals and low intake of cruciferous vegetables associated with 4-fold increase in risk for colorectal cancer.	No portion size estimates, no documentation of number of cases with dietary changes during reference period. No analysis possible for individual nutrients although data are suggestive of a dietary fat effect. Time between diagnosis and interview of cases not documented.
Increased risk with increasing intakes of calories, fat, carbohydrate, and iron. Decreased risk with increasing intake of carotenoids, vitamin C, and dietary fiber from vegetables. For ♂ there was a 2-fold increase in risk associated with retinol intake and decreased risk for carotenoids. The same held for ♀ although not significantly. For ♂ fat was most strongly associated with risk; for ♀ the association between fat and risk was not as strong. No association between intake of vitamin E and risk. Associations between diet and risk of rectal cancer were not affected by either smoking or alcohol intake.	Reliance on retrospective food-frequency interviews. No data on use of supplements or stage of disease (except that "only relatively alert, healthy subjects could tolerate the 2.5 hr. interview"). Well-conceived study.

(continued)

APPENDIX TABLE *(continued)*

Study	Type/Location	Subject Number and Description	Methods
Gerhardsson de Verdier et al., 1990	Case–control Stockholm, Sweden	569 total cases (352 *colon cancer*, and 217 *rectal cancer*). 512 controls (referents) randomly selected every 4 mo during the case recruitment period (1986–1988) and stratified by yr of birth (4 categories) and sex.	Cases filled out a questionnaire at the hospital as soon after diagnosis as possible; when necessary, cases were assisted in filling out the form. 19% of cases and all controls received the questionnaire by mail (supplemented by telephone to fill in missing items). Frequency of intake of items from 55 food categories were ascertained. The reference period was the previous 5 yr. Portion sizes were estimated from photographs. Anthropometric history was collected and body-mass index (BMI) computed.
Graham et al., 1988	Case–control New York	428 cases of *colon cancer* (CC). 428 controls matched for age, sex, and neighborhood.	All subjects given a structured 2.5-hr interview similar to that used by Freudenheim et al. (1990). No reference period was noted for the diet data. No surrogates were used.
Kune et al., 1987	Case–control Melbourne, Australia	715 cases of *colorectal cancer*, CRC (392 colon cancer, 323 rectal cancer) all histologically-confirmed new cases. 727 age- and sex-matched community controls. 159 hospital controls.	300-item food-frequency questionnaire used to ascertain usual daily consumption. Serving sizes were estimated by subjects. Calculated average weekly amounts adjusted for seasonal variations. Reference period was the previous 20 yr. Data included use of vitamin supplements.
La Vecchia et al., 1988	Case–control Italy	339 cases of *colon cancer* (CC). 236 cases of *rectal cancer* (RC). 778 hospital controls admitted for acute, non-neoplastic or digestive disorders.	All subjects given a questionnaire to obtain data on: SES, smoking, alcohol, coffee and other methylxan-thine-containing drinks, personal and family health history, and use of selected drugs. 29-item food-frequency questionnaire. Reference period was an unspecified period before current hospital admission. Subjects also asked to report changes over previous 10 yr.
Neoptolemos et al., 1988	Case–control Birmingham, U.K.	49 cases of *colorectal cancer*. 49 hospital controls matched for age and sex and admitted to same hospital as cases with benign disease.	Diet was assessed with 7-d recall obtained during hospitalization on the d before surgery. Although not stated this was presumably designed to reflect normal intake at home. Overnight fasted blood samples were collected for analysis of fatty acids in red blood cells (RBC). Adipose tissue biopsies were also collected for fatty acid analysis.
Slattery et al., 1988	Case–control Utah	229 cases of *colon cancer* (119 ♀, 110 ♂). 384 controls (204 ♀, 180 ♂) recruited by random digit dialing and matched for age (± 5 yr).	All subjects interviewed at home. Diet data were collected with food-frequency questionnaire. Amount, frequency, and method of preparation were ascertained. The reference period was 2 yr prior to diagnosis for cases and 2 yr prior to interview for controls. The same reference periods were used to determine normal exercise patterns including leisure time activities and occupational activity. Calories expended were estimated.

Results	Comments
There was an increased risk associated with total energy ($p < 0.06$ colon, 0.05 rectum), protein ($p < 0.05$ colon, 0.05 rectum), total fat ($p < 0.05$ colon, 0.05 rectum), monounsaturated fat ($p < 0.05$ colon, 0.05 rectum), and polyunsaturated fat ($p < 0.44$ colon, 0.05 rectum). Results were the same across sexes. High-fiber diet was inversely related to risk of colon cancer in ♂ and rectal cancer in both ♂ and ♀.	Variable reference period with respect to diagnosis and variable data acquisition procedure among cases. Long retrospective period for diet collection. No analysis for any other potential risk factors or demographic variables presented.
Risk of CC was positively associated with increasing intake of total fats (predominantly animal fat) and total calories. No significant risks associated with intake of protein, vitamin A from vegetables and fruits, carbohydrates, vitamin C, cruciferous vegetables, calcium, or phosphorous. There was significantly reduced risk associated with high intakes of tomatoes, peppers, carrots, onions, and celery.	No reference period for food-frequency questionnaire given. No data on supplement use.
There was a dose-dependent inverse relationship between fiber, vitamin C, β-carotene, total vegetables, and cruciferous vegetables. β-carotene was highly correlated with vegetable intake. Dietary retinol had no independent association with risk of CRC. Dietary vitamin C was protective at intakes > 230 mg/d. Vitamin supplements were highly protective. High fat was a contributing factor in the overall risk factor model (especially for ♂).	Long retrospective diet period. Supplement data not clearly presented (multivitamins or individual, quantity or interaction with diet).
Risk of both CC and RC was inversely related to intake of green vegetables, tomatoes, melon, and coffee. There was also an inverse relationship between risk and indices of carotenoid and vitamin C intake. Consumption of pasta and rice or beef/veal associated with increased risk of both cancers.	No supplement data, variable reference times between cases and controls, no population-based control. Diet database was small (only 29 items). Individual nutrient estimation unreliable due to lack of portion size information. No biochemistry. No descriptive data or comparisons to normal standards of intake.
No difference between groups for dietary intake or adipose tissue content of fatty acids. There were some differences in correlation between dietary fatty acid intake and RBC levels in cases.	Questionable reliability of 7-d recall as a tool for dietary assessment. Variable times between diagnosis of cancer and study. Small sample size. The study was designed to validate the use of RBC fatty acid profiles as a diagnostic tool; it was not designed to assess nutritional factors associated with colorectal cancer.
Calories, protein, and fat were associated with ↑ risk of colon cancer. Total physical activity was protective in both ♂ and ♀. Intense physical activity was most protective in ♂. Physical activity was not a confounder for the relation of diet in this study, and dietary intake did not confound the relation between physical activity and colon cancer risk. Data analysis suggested that physical activity modifies colon cancer risk associated with diet. The combination of high activity and low intake of calories, fat, and protein was protective.	Food-frequency questionnaire not described. Questionable external validity as study sample was largely composed of Mormons who eschew cigarettes, alcohol, and coffee.

(continued)

APPENDIX TABLE   (*continued*)

Study	Type/Location	Subject Number and Description	Methods
Tuyns et al., 1988	Case–control Belgium	453 cases of *colon cancer* (CC). 365 cases of *rectal cancer* (RC). 2851 controls. All subjects were from same 2 provinces and adjusted for age and sex.	All subjects interviewed about diet using food-frequency questionnaire. Reference period for cases 1 wk period prior to onset of disease, controls current intake. Portion sizes were estimated using food models (pictures). Cases interviewed in hospital, controls at home.
West et al., 1989	Case–control Utah	231 cases of newly (within 6 mo) diagnosed *colon cancer* (CC). 391 controls matched by age (± 5 yr), sex, and county of residence.	All subjects were interviewed in their homes. Questionnaire consisted of demographic, health history, current height and weight (2 yr before interview), computed body-mass index, physical activity, and dietary data. 99-item food-frequency questionnaire. Reference period was "2–3 years prior to the interview." Portion sizes were estimated with food models.
Whittemore et al., 1990	Case–control USA., China	905 cases of *colorectal cancer* (473 from North America, 432 from China). 2488 controls (1192 Chinese Americans from N. America, 1296 from China). Subjects were identified through cancer registries. Controls in China were selected from same neighborhood as cases and matched for age and sex (± 5 yr). Most of the N. American cases and controls were born in Asia.	All subjects interviewed about demographic characteristics, diet, physical activity, menstrual factors, and residential patterns. 84-item food-frequency questionnaire was used for diet analysis. There were additions in the Chinese version to reflect cultural patterns, e.g., more soybean products and indigenous fruits and vegetables. It also excluded cheeses, mayonnaise, cream sauces, and creamed dishes. Food models were used to estimate portion sizes. Reference yr was the yr prior to diagnosis for cases and the yr before interview for controls.
Willett et al., 1990	Prospective cohort USA	150 cases of *colon cancer* selected over a 6-yr period (1980–1986). 88,601 controls. All subjects were selected from a cohort of 88,751 ♀.	The cohort was from those ♀ in the "Nurses Health Study," who had responded to a diet questionnaire containing 61-item food-frequency questionnaire. Reference period was yr prior to questionnaire. Common unit of portions were used to estimate portion sizes. All analyses adjusted for energy.

Results	Comments
Inverse association between intake of maize, soybean, and sunflower oils and risk. No effect for butter, margarine, or fatty meats. Intake of retinol and vitamin B2 was higher in cases; intakes of β-carotene and vitamin C were lower in cases. Significant positive associations were found for retinol, oligosaccharides; negative associations for fiber, linoleic acid, thiamine, and iron. After adjustment for age, sex, province and caloric intake, retinol was positively associated with CC and RC; significant negative associations with fiber, thiamine, vitamin B6, iron, and vitamin C (for RC only).	Retrospective data collection. Differences in reference period between controls and cases. Group differences by province and sex. No biochemistry, supplementation data, descriptive data on intake, demographics, smoking, alcohol, medical histories, or comparisons to normal standards for intake. Possible bias from place of interview; hospital for cases, home for controls. There was no discussion of the food sources of retinol that might have contributed to its effect. No discussion of relationship of foods and outcomes, i.e., grains as sources of thiamine, fiber, etc.
In ♀ total fat and energy intake were associated with ↑ risk. In ♂ total fat, poly- and monounsaturated fat, energy, and protein were associated with ↑ risk. There were site-specific differences in risk associated with intake of fat and protein in ♂. Significant protective effects of β-carotene in ♂ and ♀; cruciferous vegetables in ♂; fiber was protective in ♀. No association between CC risk and intake of vitamin C or A after adjustment for age, BMI, fiber, and energy intakes.	Unknown relationship between reference period and time of diagnosis in cases. No biochemistry, comparisons to intake standards or descriptive statistics. No data for SES, alcohol, smoking, or supplement history.
In Chinese-American participants there was significant risk associated with duration of residence in N. America. Cases tended to be more westernized than controls. In both continents, cases ate more total calories, protein, fat, and cholesterol than controls. Risk of cancers of both colon and rectum was associated with food energy from fat, protein, carbohydrate, and total energy for both sexes and both sample sets. In multivariate analysis only saturated fat was significantly associated with risk for colorectal cancer. This latter effect was stronger in the N. American sample, reflecting a greater intake of meat and dairy products. There was a significant protective effect of vegetable consumption among Chinese-American ♂ and ♀ and in Chinese ♂. Fruit was not associated with any changes in risk in any group. Sedentary lifestyle was also a significant risk factor. The differences between continents were due to longer duration of high-risk lifestyles in the western sample. Physical inactivity + diet high in saturated fat were estimated to account for 60% and 40% of colorectal cancer incidence among Chinese-American ♂ and ♀, respectively.	Variable reference period for cases (time since diagnosis was not documented). Possible overestimation of energy expenditure as estimated energy output exceeded input on both continents.
Total fat, saturated and monounsaturated fats, and animal fats were all associated with ↑ risk of colon cancer. Intake of beef, pork, or lamb as main dish was highly related to risk as was the ratio of intake of red meat to intake of chicken and fish. Fish and chicken without skin offered protection.	Conclusion presumes animal fat is major contributor to risk. No analysis for protein intake or other sources of saturated fat, e.g., dairy products. No documentation of relationship between diagnosis and questionnaire in cases. No presentation of any other risk factors or confounders.

(continued)

APPENDIX TABLE   (*continued*)

		III. Pancreatic Cancer	
Study	Type/Location	Subject Number and Description	Methods
Falk et al., 1988	Case–control Louisiana	363 cases of *pancreatic cancer* (PC). 1234 hospital-based controls (HC) matched on hospital of admittance, race, sex, and age (± 5 yr).	All subjects were given an interview to obtain data on smoking, occupational and residential history, alcohol use, family health history, medical history, leisure time activities, and diet. A 59-item food-frequency questionnaire was used. The reference period was the time (unspecified) prior to diagnosis or onset of symptoms. Means for estimation of portion sizes were not described. >50% of cases were unable to be interviewed; surrogates (next of kin, usually a spouse) were used. 3% of controls were unavailable.
Farrow et al., 1990.	Case–control Washington	148 married male cases of *pancreatic cancer* diagnosed between 1982–1986. 188 married ♂ controls randomly selected and frequency-matched by age (± 5 yr).	Data was collected from surrogates (wives) in 2 steps. A telephone interview to collect demographic data, medical and occupational history, and use of tobacco, alcohol, coffee, and vitamin supplements. Dietary questionnaire was mailed and contained a 135-item food-frequency questionnaire. Reference period was 3 yr prior to diagnosis.
Ghadirian et al., 1991	Case–control Montreal, Canada	179 cases of *pancreatic cancer* recruited from 19 hospitals for the French-speaking in Montreal. 239 controls matched for age (± 5 yr), sex, and residential area. Controls randomly selected from same phone book as cases.	200-item food-frequency questionnaire. Subjects asked about amount consumed. Criteria for portion sizes not documented. Reference period for case–control matches was the yr prior to diagnosis for cases. Controls interviewed within 3 mo of cases. Other data collected included: medical history, occupation, alcohol and smoking habits, medical history, dietary supplement use, and family health history.
Howe et al., 1990b	Case–control Toronto, Canada	249 cases of newly-diagnosed *pancreatic cancer*. 505 controls matched for age (± 5 yr) and sex. 45% and 31% of eligible cases and controls respectively were included in the study.	Interviews for all subjects done at home; for cases within 3 mo of diagnosis. In 194 (78%) cases data were collected from proxy interviews primarily with spouse. For each case proxy there was a control proxy interview. Data collected included: demographics, smoking, coffee, tea, and alcohol consumption. 200-item food-frequency questionnaire. Reference period was "1–2 years before interview, in order to overcome any changes in diet among the cases due to the onset of their disease." No reference period was given for controls. Portion sizes were estimated with the aid of physical food models.
La Vecchia et al., 1990	Case–control Milan, Italy	247 cases of *pancreatic cancer* (159 ♂, 88 ♀). 1089 hospital-based controls (800 ♂, 289 ♀) admitted to same hospitals as cases for acute non-digestive or non-neoplastic diseases unrelated to alcohol or tobacco.	All subjects interviewed about sociodemographics, smoking habits, alcohol and coffee consumption, and medical history. 14-item food-frequency questionnaire. Reference period for diet collection was not reported. Procedure for portion size estimation not reported.

III. Pancreatic Cancer

Results	Comments
Pork products (bacon, ham, sausage, cold cuts, and unprocessed fresh pork) and rice were significantly associated with risk. Dairy foods were positively associated in ♂. Fruit consumption (fresh and juice) was inversely related with PC; fruit also conferred a protective effect against intake of pork products. There was a smaller non-significant inverse association with vegetable intake. No differences in risk associated with vitamin A, retinol, or carotene intakes. Trend analysis indicated increased risk with vitamin A in both sexes (significantly in ♂); there was a ↓ trend in risk associated with carotene in ♂. After adjustment for fruit intake, a non-significant inverse association was found for ♂ in highest levels of carotene index. Risks associated with consumption of fruits and with an index of vitamin C showed significant decreasing gradients across sexes. Cigarette smoking was a strong risk factor for PC.	Control diet of unknown quality used as reference. No descriptive data reported nor comparisons of diet to reference standard, i.e., RDA. No community-based control group. Unknown time period between time of interview and diagnosis and/or onset of symptoms. Controls' diet response reflective of recent intake patterns. No data on supplement use. No biochemistry. No testing for potential interactions between smoking and vitamin C index or fruit consumption. Lack of portion size estimation prevented quantification of individual nutrients, i.e., total calories, fat, protein.
No association between PC risk and intake of vitamin A or total fat, saturated fat, cholesterol, ω-3 fatty acids, or vitamin C. No difference between groups in their use of supplemental multivitamins, vitamin A, or vitamin C	Reliability and validity of data acquisition is questionable. Reliance on retrospective data collected from surrogates. Reference period was 3 yr prior to interview.
↑ risk associated with total energy. Cases ate more than controls and ♂ ate more than ♀. Significant ↑ in risk associated with total and saturated fats and cholesterol. Analyses were adjusted for age, sex, response status, cigarette use, and total energy intake.	Proxy interviews were used in 75% of cases who were either too ill or recently deceased (within 12 mo of study). 17% of controls required proxies due to death between time of diagnosis of matched case and his/her time of interview. Cases interviewed before histological confirmation of diagnosis.
Proxy data were different from data derived directly from subjects. There was no demonstrable effect from intake of total fat or its components. Total calories was associated with increased risk. Carbohydrate was the component of caloric intake that had the most significant contribution to risk. Fiber intake from fruit, vegetable, and cereal sources was inversely associated with risk.	High rate of non-compliance in recruitment of both cases and controls. Majority of data from cases was from proxy interviews. No reference period was given for controls. Variable reference period for cases.
Significantly decreased risk associated with fruit intake, fish, and oil intake. Insignificant trend for increased risk associated with meat, eggs, ham, and margarine intake.	Small data set for food-frequency analysis. Unknown and variable reference period for diet assessment. Time between diagnosis and interview was not defined or controlled. No community-based controls. Analysis of contribution of individual nutrients not possible.

(continued)

APPENDIX TABLE   (*continued*)

Study	Type/Location	Subject Number and Description	Methods
Mills et al., 1988b	Cohort California	Study population was 34,198 non-Hispanic Seventh-Day Adventists > 25 yr of age. 40 cases of death from *pancreatic cancer* (PC) occurring during the follow-up period of 1974–1982.	All subjects completed a lifestyle questionnaire; details of which were not supplied.
Olsen et al., 1989	Case–control Minnesota	212 cases of white ♂ deaths from pancreatic cancer. 220 controls white ♂.	Surrogates were interviewed for all subjects. Reference period was 2 yr prior to interview or death. Food-frequency questionnaire of unknown scope. Portion sizes not estimated.
Zatonski et al., 1991	Case–control southwest Poland	110 cases of *pancreatic cancer*. 195 controls randomly selected from same residential area and matched for age (± 5 yr) and sex.	78 (71%) of case interviews were with proxy; none of the controls were done by proxy. All except 5 cases were interviewed at home. The questionnaire data included: lifestyle factors such as demographics and SES factors, tobacco use history, alcohol, tea, and coffee consumption patterns, and medical history. 80-item food-frequency questionnaire. Reference period was 1–2 yr prior to interview. Portion sizes estimated with drawing models. Average daily intake of individual nutrients was estimated.

IV. Prostate Cancer

Study	Type/Location	Subject Number and Description	Methods
Hsing et al., 1990	Cohort/case–control USA	149 cases of fatal *prostate cancer*. 17,633 controls used for computation of food-consumption quartiles. Subjects were from a pool of 26,030 holders of Lutheran Brotherhood Insurance selected in 1966 for a mortality study.	68.5% of the original cohort completed questionnaires. Comparisons of respondents to nonrespondents showed no differences in age, residence, or policy status. Questionnaire included data on demographics, alcohol and tobacco use, and diet history. Subjects asked about current (1966) intake of 35 food items. Portion sizes were estimated from survey data (NHANES II).
Kolonel et al., 1988	Case–control Hawaii	452 cases of histologically-confirmed *prostate cancer* (PC). 899 age-matched controls. Subjects > 65 were randomly selected from a central insurance registry; those < 65 selected with random-digit-dialing.	All subjects given an extensive home interview to collect data on dietary, occupational, medical, social, and demographic histories. 100+-item food-frequency questionnaire was used. Reference period was a usual mo prior to onset of the disease for cases and a corresponding period for controls. Portion sizes were estimated with the use of colored pictures in 3 different portion sizes and common measuring tools (spoons, cups). Surrogates were used for those subjects who could not be interviewed.

Results	Comments
Current use of meat, poultry, or fish was associated with increasing risk. There was a significant increase in risk associated with increasing consumption of eggs. Intake of vegetarian protein products, legumes, and dried fruits was significantly inversely related to risk. No relationship between risk and intake of other fresh fruit, canned or frozen fruit, fresh citrus fruit, fresh winter fruit, green salads, or cooked green vegetables. These results were age- and sex-adjusted.	Problems include no comparison group, no data on quality of diet, no details on diet data, no data on individual nutrients, no data on supplement use, no biochemistry, and no demographics.
↑ risk associated with intake of beef and pork; ↓ risk associated with cruciferous vegetables	Long retrospective relying on surrogate recall. Design did not allow for estimation of individual nutrient contribution.
Significant trend towards ↑ risk associated with cholesterol intake. There was a significant inverse relationship between vitamin C intake and risk. There was a non-significant ($p = 0.10$) inverse trend for ↓ risk with ↑ total fat. The mono- ($p < 0.02$) and polyunsaturated ($p < 0.06$) fat contributed to this inverse relationship. There was a significant ↑ risk associated with carbohydrate intake. There was a trend towards an ↑ risk with ↑ total calories. However, the use of proxy interviews may have resulted in an underestimation of actual intakes. There was no adjustment in nutrient analyses for total calories.	Most of cases' data were collected from proxy interviews; none of the controls were done by proxy. Period between diagnosis and interview was variable and not controlled. Cases and control interviews were not matched for reference period interval.

IV. Prostate Cancer

No significant trends were associated with total vitamin A, retinol, or β-carotene intake. When analyzed by age the group diagnosed <75 yr had an ↑ risk associated with ↑ intake of total vitamin A. In those ≥75 the trend was reversed. This pattern held true for retinol and β-carotene. There were no changes in risk associated with intake of any of 9 food groups or any individual foods.	Self-selected population. No comparison with general population, no data on mean intakes, no supplement data. The vitamin A differences in the 2 age groups could have reflected a difference in the type of foods eaten; this was not tested. Very limited food items in food-frequency questionnaire (it lacked some major sources of vitamins, e.g., liver, broccoli, spinach, and melons). Age analysis was only reported for the vitamin A intakes, not for smoking, alcohol consumption, or other foods. In 58 of the 149 fatalities prostate cancer was not the primary cause of death. It was not clear whether prostate cancer was the primary diagnosis.
Older cases consumed significantly more saturated fat, total vitamin A, and zinc than age-matched controls. These differences were reflected in increased risk associated with saturated fat and zinc. There was a significant increase in risk with the highest quartile of total vitamin A intake as well as a trend towards increased risk. Similar finding with respect to total carotenes and β-carotene. No difference between younger subjects and their matched controls. There were no associations between risk and total or food sources of vitamin C. No differences found in potential confounding variables: SES, marital status, anthropometrics, family history. No significant interactions between nutrients	Total vitamin A and total zinc included supplements. The supplements were not characterized as either individual or multivitamins/minerals. At the time of the study β-carotene was not available in Hawaii as a supplement. The older cases consumed more of all forms of vitamin A than younger cases with the exception of food sources of retinol. This would indicate a greater use of supplements or greater intakes of carotene-rich foods. The duration of supplement use was not reported.

(continued)

APPENDIX TABLE   (*continued*)

Study	Type/Location	Subject Number and Description	Methods
Mettlin et al., 1989	Case–control Buffalo, NY	371 cases of histologically confirmed *prostate cancer*. 371 control patients with no history of cancer, matched by age. 12.1% of controls had benign prostatic hyperplasia. There were a total of 76 different diseases in this group.	All patients admitted to the Roswell Park Memorial Institute are given a lifestyle questionnaire including a 45-item food-frequency checklist. Reference period for all patients was the period preceding the onset of current illness (admission?). Portion sizes were estimated from standard food tables.
Ohno et al., 1988 Oishi et al., 1988	Case–control Japan	100 cases newly diagnosed of *prostate cancer* (PC). 100 controls with benign prostatic hyperplasia (BPH). 100 hospital controls without BPH, other malignancies, liver disease, or hormonal disorders. All subjects were matched for hospital, age (± 3 yr) and date of admission (± 3 mo).	Data collected by interview upon admission to hospital included birthplace, occupational history, marital history, religion, body type, medical history, sex-life, and dietary practices. Food-frequency questionnaire assessed dietary habits during the period 5 yr prior to current admission. Photographs were used to estimate portion sizes.
Ross et al., 1987	Case–control California	179 "black" cases (BPC) of *prostate cancer* (PC) diagnosed between 1977–1980. 142 "black" controls (BC) matched for age (± 5 yr) and residence. 142 "white" cases (WPC) of PC diagnosed between 1972–1982. 142 "white" controls (WC).	Interviews usually done at home (all WPC and WC) or occasionally at a mutually convenient location. A food-frequency questionnaire containing 20 categories of foods was used to estimate intake of fat, protein, or vitamin A. Reference period was time of diagnosis. Portion sizes estimated from common portion sizes.
Severson et al., 1989	Cohort/case–control Hawaii	174 cases of newly-diagnosed malignant *prostate cancer* divided into overt PC (OPC) and latent cancer (LPC). Cohort consisted of 7999 ♂ of Japanese ancestry.	All subjects were interviewed between 1965–1968 about demographics, marital, smoking, occupational, residence, education, alcohol use, and medical history. 23-item food-frequency questionnaire and 24-hr recall. Reference period was time of initial examination to time of diagnosis.
Slattery et al., 1990 West et al., 1991	Case–control Utah	362 cases of histologically-confirmed *prostate cancer*. 685 controls matched by age (± 5 yr). Controls identified through random-digit-dialing technique.	A 2-part questionnaire, 1 a mailed self-administered report on adolescent diet, body size, age of voice change, and the other information about adolescent years (age 12–18), limited medical information, and family history of prostate cancer. Second part was an at-home interview to obtain data about demographics, age, marital status, religious preference, education, income, medical history, and dietary history. Adolescent data included a food-frequency questionnaire about consumption of 23 food groups. The adult part included a 183-item food-frequency questionnaire. Portion sizes for adults were estimated with the use of visual aids and food models. The reference period was 3 yr prior to cancer diagnosis or any medical symptoms that might have caused a change in diet; for controls the reference period was 3 yr prior to interview.

Results	Comments
No differences in age, marital status, education, weight, and height. There was a geographical difference. Increased consumption of high-fat milk was associated with increased risk. There was a non-significant trend towards increased risk associated with fat intake. There was a significant reduction in risk associated with the highest level of intake of β-carotene in ♂ < 68 yr but not in subjects > 68 yr. Age- and resident-adjusted risk for highest level of β-carotene for the combined age groups shows a protective effect.	No supplement data, no population-based controls. Diet data collected during time of duress for most subjects. Variable time between first diagnosis and hospital admission.
Low intakes of vitamin A (retinol and β-carotene) were associated with increased risk. The risk reduction associated with vitamin A and β-carotene was seen in older (70–79 yr) but not younger (50–69 yr) ♂. Vitamin A and β-carotene from green/ yellow vegetables were significantly protective. There was no association between risk and any other nutrients.	No supplement data, confusing statistics, lack of community-based controls. Long retrospective period, 5 yr. No smoking data.
Fat intake was a risk factor for both groups, but more so in blacks (p < 0.05). High intakes of pork were associated with ↑ risk, significantly so in blacks. Significant differences between races for sexual practices and incidence of venereal disease. Venereal disease (+) and circumcision (–) were significantly associated with risk in both groups. Vitamin A consumption was inconsistently related or unrelated to PC risk in both groups.	57% response rate for black cases. Variable and long reference period. Limited items on food-frequency questionnaire. Portion sizes estimated from food tables. No supplement use data. Groups differed demographically. BC were apparently not matched to BPC group demographically. There were no statistical adjustments made for any confounding variables in the diet analysis.
Individual nutrients not evaluated. No relationship between intake of total fat and protein. Intake of certain types of foods, e.g., seaweed (+) and rice (–), were associated with risk.	Reference period unclear and variable. No supplement use data. No biochemistry. Limited nutrient data. Not designed to assess specific nutrients. No comparison to general population, limited to traditional Japanese type diet.
There was little correlation between adolescent and adult intakes. There was a ↓ consumption of eggs, whole milk, butter, white bread, cereals, and candy in adults when compared to adolescent diets. As adult subjects consumed more red meat, fish, 2% milk, cheese, yogurt, ice cream, margarine, fruits and fruit juices, vegetables, and whole wheat bread than when they were adolescents. Adolescent diets high in saturated fats were not associated with ↑ risk; however, adult consumption of saturated fat was significantly associated with ↑ risk especially for aggressive prostate tumors.	75% of both cases and controls were Mormons and all subjects were Caucasian. Long retrospective diet reference period. No proxy interviews.

(*continued*)

APPENDIX TABLE   *(continued)*

		V. Other Cancer Sites	
Study	Type/Location	Subject Number and Description	Methods
Goodman et al., 1988	Case–control Hawaii	326 cases (226♂, 100 ♀) of *lung cancer.* 865 controls (597♂, 268♀) selected by random-digit-dialing and random selection from list of participants in the Hawaii State Health Surveillance Program. To supplement controls >65 subjects were selected from registries of the Health Care Financing Administration.	A structured interview was used to collect the following data: demographics, anthropometric data, a dietary history including the use of vitamin supplements, a lifetime history of tobacco use, coffee and alcohol consumption, and occupational exposure history. A food-frequency questionnaire was used. Reference period was a usual mo before the onset of symptoms or diagnosis for the cases and during the corresponding time period for the controls. Portion sizes were estimated with the use of photographs illustrating the 3 most representative serving sizes.
Jain et al., 1990	Case–control Toronto, Canada	839 cases of lung cancer; matched pairs of ♂ and ♀. 772 population-based controls, sex-matched to case pairs. Also matched for age (± 4 yr) and borough of residence. <33% refusal by eligible controls. Initial contact of subjects was by mail.	All subjects interviewed to gain data about SES factors, lifetime residences, occupational history, and detailed smoking history. 81-item food-frequency questionnaire emphasized vitamin and cholesterol intake. Subjects were asked to approximate portion sizes using reference food models. Data collected on use of vitamin and other nutritional supplements. Reference period was 1 yr prior to interview for all subjects. Proxy interviews (primarily spouses) were used for 34% of cases. Time between interview and diagnosis in cases was not reported.
Franceschi et al., 1991	Case–control northeast Italy	302 cases (266 ♂, 36 ♀) of *cancer of the oral cavity and pharynx.* 699 hospital-based controls (549 ♂, 150 ♀). Patients with cancer of the nasopharynx were excluded. No individual matching. All subjects were from the same cachement area.	All subjects given a standard questionnaire to obtain information abut SES factors, smoking habits, alcohol-consumption history, family and personal health history, and history of selected drug use. 40-item food-frequency questionnaire. Reference period was weekly consumption before the onset of the disease which led to the current admission. Reported changes in diet were infrequent, therefore recent diet was used. Procedure for estimation of portion size was not reported.
Shu et al., 1989	Case–control Shanghai, China	172 cases of epithelial ovarian cancer. 172 cases matched for age (± 5 yr) and residence.	All subjects interviewed about demographics, reproductive history, personal and family health histories, occupational history, and diet. 63 indigenous item food-frequency questionnaire about normal adult consumption. Subjects were asked to estimate portion sizes.
Slattery et al., 1989	Case–control Utah	85 cases of primary ovarian cancer. 492 population-based controls matched for age.	All subjects interviewed by women in person at home. Data collected included demographics, smoking history, medical history, contraceptive use, pregnancy history, and anthropometrics. 183-item food-frequency questionnaire used to obtain usual adult dietary habits. No reference period given. Subjects estimated portions consumed.

V. Other Cancer Sites

Results	Comments

A significant association between dietary cholesterol and lung cancer risk in ♂ but not in ♀. The significant trend held across ethnic groups.
The cholesterol effect was limited to current heavy cigarette smokers and to squamous and small cell types of lung cancer.
Similar effects were found for total and saturated fat. However, since saturated fat was so highly correlated with cholesterol intake, the effects of these nutrients could not be separated.

Variable time periods for reference period for cases.
No data presented regarding other nutrients or supplement use.
Among cases ≈30% were proxy interviews; ≈7% of control data was supplied by proxy interviews.

Significant ↑ risk (especially adenocarcinoma) associated with cholesterol intake.
Significantly ↓ risk associated with increased intake of vegetables.
No association between risk and total vitamin A, retinol, vitamin C, or fruit.
There was an irregular nonsignificant ↓ risk associated with β-carotene.
In the small number of supplement users, there was a significant inverse relationship between vitamin A and risk. (The form or amount of vitamin A was not available.)

Large portion of cases used proxy interviews.
52% of ♀ case interviews were by spouses.
Unknown time period between diagnosis and interview in cases could have resulted in long retrospective reference period.
Most of the cases (92.5%) were smokers as opposed to 61% of controls.

Significant risk factors included smoking and alcohol consumption.
Bread, pastry, salami, sausages, butter and sugar were positively associated with risk, while total consumption of vegetables and fresh fruit, apples, citrus fruits, and whole-grain bread or pasta were inversely associated with risk. After adjustment for non-nutrient risk factors, these foods were no longer significantly associated with risk. Adjusted risk ratios for frequent consumption of pasta or rice, polenta, cheese, eggs, and pulses were significantly associated with ↑ risk; whereas frequent consumption of carrots, fresh tomatoes, and green peppers was inversely related to risk.
Significantly ↑ risk associated with total and saturated fat (from animal origin).
There was no association between risk and vegetable fat.
No effect of dietary vitamin A or β-carotene.

No community-based controls.
Variable time periods between onset of symptoms and hospitalization in both cases and controls could have resulted in variability in reference period.
Lack of portion size estimation precluded the analysis of individual nutrients.
Lack of individual nutrient data prevents generalizability to other population groups and limits analysis to effect of indigenous foods studied.

No time frame between interview and diagnosis given.
No reference period given for cases.
No biochemistry, no supplement data, no descriptive statistics or comparisons to known standards of intake.
Groups were not matched for SES, cases were more educated.

There were no associations between risk and intakes of total calories, fat (saturated, mono- or polyunsaturated), protein, fiber, or vitamins A or C. After adjustment for age, number of pregnancies, and the body-mass index, there was significantly reduced risk associated with β-carotene intake.

Used nutrient analysis rather than food groups.
No supplement data.
Low response rate in cases.
51% of eligible cases completed the interview compared to 74% of eligible controls.

(*continued*)

APPENDIX TABLE   *(continued)*

Study	Type/Location	Subject Number and Description	Methods
La Vecchia et al., 1989	Case–control northern Italy	163 cases of histologically-confirmed (within 1 yr before interview) *bladder cancer* (total pool eligible not given). 181 hospital controls (HC).	All subjects given interviews to obtain information about SES factors, smoking, alcohol, coffee and other methylxanthine consumption habits, personal and family health history, and specific medication history. Subjects were asked about frequency of consumption of 10 food items. Reference period for cases was the period before onset of symtoms; none was given for controls.
Steineck et al., 1990	Case–control Stockholm, Sweden	418 cases of urothelial cancer and/or squamous cell cancer of the lower urinary tract (renal pelvis, bladder, ureter, urethra). 511 sex- and age-stratified randomly selected controls.	Questionnaire was mailed to all subjects and included health history, drug use, occupation, smoking, and "life events," diet. Surrogates were not used. 56-item food-frequency questionnaire. Reference period was dietary habits 3 yr prior to interview. Portion sizes were estimated with the use of photographs. Separate questions about supplement use; specifically vitamins A, B, and C and "other kinds of supplements and tonics." Study conducted 1985–1987, supplement use data after 1981 was ignored.
Franceschi et al., 1989	Case–control northeast Italy	208 cases of *non-Hodgkin's lymphoma* (110♂, 98 ♀) diagnosed 2 yr prior to interview. 401 hospital-based controls (215 ♂, 186 ♀) from the same cachement area.	All subjects questioned about SES indicators, smoking history, alcohol and methylxanthine (e.g., coffee, tea, cola) beverage consumption, and frequency of consumption of 14 selected food items. Neither reference period nor method of portion size estimation was reported.
Mettlin et al., 1990	Cross-sectional New York	3334 cases of cancer. Sites included: 163 oral cavity, 115 stomach, 504 colon, 312 rectum, 542 lung, 848 breast, 231 uterus, 233 cervix, 442 prostate, 178 bladder. 1300 controls seen at the same hospital.	All patients answered questions about smoking, alcohol use, diet, occupation, family health, residence, and personal medical history. Specific emphasis of this study was on the frequency of consumption of whole milk, 2% milk, and skim milk during the period immediately preceding current illness.
Hursting et al., 1990	Cross-sectional International (20 countries)	Average cancer incidence data for breast (♀), cervix, prostate, colon (♂ and♀) and lung (♂and♀) for the yr 1973–1977 were taken from Cancer Incidence in Five Continents (20 countries included in analysis). Incidence rates were truncated to ages 35–64 yr.	Estimates of per capita disappearance of total fat, poly- and monounsaturated fat, saturated fat, fish n-3 and n-6 polyunsaturated fat, and total calories, and dietary and crude fiber for the 20 countries included in the analyses were calculated or taken directly from Food Balance Sheets published by the United Nations Food and Agricultural Organization and concurrent with the incidence data. Per capita lipid consumption was calculated from grams of fat contained in 68 fat-containing foods.

Results	Comments
There was no association between intake of fat and cancer risk. The frequency of consumption of green vegetables and carrots was significantly lower in cases. Estimated intakes of carotenoids and total vitamin A but not retinoids were significantly less in cases than controls. There was increased risk for BC associated with estimated low intakes of both carotenoids and retinol. Protective effect was stronger in current smokers. No effect from either fruit or vitamin C.	Reference period was at least 2 yr before interview for cases. Very limited number of items (10) on food-frequency questionnaire. Lack of portion size estimation precluded the analysis of individual nutrients. Lack of individual nutrient data prevents generalizability to other population groups and limits analysis to effect of indigenous foods studied. No supplement use data. No community-based controls.
Total fat and fried foods were significantly associated with increased risk. Supplemental intake of vitamin A (uncharacterized as to form or amounts) was inversely associated with risk.	The nature of the collection of the dietary data set was not clearly delineated. An apparently long retrospective period between diet and supplement use reference period and study interview. Vitamin supplements broadly categorized, e.g., vitamin B or vitamin A.
Consumption of milk, liver, butter, oil (primarily polyunsaturated), and methylzanthine beverages were associated with risk. Consumption of whole grain bread and pasta was inversely related to risk.	No reference period given, however cases were diagnosed within 2 yr of interview indicating a long retrospective recall. Limited food-frequency database.
Elevated risks for frequent consumption of whole milk relative to not drinking milk were found for cancers of the oral cavity, stomach, colon, rectum, lung, bladder, breast, and cervix. Drinking reduced fat milk was associated with significant risk reduction for oral and cervical cancers. Drinking whole milk exclusively was related to significant risk for cancer of the oral cavity, stomach, rectum, lung, and breast.	There was no defined and matched reference period. No other data for nutritional intake was presented. Milk consumption was not evaluated within the context of other dietary or nondietary risk factors. No community-based controls.
Total fat intake was strongly associated with cancer of the breast, colon, and prostate even after adjustment for total calorie intake. Cancers of the lung and cervix were not correlated with dietary fat intake. Saturated fat was positively associated with incidence of cancers of the breast, colon, and prostate and polyunsaturated fat was associated with incidence of breast and prostate cancers but not colon cancer. Fiber intake, when included in the analysis, affected the magnitude of the fat cancer correlations, particularly between total fat and colon cancer.	No direct measure of intake. No comparison with other population groups. No analysis by sex. No control for demographic or other potential confounders that might exist within or between countries. The estimated per capita intakes of nutrients studied appear well above data of national survey such as NHANES II. Use of disappearance data does not account for wastage, e.g., fat trim or discarded cooking oil, thereby creating the possibility of overestimation of intake.

Lipids and Cancer: An Update

Kenneth K. Carroll, Ph.D.

Since the original review was completed in 1991, there has been continued strong interest in the role of dietary lipids in cancer. A number of additional reviews have been published, some of which were developed from presentations at scientific meetings. These include reviews focusing on breast cancer (Boyd, 1993; Carroll, 1991, 1992; Chlebowski et al., 1992; Cohen et al., 1993; Dao and Hilf, 1992; Dwyer, 1992; Fernandez and Venkatraman, 1992; Harris et al., 1992; Kinlen, 1991; Welsch, 1992a; Wynder et al., 1992c); colon cancer (Reddy, 1992; Wynder et al., 1992a); pancreatic cancer (Roebuck, 1992) and prostatic cancer (Boyle and Zaridze, 1993; Rose and Connolly, 1992). Other reviews deal more generally with dietary lipids and cancer (Doll, 1992; Greenwald, 1992; James and Ralph, 1992; La Vecchia, 1992; Roberfroid, 1991; Weinstein, 1991) or with specific dietary lipids, such as those enriched in n-3 and n-6 polyunsaturated fatty acids (Cave, 1991a,b; De Vries and van Noorden, 1992; Galli and Butrum, 1991; Man-Fan Wan et al., 1991; Simopoulos, 1991). A considerable number of new reports on epidemiological studies have been published and these will be considered under the headings used in the original review.

Correlational Studies

Kesteloot et al. (1991) found that the well-known intercountry differences in cancers of various sites were significantly correlated with intake of dairy fat plus lard. The findings were interpreted as supporting an important role for saturated fat in cancer promotion. A more recent study from the same laboratory (Sasaki et al., 1993) showed a highly significant positive correlation between intake of animal fat minus fish fat and breast cancer mortality in women over 50. There was also a significant positive relationship between the change with time in animal fat minus fish fat and breast cancer mortality. Whenever significant, dietary fish fat intake correlated negatively and vegetable fat correlated positively with breast cancer mortality.

The mortality rate for breast cancer is lower in Southern Italy than in Northern Italy or the U.S.A. This is associated with lower intakes of both saturated and polyunsaturated fat in Southern Italy (Taoli et al., 1991a).

In a study covering 65 counties in China, breast-cancer mortality in women over 55 was compared with lipid intake measured by a dietary survey and various indicators of lipid intake, such as plasma total and LDL cholesterol (Marshall et al., 1992). The results provide modest support for a link between lipid intake and risk of breast cancer, and indicate that the association of fat intake with risk does not appear to be a result of confounding by calorie intake.

Cancer incidence rates among Chinese in Shanghai and Americans in Connecticut showed quite large differences for cancers at different sites, ranging from 26-fold for prostate cancer and tenfold for breast cancer to fourfold for colon cancer and twofold for rectal cancer (Yu et al., 1991). The incidence rates for Shanghai are 20–30 percent higher than in China as a whole and thus are not representative of the entire Chinese population.

A comparison of Chinese and Chinese-American diets in small groups of subjects indicated that the latter are higher in fat and protein and lower in carbohydrates (Yeung et al., 1991). Feces of the Chinese-Americans contained more cholesterol and bile acids and their urine contained more 3-methyl-histidine and malonaldehyde. It was suggested that these dietary differences may be responsible for the fourfold higher risk of colorectal cancer in Chinese-Americans.

Other studies have indicated a correlation between fat intake and cancers of various sites. Henderson (1992a) summarized the results of a series of analyses of international variations in annual incidence rates of reproductive organ and gastrointestinal cancers in relation to dietary fat and calculated that a 50 percent reduction in fat consumption among the U.S. population aged 55–69 years could reduce the incidence of these cancers 29–83 percent. Two studies, one comparing Northern and Southern Italy (Taoli et al., 1991b) and the other comparing the U.S.A. and Japan (Wynder et al., 1992b) have provided evidence supporting earlier evidence from intercountry data of a positive association between lung cancer mortality and fat intake. In a correlational study based on data from 59 countries, stepwise regression results for oral cancer showed increased risk from vegetable oil and excess animal fat. For esophageal cancer, stepwise results indicated increased risk for vegetable oil consumption (Hebert et al., 1993).

Migrant Studies

A study of cancer in migrants to Argentina from other Latin American countries, Europe and Asia has been reported by Matos et al. (1991). For cancers of the colon and breast, most countries of origin had lower mortality rates than Argentina and the rates in the migrants tended to converge towards that of the Argentina natives. It was suggested that the high mortality from breast and colon cancer in Argentina may be related to high consumption of animal fat compared to that of most of the migrants' countries of origin.

Incidence rates of colon and rectal cancer for Chinese-Americans in San Francisco were about the same as the rates for Americans in Connecticut, whereas the rates of postmenopausal breast cancer and prostate cancer of Chinese-Americans were intermediate between those of Shanghai Chinese and Connecticut Americans. This indicates that environmental factors have a more gradual effect on cancers of the breast and prostate compared to cancers of the colon and rectum (Yu et al., 1991).

Time-Trend Studies

Cox and Little (1992) have analyzed the trends for age-standardized mortality and incidence rates of colorectal cancer for males and females in New Zealand over the past 30 years. The rates increased in men and women aged 40–74 over this period but decreased in the younger age groups. Breast cancer mortality increased in both age groups and breast cancer incidence was similar, except for a decline in the younger age group towards the end of the period. It was suggested that these trends are related to environmental influences, such as changes in dietary fat consumption, and that a significant proportion of the lifetime risk of colorectal cancer may be determined before age 30.

Trends in cancer mortality in Europe (La Vecchia et al., 1992a–c) and in the Americas (La Vecchia et al., 1993) have recently been published. For Europe, these provide mortality data for 27 cancer sites or groups of sites, plus total cancer mortality in 28 countries over the period 1955–1989. For the Americas, similar data are presented for 14 Central and South American countries, plus the U.S.A. and Canada, for the same time period. The data are presented with a minimum of comment but can be useful for those who wish to compare them with environmental factors, such as dietary fat intake.

Cohort Studies

In an eight-year follow-up of their cohort of approximately 90,000 nurses, Willett et al. (1992) continued to find no evidence of a positive association between dietary fat and breast cancer, even though the range of fat intake was somewhat greater and a more detailed and precise dietary questionnaire was used.

Graham et al. (1992) followed 18,556 postmenopausal women in New York State from 1980 to 1987 and found no increase in risk of breast cancer related to intake of calories, vitamins A, C or E or dietary fat. In a further report on a cohort of 56,837 women enrolled in the Canadian National Breast Screening Study over the period 1982–1987, Rohan et al. (1993) observed modest reductions in risk with increasing intake of retinol, β-carotene and vitamin C, but no association with vitamin E. Another prospective cohort study of 62,573 postmenopausal women in The Netherlands from 1986 to 1989 showed no significant association between total fat intake and risk of breast cancer (Van den Brandt et al., 1993). There was some evidence of a weak positive relationship with saturated fat, but not for other types of fat or cholesterol.

In a population-based study in Denmark, 1,744 patients diagnosed with breast cancer in 1983–94 were followed until mid-1990. No significant association was found between survival, reproduction or hormonal risk factors and environmental factors, including dietary variables (Ewertz et al., 1991).

Holm et al. (1993) interviewed 240 women, aged 50–65 years with stage I–II breast cancer, about their dietary histories and followed them for 4 years. Of the total, 209 were postmenopausal. The 30 patients with estrogen-receptor-rich tumors who had treatment failure reported higher intakes of total fat, saturated fatty acids and polyunsaturated fatty acids than the 119 patients with estrogen-receptor-rich tumors who did not have treatment failure. No association between dietary habits and treatment failure was found for women with estrogen-receptor-poor cancers.

Giovannucci et al. (1992) used data from the Health Professionals Follow-Up Study to investigate relationships between diet and colorectal adenomas. The results showed a positive association with saturated fat after adjustment for energy intake, while sources of fiber (vegetables, fruits and grains) were associated with decreased risk. Kritchevsky (1992b) analyzed data from the National Health and Nutrition Survey Epidemiologic Follow-Up Study conducted between 1971 and 1984, and found that male cases consumed more cholesterol and saturated fat whereas female cases consumed less cholesterol and fat than noncases. The findings differed somewhat, depending on whether the subjects had central or peripheral obesity. The results indicate that diet cannot explain the low-blood-cholesterol–cancer association in men.

Shekelle et al. (1991) reported an increased risk of lung cancer associated with consumption of cholesterol from eggs.

Hirayama (1992) has reviewed and presented new data on the large scale cohort study begun in Japan in 1965. Daily consumption of meat was associated with elevated risk for cancer of the stomach, colon, lung, cervix and prostate, and frequent consumption of high-fat foods with risk of breast, ovarian and pancreatic cancers. Trends in breast and colorectal cancer tended to follow those of animal fat consumption. Daily consumption of green and yellow vegetables was correlated with reduced risk for cancer of the stomach, colon, lung, cervix and prostate.

Case–Control Studies

Graham et al. (1991) found no association between dietary fat and risk of breast cancer in a case–control study conducted in New York between 1986 and 1989. On the other hand,

D'Avanzo et al. (1991) observed a positive association with butter, oil and total season-ing fat, in a study conducted in Italy.

In another case–control study in The Netherlands, early stage postmenopausal but not premenopausal breast cancer patients showed a central body-fat distribution more often than controls. This was significantly related to higher serum triglyceride levels and lower concentrations of sex-hormone-binding globulin. It was suggested that this is associated with lifestyle factors and might increase the risk of breast cancer as a result of greater bioavailability of estradiol at the tissue level (Bruning et al., 1992). Obesity and lower consumption of green-yellow vegetables and dairy products were found to be associated with increased risk of postmenopausal breast cancer in a case–control study in Japan, but there was no increase in risk associated with consumption of high-fat foods (Kato et al., 1992). Data on the fatty acid consumption of serum phospholipids from breast cancer cases and controls in Norway suggested that dietary linoleic acid may decrease risk of breast cancer. No such association was observed for n-3 polyunsaturated fatty acids of marine origin (Vatten et al., 1993). In a very recent study of postmenopausal women, London et al. (1993) observed no consistent patterns of association between breast cancer risk and any of the categories of fatty acids in subcutaneous adipose tissue.

Case–control studies of colon or colorectal cancer have been reported from Majorca (Benito et al., 1991); Italy (Bidoli et al., 1992); Argentina (Iscovich et al., 1992); England (Little et al., 1993); U.S.A. (Peters et al., 1992); Australia (Steinmetz and Potter, 1993); Greece (Trichopoulou et al., 1992); and Russia (Zaridze et al., 1993). In general, the find-ings indicate positive associations with animal products, including meat, dairy products and eggs, and negative associations with fruits and vegetables. In one study, total energy intake, contributed primarily by carbohydrate, was associated with increased risk (Iscovich et al., 1992). Another showed no association with total saturated or monounsat-urated fat after adjustment for total energy intake, though there was a positive association with polyunsaturated fat (Little et al., 1993). However, Zaridze et al. (1993) found a neg-ative association with polyunsaturated fat. These workers reported a decreased risk with high milk consumption.

A case–control study of diet and pancreatic cancer in Australia provided evidence that cases consumed more eggs, as well as sweet and fatty food items, than controls (Baghurst et al., 1991). Several nutrients derived principally from plants were associated with lower risks. Another study conducted between 1984 and 1988 in The Netherlands showed increased risk associated with consumption of eggs and fish and a protective effect from daily consumption of vegetables (de Mesquita et al., 1991) .

A case–control study of diet and prostatic cancer in Italy showed a significant positive correlation with consumption of milk but not with other dietary sources of animal fat (La Vecchia et al., 1991). In another case–control study of prostatic cancer in Spain, Bravo et al. (1991) reported that risk increased with diets rich in animal fats and meats, but not with diets rich in vegetable fats. Benito and Cabeza (1993) have recently provided an overview of Spanish studies on diet and cancer risk in which they emphasize the low incidence rates in the Mediterranean area for most tumors associated with diet and repeated observations of a protective effect of high vegetable consumption.

A case–control study in Norway (Glattre et al., 1993) and an earlier study in Hawaii (Kolonel et al., 1990) provided some evidence that the high incidence of thyroid cancer in many coastal regions is associated with greater consumption of seafood in those areas.

Further evidence that risk of lung cancer is increased by consumption of high-fat foods was provided by a population-based case–control study in Hawaii (Goodman et al., 1992). Saturated fat was associated with increased risk of bladder cancer in a multicenter case–control study in Spain (Riboli et al., 1991). Intake of vitamin E was related to a slightly reduced risk, but there was no association with retinol or carotene. In a study of diet and gastric cancer in Belgium, there was no clear association with most sources of fat, but a decreased risk was observed for oils with a high P/S ratio. Most vegetables and fresh fruit were protective (Tuyns et al., 1992).

Intervention Studies

The role of intervention trials and their place among the current approaches to breast cancer prevention have been discussed by Dwyer (1992) and Henderson (1992b, 1993). After a number of years of feasibility studies, a modified version of the Women's Health Trial has been approved for a full-scale study coordinated by the Hutchinson Cancer Centre in Seattle (Freedman et al., 1993; Whittemore and Henderson, 1993).

Other ongoing studies designed to investigate whether a low-fat diet can reduce the risk of breast cancer include one involving women with benign breast disease who show evidence of being at higher risk than the general population (Boyd et al., 1992), as well as studies in the United States and Scandinavia designed to assess the use of dietary fat reduction as a potential addition to adjuvant therapy of breast cancer patients (Chlebowski et al., 1991; Nordevang et al., 1992). Sheppard et al. (1991) have provided further documentation of weight loss in women who reduce the proportion of fat in their diet. Evidence in support of the use of a low-fat diet as adjuvant therapy for postmenopausal breast cancer patients has recently been reviewed by Cohen et al. (1993).

Assessment of Dietary Fat Intake

For intercountry correlational studies, fat intake is normally estimated from food disappearance data (e.g., FAO, 1991). The total amount of fat available for consumption is then divided by the number of people to give an estimate of per capita consumption. This provides no information on the consumption of particular individuals and overestimates the amount of fat actually consumed. However, if dietary fat is expressed as percent of total calories, the values are reasonably close to those estimated by more precise methods (Carroll, 1986), although differences have been documented (Stephen and Wald, 1990). In cases where the fat intake of different countries differs by substantial amounts, one can assume that there will not be much overlap in the fat intake of individuals in the two countries. Sasaki and Kesteloot (1992) compared the FAO data with the per person intake obtained from 52 individual dietary surveys in 19 countries and concluded that the FAO data were valid for use in epidemiologic studies. They suggested, however, that it would be better to use them expressed either as a percentage of energy or as ratios of the different dietary components.

For other types of epidemiological studies, attempts are made to estimate the dietary fat intake of individuals by means of questionnaires or interviews and are usually based on dietary recall, food frequency data or dietary records maintained over short periods of time. These methods are susceptible to a variety of errors in measurement and may also be affected by inaccuracy and bias in dietary recall (Wynder, 1992). The fatty acid composition of subcutaneous adipose tissue offers a possible objective means of assessing intake of polyunsaturated and *trans* fatty acids (London et al., 1991).

Friedenreich et al. (1991) asked a group of cases and controls from the Canadian National Breast Screening Study to complete a second questionnaire recalling their dietary intake an average of 4.6 years earlier, prior to their enrollment in the study. The mean nutrient intakes were very similar for the prospective and retrospective questionnaires and did not provide evidence of recall bias.

Hammar and Norell (1991) used a questionnaire to investigate dietary recall over a 20-year period from 1967 to 1987. They found that cases of colorectal cancer and controls had a similar tendency to overestimate or underestimate their previous food intake. In a study of dietary recall by cases and controls from a multiethnic cohort over a period of up to 8–10 years, Wilkens et al. (1992) found that recall values for macronutrients were consistently higher than original levels in both cases and controls. Of five major ethnic groups, the Japanese had the best recall of their past diets. Overall, the results suggested that differential misclassification in dietary case–control studies may pose a significant problem in some instances.

In a review of 17 studies that examined either the relative validity or reliability of retrospective dietary reporting, Friedenreich et al. (1992) found that current diet exerted a strong influence on recall of past diet: correlation coefficients between original and recalled diets decreased with increasing time interval; highest coefficients were observed for foods consumed either habitually or rarely; diet stability improved recall; and increased age was associated with poorer recall.

Analysis of 3 days of dietary records from 13,388 adults in the 1977–1978 Nationwide Food Consumption Survey by Neuhaus et al. (1991) showed that within-person variability to between-person variability for 13 nutrients was very large and would result in attenuated linear regression estimates of diet–health associations. The magnitude of the attenuation decreased with age, particularly for men, indicating that fewer days of dietary intake per person would be required to assess diet–health relationships in older compared to younger adults. Wynder and Stellman (1992) have pointed out the difficulty of detecting differences in cancer incidence related to dietary fat in situations where cases and controls are both eating a relatively high-fat diet.

Factors involved in adherence to a low-fat diet in the Women's Health Trial have been examined (Urban et al., 1992). Attendance at educational sessions and an acquired distaste for fat encourage adherence, whereas costliness of the diet in time and money, and feelings of deprivation, discourage adherence. Substitutions of specially manufactured low-fat foods are easily adopted but reducing meat consumption and reliance on fats as food flavoring requires long-term reinforcement strategies (Kristal et al., 1992). Specific changes in food choices associated with adoption of a low-fat diet have been documented by Nordevang et al. (1992b).

In another study patterned after the Women's Health Trial, no specific attempt was made to recruit women at high risk for breast cancer (Heber et al., 1992). Investigation of assessment of objective methods of adherence to the low-fat diet in this study confirmed earlier observations of weight loss and reduction of plasma cholesterol levels with little change in plasma triglycerides.

Effects of Dietary Fat on Biomarkers of Cancer Risk

A number of studies have dealt with effects of dietary fat on biomarkers of risk of breast cancer (Cohen et al., 1993). For example, Baghurst et al. (1992), using 24-hr recall data, observed significant positive association between plasma prolactin concentration and saturated fatty acid intake in a group of 249 women with a history of nonskin cancers among first-degree female relatives.

Crighton et al. (1992) studied 19 postmenopausal and 18 premenopausal women who reduced their fat intake from 37.2 to 23.2 percent and from 37.9 to 24.3 percent respectively over a 4-week period. The postmenopausal group showed a minor increase in the circulating level of sex-hormone-binding globulin and a small decrease in prolactin, but no changes in free or total estradiol. The premenopausal group showed no significant changes in any of the hormone levels investigated. Rose et al. (1992) found that reduction of dietary fat to 20 percent of calories had no effect on either sex-hormone-binding globulin concentration or distribution of estrogen in a small group of breast cancer patients followed for 6–12 months.

Anti et al. (1992) found that supplementation of the diet of patients having sporadic adenomatous colorectal polyps with fish oil to provide 4.3 g/d of eicosapentaenoic acid and 3.6 g/d of docosahexaenoic acid reduced the number of replicative S-phase cells in the upper part of colonic crypts after only 2 weeks of treatment. The reduction was main-tained for the 12 weeks of the study. These cells are considered to be a reliable marker of colon cancer risk. These authors and Wargovich (1992) have discussed the possibility that ω-3 fatty acids in fish oils inhibit cell proliferation by competing with ω-6 fatty acids, while Gonzales (1992) has considered the possibility that lipid peroxidation is a factor in growth inhibition by the highly unsaturated ω-3 fatty acids.

Geltner-Allinger et al. (1991) found no significant differences in the concentration of bile acids in the aqueous phase of feces from colon cancer patients or controls, or in rates of proliferation of colonic epithelial cells. They concluded that it may be premature to rely too heavily on either of these markers to predict risk of developing the disease. Clausen et al. (1991) observed a low ratio of formation of colonic butyrate compared to total short-chain fatty acids in patients with colonic cancer and adenomas compared to healthy controls, and suggested that this may increase the risk of colon cancer.

Dietary saturated fat has been associated with an increased risk of colon cancer and Schneider (1992) has hypothesized that this may involve inhibition of colon epithelial cell glutathione-*S*-transferase by lithocholic acid, one of the major secondary bile acids. Since glutathione-*S*-transferase detoxifies genotoxins, this could allow mutagens to per-sist in colonic epithelial cells while proliferation is stimulated by secondary bile acids.

Discussion

Further studies will undoubtedly be required to resolve the differences of opinion that exist regarding the significance of dietary fat in breast cancer (Freedman et al., 1993; Hiller and McMichael, 1990; Howe, 1990; Prentice and Sheppard, 1990; Whittemore and Henderson, 1993; Willett and Stampfer, 1990). Although intercountry comparisons show a strong positive correlation with dietary fat, which is supported by studies on experimen-tal animals (Boyd, 1993; Carroll, 1992; Doll, 1992), cohort studies and case–control stud-ies have generally given equivocal results. In particular, Willett et al. (1992) have been unable to find any association between dietary fat and breast cancer in their cohort of American nurses, although the same cohort has shown a positive correlation between dietary animal fat and colon cancer (Willett et al., 1990).

This difference may be related to differing patterns of development of cancer at these two sites. Experiments with animals have shown that mammary cancer can be induced much more readily in young animals when the mammary glands are developing (Carroll et al., 1989). The state of development of the mammary glands is probably also an important factor in human breast cancer (Russo et al., 1992). The latent period for breast cancer may thus be longer on average than for colon cancer, and this could help to explain why incidence and mortality tend to change more slowly for breast cancer than for colon cancer in studies on migrants (Berg, 1975) and in time–trend studies in countries such as Japan (Willett, 1989).

Another reason for thinking that initiation of breast cancer often occurs soon after puberty is that early menarche and longer time between menarche and first pregnancy are associated with increased risk (De Waard, 1992). Early menarche could be related to high-fat diets associated with higher energy intake, and this may also help to explain observations that taller women are more susceptible to breast cancer (Vatten et al., 1992).

Early menarche is probably a result of increased estrogen levels, which could facilitate initiation and development of preneoplastic mammary lesions (De Waard, 1992).

Obesity is also associated with increased risk of breast cancer (De Waard, 1992) and colon cancer (Colditz, 1992). The economic costs of breast and colon cancer related to obesity were estimated to be $1.9 billion for 1986 in the United States (Colditz, 1992). It has been postulated that the high incidence of hormone-related cancers of the breast, endometrium and prostate may be at least partially related to central body fat accummulation (Bruning et al., 1992).

Obesity can be exacerbated by a sedentary lifestyle and by high-fat diets because of their high energy density and the more efficient utilization of dietary fat, compared to dietary carbohydrate and protein (Donato, 1987; Tucker and Kano, 1992). Conditions that favor obesity are also likely to increase the fat content of the mammary gland and this may be particularly effective in promoting breast cancer because of its intimate association with mammary epithelial tissue, where breast cancer normally develops (Carroll and Parenteau, 1991). De Waard et al. (1992) have provided evidence of the feasibility of weight reduction as an adjuvant treatment of breast cancer in obese postmenopausal patients.

The importance of caloric intake and energy balance for cancer, as opposed to specific effects of dietary fat, is a subject of continuing debate (Jacobs, 1992). Women who participated in organized athletics in college were reported by Frisch et al. (1992) to have a lower lifetime occurrence rate of cancers of the reproductive system and breast cancer than their nonathletic classmates. The studies of Paffenberger et al. (1992) were less consistent in showing a relationship between physical activity and cancer. Evidence from experiments in animal cancer models, including effects of exercise and of dietary restriction, have emphasized the influence of caloric balance on carcinogenesis (Boutwell, 1992; Cohen et al., 1992; Kritchevsky, 1992a; Rogers, 1992; Thompson, 1992; Welsch, 1992b) but other evidence from both animal experiments (Freedman et al., 1990) and epidemiological data (Sasaki et al., 1993) continue to indicate that fat plays a role in breast cancer.

The search continues for mechanisms by which dietary fat may influence breast cancer. Dao and Hilf (1992) discuss these in terms of direct or indirect effects mediated by changes in the hormonal milieu. These are not mutually exclusive and may involve an interaction between fatty acids and hormones on mammary tumor growth. The possible role of prostaglandins is also considered. Fatty acids, hormones and prostaglandins may also be involved in the promotion of prostatic cancer, but in this case there is less evidence that dietary fat has an important influence (Rose and Connolly, 1992).

Reddy (1992) has reviewed possible mechanisms by which dietary fat may influence colon cancer. The predominant theory is that dietary fat increases the concentration of secondary bile acids in the colon, which have been shown to act as promoting agents. Pancreatic cancer can be suppressed in the rat by an increase in exercise or a decrease in caloric intake, but promotion by dietary fat appears to be only partly related to the high caloric content of fat (Giles and Roebuck, 1992; Roebuck, 1992).

Based on the totality of the scientific evidence, and significant scientific agreement among qualified experts that diets low in fat may reduce the risk of some cancers, the Food and Drug Administration (1993) has concluded that claims of certain foods relating fat reduction to reduced risk of cancer are justified.

Conclusions

Recent publications on lipids and cancer have done little to alter the conclusions reached at the time of original completion of this review. There continues to be a consensus that reducing the fat content of the diet would decrease the risk of some types of cancer, although the mechanisms involved remain unclear.

Bibliography

Anti, M.; Marra, G.; Armelao, F.; Bartoli, G.M.; Ficarelli, R.; Percesepe, A.; De Vitis, I.; Maria, G.; Sofo, L.; Rapaccini, G.L.; Gentiloni, N.; Piccioni, E. and Miggiano, G. 1992. Effect of ω-3 fatty acids on rectal mucosal cell proliferation in subjects at risk for colon cancer. *Gastroenterol.* 102:883–891.

Baghurst, P.A.; Carman, J.A.; Syrete, J.A.; Baghurst, K.I. and Crocker, J.M. 1992. Diet, prolactin, and breast cancer. *Am. J. Clin. Nutr.* 56:943–949.

Baghurst, P.A.; McMichael, A.J.; Slavotinek, A.H.; Baghurst, K.I.; Boyle, P. and Walker, A.M. 1991. A case–control study of diet and cancer of the pancreas. *Am. J. Epidemiol.* 134:167–179.

Benito, E. and Cabeza, E. 1993. Diet and cancer risk: An overview of Spanish studies. *Eur. J. Cancer Prev.* 2:215–219.

Benito, E.; Stiggelbout, A.; Bosch, F.X.; Obrador, A.; Kaldor, J.; Mulet, M. and Munoz, N. 1991. Nutritional factors in colorectal cancer risk: A case–control study in Majorca. *Int. J. Cancer* 49:161–167.

Berg, J.W. 1975. Can nutrition explain the pattern of international epidemiology of hormone-dependent cancers? *Cancer Res.* 35:3345–3350.

Bidoli, E.; Franceschi, S.; Talamini, R.; Barra, S. and La Vecchia, C. 1992. Food consumption and cancer of the colon and rectum in North-Eastern Italy. *Int. J. Cancer* 50:223–229.

Boutwell, R.K. 1992. Caloric intake, dietary fat level, and experimental carcinogenesis. In: Jacobs, M.M.; ed. *Adv. Exp. Med. Biol.,* Vol. 322. Exercise, Calories, Fat and Cancer. New York: Plenum Press. pp. 95–101.

Boyd, N.F. 1993. Nutrition and breast cancer. *J. Natl. Cancer. Inst.* 85:6–7.

Boyd, N.F.; Cousins, M.; Lockwood, G. and Tritchler, D. 1992. Dietary fat and breast cancer risk: The feasibility of a clinical trial of breast cancer prevention. *Lipids* 27:821–826.

Boyle, P. and Zaridze, D.G. 1993. Risk factors for prostate and testicular cancer. *Eur. J. Cancer* 29:1048–1055.

Bravo, M.; Castellanos, E. and del Ray Calero, J. 1991. Dietary factors and prostatic cancer. *Urology Int.* 46:163–166.

Bruning, P.F.; Bonfrer, J.M.G.; Hart, A.A.M.; Van Noord, P.A.H.; Van Der Hoeven, H.; Collette, H.J.A.; Battermann, J.J.; De Jong-Bakker, M.; Nooijen, W.J. and De Waard, F. 1992. Body measurements, estrogen availability and the risk of human breast cancer: A case–control study. *Int. J. Cancer* 51:14–19.

Carroll, K.K. 1986. Experimental studies on dietary fat and cancer in relation to epidemiological data. In: Ip, C.; Birt, D.F.; Rogers, A.E. and Mettlin, C.; eds. *Proc. Clin. Biol. Res.* Vol. 222, Dietary Fat and Cancer. New York: Alan R. Liss, Inc. pp. 231–248.

Carroll, K.K. 1991. Dietary fat as a promoter of mammary cancer: Evidence pro and con. In: Hin, C.Y.; Wai, T.N.K.; Siong, T.E. and Noor, M.I.; eds. *Proc. 6th Asian Congress of Nutrition.* Kuala Lumpur: The Nutrition Society of Malaysia. pp. 206–211.

Carroll, K.K. 1992. Dietary fat and breast cancer. *Lipids* 27:793–797.

Carroll, K.K.; Jacobson, E.A. and James, K.A. 1989. Role of dietary fat in carcinogenesis. In: Kabara, J.J. ed. *The Pharmacological Effects of Lipids III.* Champaign, IL: American Oil Chemists' Society. pp. 129–135.

Cave, W.T., Jr. 1991a. Dietary n-3 (ω-3) polyunsaturated fatty acid diet effects on animal tumorigenesis. *FASEB J.* 5:2160–2166.

Cave, W.T., Jr. 1991b. Omega-3 fatty acid diet effects on tumorigenesis in experimental animals. *World Rev. Nutr. Dietet.* 66:462–476.

Chlebowski, R.T.; Rose, D.; Buzzard, M.; Blackburn, G.L.; Insull, W., Jr.; Grosvenor, M.; Elashoff, R. and Wynder, E.L. 1992. Adjuvant dietary fat intake reduction in postmenopausal breast cancer patient management. *Breast Cancer Res. Treatment* 20:73–84.

Clausen, M.R.; Bonnen, H. and Mortensen, P.B. 1991. Colonic fermentation of dietary fibre to short chain fatty acids in patients with adenomatous polyps and colonic cancer. *Gut* 32:923–928.

Cohen, L.A.; Boylan, E.; Epstein, M. and Zang, F. 1992. Voluntary exercise and experimental mammary cancer. In: Jacobs, M.M. ed. *Adv. Exp. Med. Biol.,* Vol. 322. Exercise, Calories, Fat and Cancer. New York: Plenum Press. pp. 41–59.

Cohen, L.A.; Rose, D.P. and Wynder, E.L. 1993. A rationale for dietary intervention in post-menopausal breast cancer patients: An update. *Nutr. Cancer* 19:1–10.

Colditz, G.A. 1992. Economic costs of obesity. *Am. J. Clin. Nutr.* 55:503S–507S.

Cox, B. and Little, J. 1992. Reduced risk of colorectal cancer among recent generations in New Zealand. *Br. J. Cancer* 66:386–390.

Crighton, I.L.; Dowsett, M.; Hunter, M.; Shaw, C. and Smith, I.E. 1992. The effect of a low-fat diet on hormone levels in healthy pre- and postmenopausal women: Relevance for breast cancer. *Eur. J. Cancer* 28A:2024–2027.

Dao, T.L. and Hilf, R. 1992. Dietary fat and breast cancer: A search for mechanisms. In: Jacobs, M.M. ed. *Adv. Exp. Med. Biol.,* Vol. 322. Exercise, Calories, Fat and Cancer. New York: Plenum Press. pp. 221–237.

D'Avanzo, B.; Negri, E.; Gramenzi, A.; Franceschi, S.; Parazzini, F.; Boyle, P. and La Vecchia, C. 1991. Fats in seasoning and breast cancer risk: An Italian case–control study. *Eur. J. Cancer* 27:420–423.

De Mesquita, H.B.B.; Maisonneuve, P.; Runia, S. and Moerman, C.J. 1991. Intake of foods and nutrients and cancer of the exocrine pancreas: A population-based case–control study in The Netherlands. *Int. J. Cancer* 48:540–549.

De Vries, C.E.E. and van Noorden, C.J.F. 1992. Effects of dietary fatty acid composition on tumor growth and metastasis. *Anticancer Res.* 12:1513–1522.

De Waard, F. 1992. Preventive intervention in breast cancer, but when? *Eur. J. Cancer Prevent.* 1:395–399.

De Waard, F.; Ramlau, R.; Mulders, Y.; de Vries, T. and van Waveren, S. 1992. A feasibility study on weight reduction in obese postmenopausal breast cancer patients. *Eur. J. Cancer Prev.* 2:233–238.

Doll, R. 1992. The lessons of life: Keynote address to the Nutrition and Cancer Conference. *Cancer Res.* 52:2024S–2029S.

Donato, K.A. 1987. Efficiency and utilization of various energy sources for growth. *Am. J. Clin. Nutr.* 45:164S–167S.

Dwyer, J.J. 1992. Dietary fat and breast cancer: Testing interventions to reduce risks. In: Jacobs, M.M. ed. *Adv. Exp. Med. Biol.,* Vol. 322. Exercise, Calories, Fat and Cancer. New York: Plenum Press. pp. 155–183.

Ewertz, M.; Gillanders, S.; Meyer, L. and Zedeler, K. 1991. Survival of breast cancer patients in relation to factors which affect the risk of developing breast cancer. *Int. J. Cancer* 49:526–530.

FAO. 1991. *Food Balance Sheets, 1984–1986.* Average. Rome: Food and Agriculture Organization of the United Nations.

Fernandez, G. and Venkatraman, J.T. 1992. Possible mechanisms through which dietary lipids, calorie restriction, and exercise modulate breast cancer. In: Jacobs, M.M. ed. *Adv. Exp. Med. Biol.,* Vol. 322. Exercise, Calories, Fat and Cancer. New York: Plenum Press. pp. 185–201.

Food and Drug Administration, Department of Health and Human Services. 1993. Food labeling: Health claims and label statements: Dietary fat and cancer. *Federal Register* 58:2787–2819.

Freedman, L.S.; Prentice, R.L.; Clifford, C.; Harlan, W.; Henderson, M. and Rossouw, J. 1993. Dietary fat and breast cancer: Where we are. *J. Natl. Cancer Inst.* 85:764–765.

Friedenreich, C.M.; Howe, G.R. and Miller, A.B. 1991. The effect of recall bias on the association of calorie-providing nutrients and breast cancer. *Epidemiology* 2:424–429.

Friedenreich, C.M.; Slimani, N. and Riboli, E. 1992. Measurement of past diet: Review of previous and proposed methods. *Epidemiol. Rev.* 14:177–196.

Frisch, R.E.; Wyshak, G.; Albright, N.L; Albright, T.E.; Schift, I. and Witschi, J. 1992. Former athletes have a lower lifetime occurrence of breast cancer and cancers of the reproductive system. In: Jacobs, M.M. ed. *Adv. Exp. Med. Biol.,* Vol. 322. Exercise, Calories, Fat and Cancer. New York: Plenum Press. pp. 29–39.

Galli, C. and Butrum, R. 1991. Dietary omega-3 fatty acids and cancer: An overview. *World Rev. Nutr. Dietet.* 66:446–461.

Geltner-Allinger, U.; Brismar, B.; Reinholt, F.P.; Anderson, G. and Rafter, J.J. 1991. Soluble fecal acidic lipids and colorectal epithelial cell proliferation in normal subjects and in patients with colon cancer. *Scand. J. Gastroenterol.* 26:1069–1074.

Giles, T.C. and Roebuck, B.D. 1992. Effects of voluntary exercise and/or food restriction on pancreatic tumorigenesis in male rats. In: Jacobs, M.M. ed. *Adv. Exp. Med. Biol.,* Vol. 322. Exercise, Calories, Fat and Cancer. New York: Plenum Press. pp. 17–27.

Giovannucci, E.; Stampfer, M. J.; Colditz, G.; Rimm, E.B. and Willett, W.C. 1992. Relation of diet to risk of colorectal adenomas in man. *J. Natl. Cancer Inst.* 84:91–98.

Glattre, E.; Haldorsen, T.; Berg, J.P.; Stensvold, I. and Solvoll, K. 1993. Norwegian case–control study testing the hypothesis that seafood increases the risk of thyroid cancer. *Cancer Causes Control* 4:11–16.

Gonzalez, M.J. 1992. Lipid peroxidation and tumor growth: An inverse relationship. *Med. Hypotheses* 38:106–110.

Goodman, M.T.; Hankin, J.H.; Wilkens, L.R. and Kolonel, L.W. 1992. High-fat foods and the risk of lung cancer. *Epidemiology* 3:288–299.

Graham, S.; Hellmann, J.; Marshall, J.; Freudenheim, J.; Venna, J.; Swanson, M.; Zielezny, M.; Nemoto, T.; Stubbe, N. and Raimondo, T. 1991. Nutritional epidemiology of postmenopausal breast cancer in Western New York. *Am. J. Epidemiol.* 134:552–566.

Graham, S.; Zielezny, M.; Marshall, J.; Priore, R.; Freudenheim, J.; Brasure, J.; Haughey, B.; Nasca, P. and Zdeb, M. 1992. Diet in the epidemiology of postmenopausal breast cancer in the New York State cohort. *Am. J. Epidemiol.* 136:1327–1337.

Greenwald, P. 1992. Keynote address: Cancer prevention. *Monogr. Natl. Cancer Inst.* 12:9–14.

Hammar, N. and Norell, S.E. 1991. Retrospective versus original information on diet among cases of colorectal cancer and controls. *Int. J. Epidemiol.* 20:621–627.

Harris, J.R.; Lippman, M.E.; Veronesi, U. and Willett, W. 1992. Breast cancer. *N. Eng. J. Med.* 327:319–328, 390–398, 473–480.

Heber, D.; Ashley, J.M.; McCarthy, W.J.; Solares, M.E.; Leaf, D.A.; Chang, L.-J.C. and Elashoff, R.M. 1992. Assessment of adherence to a low-fat diet for breast cancer prevention. *Prev. Med.* 21:218–227.

Hebert, J.R.; Landon, J. and Miller, D.R. 1993. Consumption of meat and fruit in relation to oral and esophageal cancer: A cross-national study. *Nutr. Cancer* 19:169–179.

Henderson, M.M. 1992a. International differences in diet and cancer incidence. *Monogr. Natl. Cancer Inst.* 12:59–63.

Henderson, M.M. 1992b. Role of intervention trials in research on nutrition and cancer. *Cancer Res.* 52:2030S–2034S.

Henderson, M.M. 1993. Current approaches to breast cancer prevention. *Science* 259:630–631.

Hiller, J.E. and McMichael, A.J. 1990. Dietary fat and cancer: A comeback for ecological studies? *Cancer Causes Control* 1:101–102.

Hirayama, T. 1992. Life-style and cancer: From epidemiological evidence to public behaviour change to mortality reduction of target cancers. *Monogr. Natl. Cancer Inst.* 12:65–74.

Holm, L.-E.; Nordevang, E.; Hjalmar, M.-L.; Lidbrink, E.; Callmer, E. and Nilsson, B. 1993. Treatment failure and dietary habits in women with breast cancer. *J. Natl. Cancer Inst.* 85:32–36.

Howe, G.R. 1990. Dietary fat and cancer. *Cancer Causes Control* 1:99–100.

Iscovich, J.M.; L'Abbé, K.A.; Castelleto, R.; Calzona, A.; Bernedo, A.; Chopita, N.A.; Jmelnitzsky, A.C.; Kaldor, J. and Howe, G.R. 1992. Colon cancer in Argentina. II: Risk from fibre, fat and nutrients. *Int. J. Cancer* 51:858–861.

James, W.P.T. and Ralph, A. 1992. Dietary fat and cancer. *Nutr. Res.* 12:147S–158S.

Kato, I.; Miura, S.; Kasumi, F.; Iwase, T.; Tashiro, H.; Fujita, Y.; Koyama, H.; Ikeda, T.; Fujiwara, K.; Saotome, K.; Asaishi, K.; Abe, R.; Nihei, M.; Ishida, T.; Yokoe, T.; Yamamoto, H. and Murata, M. 1992. A case–control study of breast cancer among Japanese women: With special reference to family history and reproductive and dietary factors. *Breast Cancer Res. Treatment* 24:51–59.

Kesteloot, H.; Lesaffre, E. and Joossens, J.V. 1991. Dairy fat, saturated animal fat, and cancer risk. *Prev. Med.* 20:226–236.

Kinlen, L.J. 1991. Diet and breast cancer. *Br. Med. Bull.* 47:462–469.

Kolonel, L.N.; Hankin, J.H.; Wilkens, I.R.; Funnunago, F.H. and Hinds, M.W. 1990. An epidemiologic study of thyroid cancer in Hawaii. *Cancer Causes Control* 1:233–234.

Kristal, A.R.; White, E.; Shattuck, A.L.; Curry, S.; Anderson, G.L.; Fowler, A. and Urban, N. 1992. Long-term maintenance of a low-fat diet: Durability of fat-related dietary habits in the Women's Health Trial. *J. Am. Dietet. Assoc.* 92:553–559.

Kritchevsky, D. 1992a. Caloric restriction and experimental carcinogenesis. In: Jacobs, M.M. ed. *Adv. Exp. Med. Biol.,* Vol. 322. Exercise, Calories, Fat and Cancer. New York: Plenum Press. pp. 131–141.

Kritchevsky, S.B. 1992b. Dietary lipids and the low blood cholesterol–cancer association. *Am. J. Epidemiol.* 135:509–520.

La Vecchia, C. 1992. Cancers associated with high-fat diets. *Monogr. Natl. Cancer Inst.* 12:79–85.

La Vecchia, C.; Lucchini, F.; Negri, E.; Boyle, P.; Maisonneuve, P. and Levi, F. 1993. Trends of cancer mortality in the Americas, 1955–1989: *Eur. J. Cancer* 29A:431–470.

La Vecchia, C.; Lucchini, F.; Negri, E.; Boyle, P. and Levi, F. 1992a. Trends of cancer mortality in Europe, 1955–1989: I, Digestive sites. *Eur. J. Cancer* 28:132–235.

La Vecchia, C.; Lucchini, F.; Negri, E.; Boyle, P.; Maisonneuve, P. and Levi, F. 1992b. Trends of cancer mortality in Europe, 1955–1989: II, Respiratory tract, bone, connective and soft tissue sarcomas, and skin. *Eur. J. Cancer* 28:514–599.

La Vecchia, C.; Lucchini, F.; Negri, E.; Boyle, P.; Maisonneuve, P. and Levi, F. 1992c. Trends of cancer mortality in Europe, 1955–1989: III, Breast and genital sites. *Eur. J. Cancer* 28A:927–998.

La Vecchia, C.; Negri, E.; D'Avanzo, B.; Franceschi, S. and Boyle, P. 1991. Dairy products and the risk of prostatic cancer. *Oncology* 48:406–410.

Little, J.; Logan, R.F.A.; Hawtin, P.G.; Hardcastle, J.D. and Turner, I.D. 1993. Colorectal adenomas and diet: A case–control study of subjects participating in the Nottingham faecal occult blood screening programme. *Br. J. Cancer* 67:177–184.

London, S.J.; Sacks, F.M.; Caesar, J.; Stampfer, M.J.; Siguel, E. and Willett, W.C. 1991. Fatty acid composition of subcutaneous adipose tissue and diet in postmenopausal U.S. women. *Am. J. Clin. Nutr.* 54:340–345.

London, S.J.; Sacks, F.M.; Stampfer, M.J.; Henderson, I.C.; Maclure, M.; Tomita, A.; Wood, W.C.; Remine, S.; Robert, N.J.; Dmochowski, J.R. and Willett, W.C. 1993. Fatty acid composition of the subcutaneous adipose tissue and risk of proliferative benign breast disease and breast cancer. *J. Natl. Cancer Inst.* 85:785–793.

Man-Fan Wan, J.; Kanders, B.S.; Kowalchuk, M.; Knapp, H.; Szeluga, D.J.; Bagley, J. and Blackburn, G.L. 1991. Omega-3 fatty acids and cancer metastasis in humans. *World Rev. Nutr. Dietet.* 66:477–487.

Marshall, J.R.; Yinsheng, Q.; Junshi, C.; Parpia, B. and Campbell, T.C. 1992. Additional ecological evidence: Lipids and breast cancer mortality among women aged 55 and over in China. *Eur. J. Cancer* 28A:1720–1727.

Matos, E.L.; Khlat, M.; Loria, D.I.; Vilensky, M. and Parkin, D.M. 1991. Cancer in migrants to Argentina. *Int. J. Cancer* 49:805–811.

Neuhaus, J.M.; Murphy, S.P. and Davis, M.A. 1991. Age and sex differences in variation of nutrient intakes among U.S. adults. *Epidemiology* 2:447–450.

Nordevang, E.; Callmer, E.; Marmur, A. and Holm, L.-E. 1992. Dietary intervention in breast cancer patients: Effects on food choices. *Eur. J. Clin. Nutr.* 46:387–396.

Paffensberger, R.S.; Lee, I.-M. and Wing, A.L. 1992. The influence of physical activity on the incidence of site-specific cancers in college alumnus. In: Jacobs, M.M. ed. *Adv. Exp. Med. Biol.,* Vol. 322. Exercise, Calories, Fat and Cancer. New York: Plenum Press. pp. 7–15.

Peters, R.K.; Pike, M.C.; Garabrant, D. and Mack, T.M. 1992. Diet and colon cancer in Los Angeles County, California. *Cancer Causes Control* 3:457–473.

Prentice, R.L. and Sheppard, L. 1990. Dietary fat and cancer: Consistency of the epidemiologic data, and disease prevention that may follow from a practical reduction in fat consumption. *Cancer Causes Control* 1:81–97.

Reddy, B.S. 1992. Dietary fat and colon cancer: Animal model studies. *Lipids* 27:807–813.

Reddy, B.S.; Burill, C. and Rigotty, J. 1991. Effect of diets in ω-3 and ω-6 fatty acids on initiation and postinitiation stages of colon carcinogenesis. *Cancer Res.* 51:487–491.

Riboli, E.; Gonzalez, C.A.; Lopez-Abente, G.; Errezola, M.; Izarzugaza, I.; Escolar, A.; Nebot, M.; Hémon, B. and Agudo, A. 1991. Diet and bladder cancer in Spain: A multi-centre case–control study. *Int. J. Cancer* 49:214–219.

Roberfroid, M.B. 1991. Dietary modulation of experimental neoplastic development: Role of fat and fiber content and caloric intake. *Mutat. Res.* 259:351–362.

Roebuck, B.D. 1992. Dietary fat and the development of pancreatic cancer. *Lipids* 27:804–806.

Rogers, A.E. 1992. Selected recent studies of exercise, energy metabolism, body weight, and blood lipids relevant to interpretation and design of studies of exercise and cancer. In: Jacobs, M.M. ed. *Adv. Exp. Med. Biol.,* Vol. 322. Exercise, Calories, Fat and Cancer. New York: Plenum Press. pp. 239–245.

Rohan, T.E.; Howe, G.R.; Friedenreich, C.M.; Jain, M. and Miller, A.B. 1993. Dietary fiber, vitamins A, C, and E, and risk of breast cancer: A cohort study. *Cancer Causes Control* 4:29–37.

Rose, D.P.; Chlebowski, R.T.; Connolly, J.M.; Jones, L.A. and Wynder, E.L. 1992. Effects of tamoxifen adjuvant therapy and a low-fat diet on serum binding proteins and estradiol bioavailability in postmenopausal breast cancer patients. *Cancer Res.* 52:5386–5390.

Rose, D.A. and Connolly, J.M. 1992. Dietary fat, fatty acids and prostate cancer. *Lipids* 27:798–803.

Russo, J.; Rivera, R. and Russo, I.H. 1992. Influence of age and parity on the development of the human breast. *Breast Cancer Res. Treat.* 23:211–218.

Sasaki, S.; Horacsek, M. and Kesteloot, H. 1993. An ecological study of the relationship between dietary fat intake and breast cancer mortality. *Prevent. Med.* 22:187–202.

Sasaki, S. and Kesteloot, H. 1992. Value of Food and Agriculture Organization data on food-balance sheets as a data source for dietary fat intake in epidemiologic studies. *Am. J. Clin. Nutr.* 56:716–723.

Schneider, H. 1992. A factor in the increased risk of colorectal cancer due to ingestion of animal fat is inhibition of colon epithelial cell glutathione S-transferase, an enzyme that detoxifies mutagens. *Med. Hypoth.* 39:119–122.

Shekelle, R.B.; Rossof, A.H. and Stamler, J. 1991. Dietary cholesterol and incidence of lung cancer: The Western Electric study. *Am. J. Epidemiol.* 134:480–484.

Sheppard, L.; Kristal, A.R. and Kushi, L.H. 1991. Weight loss in women participating in a randomized trial of low-fat diets. *Am. J. Clin. Nutr.* 54:821–828.

Simopoulos, A.P. 1991. Omega-3 fatty acids in health and disease and in growth and development. *Am. J. Clin. Nutr.* 54:438–463.

Steinmetz, K.A. and Potter, J.D. 1993. Food-group consumption and colon cancer in the Adelaide case-control study. II. Meat, poultry, seafood, dairy foods and eggs. *Int. J. Cancer* 53:720–727.

Stephen, A.M. and Wald, N.J. 1990. Trends in individual consumption of dietary fat in the United States, 1920–1984. *Am. J. Clin. Nutr.* 52:457–469.

Taoli, E.; Nicolosi, A. and Wynder, E.L. 1991a. Dietary habits and breast cancer: A comparative study of United States and Italian data. *Nutr. Cancer* 16:259–265.

Taoli, E.; Nicolosi, A. and Wynder, E.L. l991b. Possible role of diet as a host factor in the etiology of tobacco-induced lung cancer. *Int. J. Epidemiol.* 20:611–614.

Thompson, H.J. 1992. Effect of amount and type of exercise on experimentally induced breast cancer. In: Jacobs, M.M. ed. *Adv. Exp. Med. Biol.,* Vol. 322. Exercise, Calories, Fat and Cancer. New York: Plenum Press. pp. 61–71.

Trichopoulou, A.; Tzonou, A.; Hsieh, C.C.; Toupadaki, N.; Manousos, O. and Trichopoulou, D. 1992. High protein, saturated fat and cholesterol diet, and low levels of serum lipids in colorectal cancer. *Int. J. Cancer* 51:386–389.

Tucker, L.A. and Kano, M.J. 1992. Dietary fat and body fat: A multivariate study of 205 adult females. *Am. J. Clin. Nutr.* 56:616–622.

Tuyns, A.J.; Kaaks, R.; Haeltetman, M. and Riboli, E. 1992. Diet and gastric cancer. A case–control study in Belgium. *Int. J. Cancer* 51:1–6.

Urban, N.; White, E.; Anderson, G.L.; Curry, S. and Kristal, A.R. 1992. Correlates of maintenance of a low-fat diet among women in the Women's Health Trial. *Prev. Med.* 21:279–291.

Van den Brandt, P.A.; van't Veer, P.; Goldbohm, R.A.; Dorant, E.; Volovics, A.; Hermus, R.J.J. and Sturmans, F. 1993. A prospective cohort study on dietary fat and the risk of postmenopausal breast cancer. *Cancer Res.* 53:75–82.

Vatten, L.J.; Bjerve, K.S.; Andersen, A. and Jellum, E. 1993. Polyunsaturated fatty acids in serum phospholipids and risk of breast cancer: A case–control study from the Janus serum bank in Norway. *Eur. J. Cancer* 29A:532–538.

Vatten, L.J.; Kvikstad, A. and Nymoen, E.H. 1992. Incidence and mortality of breast cancer related to body height and living conditions during childhood and adolescence. *Eur. J. Cancer* 28:128–131.

Wargovich, M.J. 1992. Fish oil and colon cancer. *Gastroenterol.* 103:1096–1101.

Weinstein, I.B. 1991. Cancer prevention: Recent progress and future opportunities. *Cancer Res.* 51:5080S–5085S.

Welsch, C.W. 1992a. Relationship between dietary fat and experimental mammary tumorigenesis: A review and critique. *Cancer Res.* 52:2040S–2048S.

Welsch, C.W. 1992b. Dietary fat, calories and mammary gland tumorigenesis. In: Jacobs, M.M. ed. *Adv. Exp. Med. Biol.,* Vol. 322. Exercise, Calories, Fat and Cancer. New York: Plenum Press. pp. 203–222.

Whittemore, A.S. and Henderson, B.E. 1993. Dietary fat and breast cancer: Where are we? *J. Natl. Cancer Inst.* 85:762–763.

Wilkens, L.R.; Hankin, J.H.; Yoshizawa, C.N.; Kolonel, L.N. and Lee, J. 1992. Comparison of long-term dietary recall between cancer cases and noncases. *Am. J. Epidemiol.* 136:825–835.

Willett, W.C.; Hunter, D.J.; Stampfer, M.J.; Colditz, G.; Manson, J.E.; Spiegelman, D.; Rosner, B.; Hennekens, C.H. and Speizer, F.E. 1992. Dietary fat and fiber in relation to risk of breast cancer. An 8-year follow-up. *JAMA* 268:2037–2044.

Willett, W.C. and Stampfer, M.J. 1990. Dietary fat and cancer: Another view. *Cancer Causes Control* 1:103–109.

Wynder, E.L. 1992. Cancer prevention: Optimizing life-styles with special reference to nutritional carcinogenesis. *Monogr. Natl. Cancer Inst.* 12:87–91.

Wynder, E.L.; Reddy, B.S. and Weisburger, J.H. 1992a. Environmental dietary factors in colorectoral cancer. Some unresolved issues. *Cancer* 70:1222S–1228S.

Wynder, E.L. and Stellman, S.D. 1992. The "over-exposed" control group. *Am. J. Epidemiol.* 135:459–461.

Wynder, E.L.; Taioli, E. and Fujita, Y. 1992b. Ecologic study of lung cancer risk factors in the U.S. and Japan, with special reference to smoking and diet. *Jpn. J. Cancer Res.* 83:418–423.

Wynder, E.L.; Taioli, E. and Rose, D.P. 1992c. Breast cancer—The optimal diet. In: Jacobs, M.M. ed. *Adv. Exp. Med. Biol.,* Vol. 322. Exercise, Calories, Fat and Cancer. New York: Plenum Press. pp. 143–153.

Yeung, K.S.; McKeown-Eyssen, G.E.; Li, G.F.; Glazer, E.; Hay, K.; Child, P.; Gurgin, V.; Zbu, S.L.; Baptista, J.; Aloe, D.; Mee, D.; Jazmaji, V.; Austin, D.F.; Li, C.C. and Bruce, W.R. 1991. Comparisons of diet and biochemical characteristics of stool and urine between Chinese populations with low and high colorectal cancer rates. *J. Natl Cancer Inst.* 83:46–50.

Yu, H.; Harris, R.E.; Gao, Y.-T.; Gao, R. and Wynder, E.L. 1991. Comparative epidemiology of cancers of the colon, rectum, prostate and breast in Shanghai, China, versus the United States. *Int. J. Epidemiol.* 20:76–81.

Zaridze, D.; Filipchenko, V.; Kustov, V.; Serdyuk, V. and Duffy, S. 1993. Diet and colorectal cancer: Results of two case–control studies in Russia. *Eur. J. Cancer* 29A:112–115.